"Wellness is critical to the purpose of the work that mental health and addictions professionals do with clients. In Clarke and Lewis' book, they are the first to center wellness in addictions counseling that flips our understanding of addiction and recovery work. Highlighting the empowerment of the individual and how their involvement in their own recovery process is part of their own wellness, *Wellness-Based Addictions Counseling* offers a positive reframing of life choices that is more about balance and less about flawlessness."

   Donna M. Gibson, *PhD, LPC, NCC, BC-TMH, Professor, Virginia Commonwealth University*

"The WBAC is a substantial addition to the field of SUD counseling. While there has been a significant increase in theoretical ways to view SUD work over the past twenty-five years, framing addiction treatment through the lens of wellness counseling moves professionals toward a much more holistic approach to treatment for clients. And the more areas of life we can help clients with, the greater the likelihood of successful treatment outcomes for more clients. The authors have functionally expanded the long held biopsychosocial concept to effectively address the entirety of client experience – the biopsychosocial, spiritual, emotional, multicultural, strengths-based, model. This is a must read for SUD counseling practitioners working with clients in today's treatment environment."

   John R. Culbreth, *PhD, LCMHCS, LCAS, CCS, Professor, University of North Carolina Charlotte, Director of the McLeod Institute on Addiction*

WELLNESS-BASED ADDICTIONS COUNSELING

This book presents a culture change in addictions treatment that places wellness at the forefront of relapse, addiction, and recovery. The authors introduce a wellness-based conceptualization of addiction and recovery including the wellness model that grounds Wellness-Based Addictions Counseling (WBAC) and the techniques of this approach.

Wellness-Based Addictions Counseling advocates for wellness as the primary variable in addiction and recovery outcomes, presents a wellness-based model of addiction and recovery, and highlights techniques for unlocking the motivational and strength-based aspects of this approach. Specifically, the authors provide wellness questions and screening tools to incorporate into the clinical evaluation and structure for creating a wellness plan and family wellness plan for the client's loved ones. Readers will learn numerous wellness-based techniques related to the mind, body, spirit, emotions, and connection that can prevent relapse and facilitate well-being. All WBAC interventions are grounded in developmental, culturally responsive, and strength-based perspectives.

Wellness-Based Addictions Counseling is essential reading for professionals who provide addictions treatment and counseling as well as scholars who conduct writing and research on addiction.

Philip B. Clarke, PhD, LCMHC, is an associate teaching professor in the Department of Counseling at Wake Forest University.

Todd F. Lewis, PhD, LPC, NCC, is a professor in the Department of Counselor Education at North Dakota State University.

WELLNESS-BASED ADDICTIONS COUNSELING

Facilitating Holistic Recovery

Philip B. Clarke and Todd F. Lewis

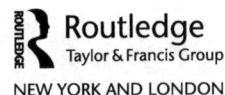

Routledge
Taylor & Francis Group

NEW YORK AND LONDON

Cover image by © Getty Images

First published 2024
by Routledge
605 Third Avenue, New York, NY 10158

and by Routledge
4 Park Square, Milton Park, Abingdon, Oxon, OX14 4RN

Routledge is an imprint of the Taylor & Francis Group, an informa business

Library of Congress Cataloging-in-Publication Data
Names: Clarke, Philip B., author. | Lewis, Todd F., author.
Title: Wellness-based addictions counseling: facilitating holistic
recovery / Philip B. Clarke and Todd F. Lewis.
Description: New York, NY: Routledge, 2024. |
Includes bibliographical references and index. |
Identifiers: LCCN 2023027498 (print) | LCCN 2023027499 (ebook) |
ISBN 9780367705909 (hbk) | ISBN 9780367362225 (pbk) |
ISBN 9781003147954 (ebk)
Subjects: LCSH: Substance abuse—Alternative treatment. |
Holistic medicine. | Mind and body.
Classification: LCC RC564 .C537 2024 (print) |
LCC RC564 (ebook) | DDC 362.29—dc23/eng/20231017
LC record available at https://lccn.loc.gov/2023027498
LC ebook record available at https://lccn.loc.gov/2023027499

ISBN: 978-0-367-70590-9 (hbk)
ISBN: 978-0-367-36222-5 (pbk)
ISBN: 978-1-003-14795-4 (ebk)

DOI: 10.4324/9781003147954

Typeset in Baskerville
by codeMantra

For my wife Denise and children Evie and Alex. Thanks for keeping me well with your love, humor, and fun during the writing of this book. I love to the moon and back! – Todd

To my biggest heroes and supporters – Rebecca, Andrew, Carolina, Jessica, Lynn, and Ray.

CONTENTS

1 WELLNESS: THE KEY TO RECOVERY   1

Introduction 1
The Addiction Field's Traditional View of Addiction 2
Addiction as a Moral Failing 2
Addiction as Disease 2
Traditional Addiction Treatment 3
Review of the Literature on Individual Dimensions of Wellness 4
The Case for a Holistic Wellness Perspective 6
Conclusion 7

2 AN OVERVIEW OF WELLNESS COUNSELING AND WELLNESS-BASED ADDICTIONS COUNSELING   11

Wellness 11
Well-Being 12
Wellness Counseling 12
Wellness-Based Addictions Counseling 15
The Wellness-Substance Use Relationship 17
WBAC is Strengths-Based and Client-Centered 18
WBAC Guidelines 18
What about Maslow? 19
How Do WBAC and the Brain Science on Addiction Co-Exist? 19
Co-Occurring Disorders 20
WBAC in Abstinence-Based Treatment Programs 21
Considerations for Implementing WBAC 21
Client Example – Eric 21
Client Background 22
Family History 22
Substance Use History 23
Conclusion 23

LIST OF FIGURES

LIST OF TABLES

LIST OF HANDOUTS

ABOUT THE AUTHORS

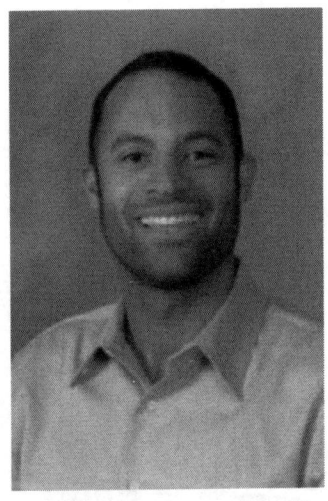

Philip B. Clarke, PhD, LCMHC, is an associate teaching professor at Wake Forest University, where he has been a faculty member in the Department of Counseling since 2011. He has been a licensed clinical mental health counselor (North Carolina) since 2006. Dr. Clarke has experience facilitating counseling groups for individuals with co-occurring mental health and substance use disorders and providing addictions counseling in a treatment study setting. He has taught a course on addictions counseling since 2011 and has published several peer-reviewed journal articles on addictions topics including relapse, spirituality and 12-Step groups, humanistic addictions counseling, and teaching approaches in addictions counseling. Dr. Clarke has received external funding for his research on wellness and co-authored a book on wellness counseling titled *Wellness Counseling: A Holistic Approach to Prevention and Intervention*.

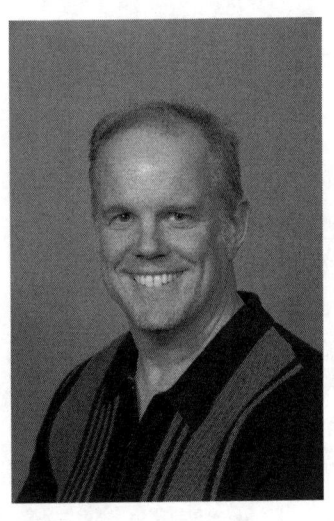

Todd F. Lewis, PhD, LPC, NCC, is a professor of counseling and counselor education at North Dakota State University. He is a licensed professional counselor and a national certified counselor. Dr. Lewis is past Treasurer and President of the International Association of Addictions and Offender Counselors (IAAOC), a subdivision of the American Counseling Association. He has served as the IAAOC representative on the Governing Council of the American Counseling Association. Throughout his career, Dr. Lewis has taught graduate-level students in motivational interviewing, substance use disorders counseling, assessment, diagnosis, treatment planning, and quantitative research methods. He has presented on these topics at numerous local, state, national, and international venues. Dr. Lewis has published numerous research articles related to substance misuse, collegiate drinking, and theoretical approaches to addictions treatment. He has twice received the Exemplary Research Award from IAAOC for his research and was the 2012 recipient of the Teaching Excellence Award from the University of North Carolina at Greensboro School of Education. In 2022, the second edition of his textbook, *Substance Abuse and Addiction Treatment: Practical Application of Counseling Theory*, was published by Cognella.

Dr. Lewis is currently a member of the Motivational Interviewing Network of Trainers (MINT). He has secured internal and external funding for his work in motivational interviewing, primarily using the approach to address health disparities within surrounding communities. In addition to his full-time faculty work, Dr. Lewis has garnered significant clinical experience where he has coordinated substance use clinical research and treatment services with clients struggling with a range of substance use and mental health issues. Currently, Dr. Lewis leads a small private practice, training, and consultation business where he counsels those struggling with mental and behavioral disorders as well as trains practitioners in the practice of motivational interviewing.

CONTRIBUTORS

M.K. Curry is completing their PhD in Counselor Education and Supervision at the College of William and Mary, where their work has included research in contemplative models of counselor supervision and practice.

Amanda L. Giordano, PhD, LPC, is an associate professor at the University of Georgia who specializes in addictions counseling. She is the sole author of a clinical reference book titled *A Clinical Guide to Treating Behavioral Addictions* and co-author of a textbook titled *Addiction Counseling: A Practical Approach*. Dr. Giordano collaborates with domestic and international organizations to provide trainings to increase awareness related to behavioral addictions. She maintains a blog called *Understanding Addiction* for Psychology Today and has been a guest on several podcasts.

Lindsay A. Lundeen, PhD, NCC, is an assistant professor at the University of Arkansas, specializing in suicide and self-directed violence counseling among special populations. She has co-authored multiple behavioral addiction-related manuscripts and has received regional and national awards for her research exploring predictors of suicidality among international collegiate students. Dr. Lundeen presents at the state, regional, and national levels, providing training on behavioral addiction, culturally responsive mental health treatment, as well as cultural and identity-inclusive suicide prevention.

PREFACE

Through our work and research about clients with substance use concerns, we have reflected both on ways to incorporate the underpinnings of wellness from the counseling profession into the addictions field and on lingering questions about addictions treatment. Why is wellness only emphasized once the person had achieved abstinence for several weeks or months? Why is wellness not central from the beginning? Have we maximized our impact as clinicians if some of our clients continue to smoke cigarettes, eat poorly, engage in minimal physical activity, and experience a dearth of meaning and purpose?

This mutual interest resulted in Todd serving as my (Phil) dissertation co-chair on a study in which we sought to answer questions such as "if someone is lower in holistic wellness, does that make them more susceptible to relapse?", "are certain elements of wellness more predictive of relapse than others?", and "can client wellness reduce their relapse risk?" Marlatt's Covert Antecedents Model (1985) of relapse, which anchored this study, was the first and only time we had observed wellness playing a starring role in conceptualizing the causes of addiction and foci of treatment. In other words, in this model, lifestyle imbalance prompted relapse rather than craving, people, places, things, etc. In this book, we hope that we have articulated a clear adaptation of wellness counseling into a treatment approach for clients with substance use disorders (SUDs).

This book is geared toward use with clients with SUDs and has been informed by our clinical experience and research about individuals with SUDs. We believe that content from this book can be meaningful in counseling clients with behavioral addictions, but you will have to determine the appropriateness of the techniques and concepts for your clients. This does lead to several points about the terminology contained in this book. The terms "substance use concerns", "substance use problems", and "substance misuse" are used interchangeably to encompass binge use and/or substance use with negative consequences that may or may not reach a diagnostic threshold for a SUD. The word "addiction" is used interchangeably with "SUD", and the term "addictive behaviors" is also utilized in this book to be inclusive of behavioral addiction or the occurrence of concurrent substance use and behavioral addiction concerns. We also vary how we describe the client's wellness goals and substance use goals given that substance use goals are a part of the client's wellness goals. To that end, we employ the terms "wellness", "holistic recovery", "wellness recovery", or "wellness plan journey". Additionally, the mind dimension of wellness is often referred to as "mental wellness" in this book and the body dimension is alternately referred to as "physical wellness".

This book begins with a chapter establishing our rationale for why a wellness-based counseling approach is needed. Chapter 2 pertains to describing the origins of wellness counseling and an overview of the philosophy and guidelines of Wellness-Based Addictions Counseling (WBAC). Chapters 3 and 4 cover the WBAC perspective and skills regarding evaluation and treatment planning and relapse prevention, respectively. In Chapter 5, we elaborate on skills and concepts for maximizing client strengths in addressing their addictive behaviors. Chapter 6 covers development, culture, and context which are the lenses through which we view the five dimensions of wellness (mind, body, spirit, emotion, and connection of Chapters 7 through 11). The final chapter is on strategic ways to foster wellness in the individual family members/loved ones of those with substance use concerns, stimulating their support for the client's wellness plan, and developing a family wellness plan that encourages shared wellness.

For purposes of depth and consistency, we predominantly use one client to illustrate the WBAC skills and concepts. Eric is a fictional client based on multiple clients and insights that we have had in our clinical, supervision, and research experiences related to addiction. No client names or identifying information are included in this book. We will provide substantial details about this fictional client in Chapter 3 so that when you see examples applying WBAC with Eric in future chapters, you will have prior information about him as context for your learning. We recognize that there are numerous endeavors you can pursue to continue your growth and knowledge as a clinician. Hence, we are grateful that you have elected to read of this book. We have included several handouts over the course of the book that can be incorporated with clients as well as practical skills and techniques that will help you place wellness at the center of your work with clients struggling with addictions.

REFERENCE

Marlatt, G. A. (1985). Relapse prevention: Theoretical rationale and overview of the model. In G. A. Marlatt & J. R. Gordon (Eds.), *Relapse prevention: Maintenance strategies in the treatment of addictive behaviors* (pp. 3–70). Guilford Press.

ACKNOWLEDGMENTS

The writing of this book has taken years longer than anticipated. However, the passion for this subject matter has never wavered. The foundation of the content planning and writing was through conversation with each other in which we shared ideas, experiences, and encouragement. We wish to thank several individuals who helped us in completing this book. First, we would like to thank our editorial team including Amanda Savage and Katya Porter for their patience and resourcefulness during the writing and publishing process. We are grateful to the individuals who agreed to be interviewed to share their feedback on wellness, addiction, and recovery. Those individuals include Robin Silver, Jack Register, LCSW, LCAS, CCS, CCTP, Caroline Tisdale, LCSW, LCAS, CSI, CCTP-II, RYT200, and Caroline Pegram, LCSW, TCTSY-F Somatic Therapist. Thank you, Sara Oberle, for designing the figure for the five-dimension model of Wellness-Based Addictions Counseling; Kelsey Catherwood for assistance with organizing the figures, tables, handouts, and table of contents; MK Curry for developing several experiential activities included in this book; and Amanda Giordano and Lindsay Lundeen for co-authoring the spiritual wellness chapter. We would again like to express gratitude to our families for the remarkable support they provided.

CHAPTER 1

WELLNESS: THE KEY TO RECOVERY

INTRODUCTION

Substance addiction involves introducing a chemical into our bodies with the conscious or sub-conscious goal of feeling more well. Substance use is deceptive in the short-term wellness benefits that it provides. Yes, you heard us correctly. Substance use can yield temporary wellness. For the divorcee who is trying to forget the pain of sharing custody of his kids and adjusting to life alone, the drink or the drug does initially help. For the high-powered businesswoman who rarely gets a break, the drink or the drug provides a respite. For the person who has struggled with homelessness for the past five years and who has burned bridges with friends and family, the drink or the drug temporarily makes the current situation easier to forget.

Over time though, this ephemeral wellness gives way to an imbalance and decline in wellness. The hangover makes it difficult to function and excel at work. The scales have tipped, the balance is "off", and overall wellness suffers. We believe that there are multiple components that make a person well and that indicate wellness and addiction recovery above and beyond the results of a urine drug screen. We believe that addiction develops in large part due to deficits in wellness. These deficits can snowball on a person because the components of wellness are interconnected (Myers & Sweeney, 2005). Thus, as one area of wellness declines, so do other areas of wellness. The downward spiral of addiction continues to chip away at wellness, while low wellness feeds one's appetite to engage in substances or behaviors addictively.

This perspective enables the identification of a path forward into recovery: to situate wellness at the center of one's recovery provides the best chance to achieve harm reduction or abstinence goals while living a fulfilling life. Wellness serves as a foundation for recovery while one finds their footing. The person in recovery now has something to move toward (wellness goals) rather than solely something to avoid (use of the substance). The individual learns that establishing a wellness foundation reduces the risk of cracks developing in the framework of the recovery they are building. This requires the integration of wellness into SUDs treatment and the recovery process. Our intention with this book is to detail a new addictions counseling approach based on wellness models and wellness counseling called Wellness-Based Addictions Counseling (WBAC).

Addictions treatment providers have made strides in incorporating aspects of wellness as a supplement to treatment; however, minimal interventions utilize holistic or multidimensional wellness as their driving force for conceptualizing their clients' addiction *and* in directing how they address the addiction from session to session. With wellness on the periphery of addiction treatment, its impact is softened. The message to clients is that wellness plays a secondary role in their recovery. WBAC seeks to amend this message, sending a clear communication to clients that *wellness is the key to recovery*. In other words, wellness challenges helped create the addiction problem and wellness changes can ameliorate the problem. Before we discuss facets of WBAC and how to actualize the approach, it is important to justify the need for such an approach. To that end, we will explore how addiction providers, researchers,

DOI: 10.4324/9781003147954-1

and clients view and treat addiction. We will also examine evidence of the need for WBAC including what the literature reveals on the relationship between wellness and addiction.

THE ADDICTION FIELD'S TRADITIONAL VIEW OF ADDICTION

A review of the history of addiction in the United States provides a fascinating look into the shifting and, at times, contradictory views of those struggling with addiction and the addictive process and how perspectives on addiction closely follow trends in political, social, and cultural movements of the day. Traditional views of addictive behavior generally fall into two overarching camps (Thombs & Osborn, 2019): addiction as a moral failing and addiction as disease. Let's take a brief look at each of these perspectives, which will help us better understand "traditional" treatment approaches.

Addiction as a Moral Failing

Proponents of this view argue that substance addiction is "sinful" and that people who misuse substances engage in "willful misconduct". That is, they know full well what they are doing and thus make the choice to imbibe alcohol and/or drugs. This "moral model" of addiction has a long history in the United States and has served as the foundation for our penal system and many treatment programs for decades (Lewis, 2014).

As the name implies, the moral model has religious undertones; the sinful nature of addiction requires religious and/or spiritual intervention. An addicted individual, instead of seeking a higher power for fulfillment, turns to drugs or alcohol to fill an existential void (Lewis, 2014). Interventions from this model include making better choices, strengthening spiritual lives, and punitive measures for wrongdoing such as prison. Unfortunately, the moral view is so ingrained in our society that addiction has become synonymous with guilt and shame.

Addiction as Disease

The disease concept (or disease model of addiction) is probably the most popular viewpoint of addiction today in the United States, especially within treatment communities (Thombs & Osborn, 2019). This model suggests that SUDs are the result of an underlying disease process, like other chronic diseases. There is certainly merit to this line of thinking on both genetic and biological grounds (Thombs & Osborn, 2019). First, research into the genetic origins of addictions has produced convincing evidence of familial transmission of substance use problems (Volkow & Baler, 2014). In addition, the brain has been shown to alter its functioning after significant exposure to substances, suggesting that a disease process develops after one ingests substances (Thombs & Osborn, 2019). Psychosocial variables, such as personality, unconscious motives, choice, and mental health struggles, are thus given secondary importance to the onset and maintenance of addiction. The emergence of the disease concept has had an enormous influence on treating addiction; stakeholders, politicians, and society at large are more willing to direct resources to help those they believe suffer from a disease compared to those who willfully engage in misconduct. As such, the disease model, or elements of it, runs through most contemporary treatment programs within the United States.

The addiction as disease concept is in direct contrast to the moral weakness argument. Indeed, it is responsible for moving alcohol and drug addiction out of the moral realm, which in turn helps clients overcome their guilt and fully engage in treatment; there is less stigma attached to a disease process compared to a moral failing. Although the disease model has a firm establishment within the medical and treatment communities, it has been challenged on both philosophical and scientific grounds (Thombs & Osborn, 2019). Philosophically, Fingarette (1988) called into question one of the major arguments of the addiction as a disease idea: that ingestion of alcohol and drugs leads to physiological *loss of control*. That is, as a result of imbibing alcohol or drugs, some underlying physical mechanism causes the person to lose control of their drinking and using. This hypothesis implies that loss of control happens only when substances enter the system. However, if this were the case, we would not see evidence of craving when substances are *not* in the body. Clearly, those abstaining from substances continue to experience craving for drugs even though there is no trace of a substance in their system (Fingarette). In addition, studies (e.g., Marlatt, Demming, & Reid, 1973) on this topic have failed to establish a loss of control phenomenon; even participants with alcohol use disorders who were given small doses of alcohol were able to moderate their drinking and did not lose control, as the disease model would predict.

Throughout much of United States history, interested stakeholders, and society at large, viewed substance addiction as both a moral weakness (van Wormer & Davis, 2003) and an inherent disease process, with each viewpoint getting more focus depending on cultural, political, and economic winds of the time. This "hybrid" conceptualization of addiction is still present today, permeating drug enforcement and treatment programs throughout the United States (Thombs & Osborn, 2019). For example, in many states, relatively minor drug offenses (e.g., marijuana possession) result in punitive consequences such as community service, steep fines, and jail time. On the one hand, these consequences clearly align with the "addiction as a moral failing" perspective. On the other hand, drug courts often hand down sentencing where addicts are sent to treatment facilities as a condition of their sentence. This, of course, aligns more with the "addiction as disease" mentality.

Traditional Addiction Treatment

Although we have not set out to provide a thorough history of addiction treatment in this chapter, what we mean by "traditional" treatment probably traces back to the post-prohibition era (after 1933) where the disease concept of addiction gained greater notoriety and acceptance. During this time, the advent of Alcoholics Anonymous (AA) (and its corollaries, e.g., Narcotics Anonymous) further influenced moving away from moral reasoning to addiction as a disease; however, the term "disease" is conceptualized. E. M. Jellinek's classic analysis, *The Disease Concept of Alcoholism* (1960), solidified the disease model perspective.[1] As such, Jellinek's work and the growing popularity of AA, supported by accumulating academic research, provided a path for addiction treatment moving forward. Two important groups began to support the addiction as disease concept: Congress and the medical community. Now that addiction was conceptualized as outside of one's control, government funding was provided to enhance SUD treatment within the medical community.

A classic example of traditional treatment is the Minnesota Model (MM), still practiced today. MM has had a strong influence in both inpatient and outpatient settings (Stevens & Smith, 2013). Pioneered by Hazelden (formed in 1949), the MM promotes two overarching goals: total abstinence from substances and improving (or returning to) one's life by establishing positive lifestyle habits and skills. AA and other 12-step mutual help groups are a key component of the program. The MM emphasizes spiritual growth, personal responsibility for one's recovery, connecting with others, and promoting life skills (Stevens & Smith, 2013).

Traditional addiction practices also have a darker side, emphasizing harsher forms of confrontation than what is commonly used today (although, sadly, some elements of these early programs still permeate treatment programs). This confrontational approach operated under the following assumptions: (a) individuals with SUDs have an inner defect, and it is the therapist's job to set them straight, (b) individuals with SUDs do not have the capacity to help themselves or offer anything useful in therapy, (c) the pervasiveness of denial requires harsh confrontation, and (d) clients must first admit they are "defective", given their addiction, in order for change to take place. There were two obvious problems with this approach. First, it was not very effective in helping people stop or cut down substance use. Second, too much confrontation tends to engender greater resistance, serving as a major impediment to change. That is, harsh confrontations, beating down denial, and arguing only seemed to embolden clients to dig in their heels. In addition, the idea that one must admit that they are an "addict" or "alcoholic" in order to improve has no empirical support (Miller, Rollnick, & Moyers, 1998).

REVIEW OF THE LITERATURE ON INDIVIDUAL DIMENSIONS OF WELLNESS

Research on holistic wellness as a factor in SUD symptomology is limited. However, the impact of individual wellness dimensions on addiction is more prevalent in the literature. Low mind, body, spirit, emotion, and connection (social), developmental, cultural, contextual wellness can predispose someone to substance use problems, and conversely, addiction can negatively impact these wellness dimensions. In terms of mental wellness, addiction affects the brain. The brain's response to substance use results in pleasure but not without inflicting consequences. The brain changes necessitate a person to use more of the substance in order to avoid aversive physical and psychological symptoms. Furthermore, the ability to experience pleasure, make decisions, and self-regulate becomes compromised starting at the brain level (Perry & Lawrence, 2017).

A myopic focus on substance use with concurrent neglect of mentally stimulating activities (e.g., absence of meaningful employment) reduces mental wellness. Conversely, positive attention to the mind improves wellness in this dimension and overall. For example, researchers studied the brains of participants with opioid use disorders who received mindfulness as a part of their overall addiction treatment compared to those who did not (Fahmy et al., 2018). There were differences in the brains of the two groups of participants by the end of the study with mindfulness participants exhibiting increases in size of parts of the brain responsible (in part) for decision-making and motivation.

Substance use has profound effects on physical wellness. Researchers and clinicians are aware of the acute and chronic damage that can be caused from substance use in the brain and throughout the body. Self-reported mental and physical quality of life is noticeably lower for individuals with opioid use disorders than for those not diagnosed with opioid use disorder even when sustained remission has been achieved (Rhee & Rosenheck, 2019). Individuals in recovery who have a bad night of sleep may experience stronger cravings (Lydon-Staley et al., 2017). Jeynes and Gibson (2017) stated that "There appears to be a consensus in the research literature that subjects with alcohol use disorders [AUD] and drug use disorders [DUD] are often malnourished and nutrient deficient…" (p. 235).

What is remarkable is how the brain and body can improve through treatment and recovery. When nutrition information and interventions are incorporated into addiction treatment (as part of a focus on physical wellness), issues related to mental, medical, and interpersonal health decrease (Grant, Haughton, & Sachan, 2004). Exercise can also serve as an avenue to recovery and alleviate some of the problems caused by substance use. Studies of exercise approaches integrated into addiction treatment indicate correlations between physical activity and decreased substance use (Wang, Wang, Wang, & Zhou, 2014).

The ability to use emotions as a guide to understanding ourselves and others may be a liability for some individuals with SUDs. Proponents of the self-medication hypothesis of co-occurring disorders (that the pathway to developing both a mental health disorder and SUD is through using substances to "treat" the mental health symptoms [Miller, Forcehimes, & Zweben, 2019]) might argue that emotions are at the crux of SUDs, rendering the high prevalence of mental health disorders in people with SUDs. Creators of the Relapse Prevention (RP) approach have identified emotions that trigger relapse including cravings, "enhancement of positive emotional states", and "coping with frustration and anger" (Marlatt, Parks, & Witkiewitz, 2002, p. 11). It is difficult to discern the extent to which these emotion wellness challenges are the cause or consequence of substance use. However, it is becoming increasingly clear that people with SUDs are more likely than people not diagnosed with a SUD to struggle to know what they are feeling, manage what they are feeling, and convey what they are feeling (Dingle, Neves, Alhadad, & Hides, 2018).

Positive emotions are inversely related to craving (Lydon-Staley et al., 2017). Thus, emotional wellness skills that can be facilitated through interventions such as Dialectical Behavior Therapy, for example, have been shown to improve emotion regulation and substance-related outcomes (Cavicchioli et al., 2019). However, meta-analytic data suggests that attending treatment only precipitates small declines in negative affect and may not promote positive emotions (Kang, Fairbairn, & Ariss, 2019).

Recovery may be an impossible task to sustainably do alone. Twelve-step and mutual help group programs like AA have approximately 2,130,419 members and 125,352 groups across the globe (https://www.aa.org/assets/en_US/smf-132_en.pdf). SUDs, as noted in the DSM-5-TR (APA, 2022) criteria, can lead to a shrinking of one's social system to primarily people who use and misuse substances and is also associated with social strain. Think of the bridges that have been burned by the clients you have worked with. I (Phil) recall co-facilitating multi-family groups for individuals with SUDs and their families and that it was hard for several clients to identify a family member or friend to attend the group with them.

Social wellness is further complicated by potential social skills impairment (Dingle et al., 2017) and attachment wounds (Luke, 2017). Relationships impact the ability of individuals with substance use issues to make constructive changes to their use. The chance of sustaining drug or alcohol cessation for people with SUDs sharply declines if they perceive their spouse or partner also misuses substances and if the relationship causes them stress (Tracy, Kelly, & Moos, 2005). However, the effectiveness of 12-Step groups (e.g. Timko & DeBenedetti, 2007) and other interventions that bolster social support such as community reinforcement approaches (Meyers, Villanueva, & Smith, 2005) are a testament to the importance of social wellness in recovery.

Religious beliefs and practices and a sense of meaning and purpose are a key component of wellness and addiction recovery. Spirituality is central to 12-Step programming and is evident upon reviewing the 12 steps which include beliefs ("Came to believe that a power greater than ourselves could restore us to sanity") (Alcoholics Anonymous [AA], 1981, p. 25) and practices ("Sought through prayer and meditation to improve our conscious contact with God, as we understood Him, praying only for knowledge of His will for us and the power to carry that out") (AA, 1981, p. 96). Religious beliefs and spirituality for individuals who have completed SUD treatment or attended 12-Step meetings are a positive factor in addressing substance misuse (Kelly & Eddie, 2020). For example, Sliedrecht, Waart, Witkiewitz and Roozen (2019) discovered that spirituality is correlated with decreased occurrence of alcohol relapse in seven out of ten studies as was "life purpose" in six studies on alcohol relapse. Clearly, spiritual wellness plays an important role in the recovery process.

THE CASE FOR A HOLISTIC WELLNESS PERSPECTIVE

What's missing in the mental health and addictions literature is the research on the interconnection among these wellness dimensions. How do these components interact with each other and therein contribute to or detract from one's wellness and recovery? How do these components combine in a way that changes the likelihood of relapse? We published a study exploring wellness individually and holistically as well as how it relates to one's ability to regulate their emotions and mitigate relapse (Clarke et al., 2020). Even though our ability to detect a strong impact of wellness on relapse was limited due to the cross-sectional nature of the study, we still found strong relationships between each dimension of wellness and the ability to manage one's feelings. This is particularly relevant given the literature cited above on the ties between emotion regulation and substance use. We also discovered that one's physical wellness, in a small way, was predictive of relapse for individuals currently involved in SUDs treatment (Clarke et al., 2020). Namely, that greater physical wellness was associated with decreased odds of relapse.

Individuals living with SUDs have made a clear statement that recovery is a holistic process. William White, a leader in the addiction field noted that "Most recovered and recovering people define recovery in terms of the resolution of AOD problems and the progress toward global health (physical, cognitive, emotional, ontological, relational, educational/ occupational, financial, and legal)" (White, 2007, p. 234). White's point here is substantiated by a study to ascertain the definition of recovery from over 9,000 individuals with SUDs (Kaskutas et al., 2014). More than 90% of study participants desired for the following clauses to be in the definition:

> being honest with myself, handling negative feelings without using drugs or alcohol, being able to enjoy life without drinking or using drugs like I used to…a process of growth and development, reacting to life's ups and downs in a more balanced way than I used to, taking responsibility for the things I can change.
>
> (Kaskutas et al., 2014, p. 1008)

Has the addiction treatment field heeded the recommendations of its consumers?

The Substance Abuse and Mental Health Services Administration (SAMHSA) is a federal organization that supports persons with SUDs, SUD researchers, and treatment providers. SAMHSA defines recovery from mental disorders and SUDs as "A process of change through which individuals improve their health and wellness, live a self-directed life, and strive to reach their full potential" (SAMHSA, 2012, p. 5). One of SAMHSA's "10 Guiding Principles of Recovery" that are linked with this definition includes that "recovery is holistic" meaning it "encompasses an individual's whole life, including mind, body, spirit, and community" (2012, p. 5). SAMHSA espouses that

> Recovery occurs via many pathways—Individuals are unique with distinct needs, strengths, preferences, goals, culture, and backgrounds—including trauma experience—that affect and determine their pathway(s) to recovery. Recovery is built on the multiple capacities, strengths, talents, coping abilities, resources, and inherent value of each individual.
>
> (2012, p. 5)

WBAC is clearly aligned with this holistic perspective on recovery.

Whereas strength-based approaches are increasingly used in schools and mental health counseling, there remains a deficit of such approaches in the addictions field. However, it is clear that every client with a SUD has strengths to be mined and that approaches that capitalize on this hold great potential. For example, Solution-Focused Brief Therapy (SFBT) for parents who had lost custody of their children due to their substance use was equivalent to Motivational Interviewing (MI) and Cognitive-Behavioral Therapy (CBT) in reducing substance use and its corresponding problems as well as alleviating traumatic stress (Kim et al., 2018). WBAC intentionally incorporates a strength-based perspective, drawing from SFBT, positive psychology, and MI (among other approaches), to build on client strengths in the service of a meaningful recovery.

Further, persons with co-occurring disorders (concurrent mental health disorder and SUD), trauma, and medical issues along with the SUD are the norm, rather than the exception. The 2021 National Survey on Drug Use and Health stated that of the 44 million adults with a SUD, 19.4 million had a co-occurring disorder (SAMHSA, 2022). Because the likelihood of incurring a SUD rises noticeably in conjunction with reports of higher numbers of adverse childhood experiences (LeTendre & Reed, 2017), clinicians should be mindful of the role of trauma in the conceptualization and treatment of all individuals with SUDs. In addition to the importance of reducing or eliminating substance use for an individual with SUDs, a holistic approach is needed, taking into account past traumatic experiences, to help the individual address the full context of their life. Otherwise, relapse or debilitating mental health concerns can derail the person's life and recovery. Although WBAC is not a trauma-based approach, it does operate with trauma sensitivity, keeping in mind the importance of addressing these issues as part of a holistic recovery.

Family members often get lost in the narrative about the ravages of addiction. We must remember the mental and physical health damage that can arise for not only the addicted family member but also the loved ones of someone with a SUD. Hence, WBAC is also geared toward empowering family members and loved ones with their own wellness. The indirect results of family and loved one wellness can be a positive influence and can facilitate natural and logical consequences for the addicted individual.

CONCLUSION

In this book, we present WBAC as an exciting approach that works with the client not only to help them stop drinking or using but also to enhance wellness so they can thrive in recovery. WBAC is one of the first approaches that fully integrates wellness throughout the addiction treatment process. Before we describe WBAC, we will expound on the literature on wellness counseling. Clinicians need to be aware of the models of wellness and the procedures involved in wellness counseling that undergird WBAC. From there, we will explore common topics on addictions counseling such as assessment, treatment planning, and RP, all from a WBAC perspective. We then journey through cultivating client strengths and the different components of wellness and their unique relation to addiction including mind, body, spirit, emotion, connection, developmental, cultural, and contextual wellness. We conclude the book with the WBAC approach to family care. Throughout all chapters, we offer a bevy of interventions to help clients cut down or abstain from substance use, strengthen their recovery, and embrace a wellness lifestyle.

NOTE

1   Interestingly, according to van Wormer and Davis (2003), Jellinek never said that alcoholism was a disease but "like" a disease. Indeed, the disease conceptualization of addiction has been challenged on many fronts (see Thombs & Osborn, 2019).

REFERENCES

Alcoholics Anonymous World Services (1981). *Twelve steps and twelve traditions.* Alcoholics Anonymous World Services.

American Psychiatric Association. (2022). *Diagnostic and statistical manual of mental disorders* (5th ed., text rev.). https://doi.org/10.1176/appi.books.9780890425787

Cavicchioli, M., Movalli, M., Vassena, G., Ramella, P., Prudenziati, F., & Maffei, C. (2019). The therapeutic role of emotion regulation and coping strategies during a stand-alone DBT skills training program for alcohol use disorder and concurrent substance use disorders. *Addictive Behaviors, 98.* https://doi.org/10.1016/j.addbeh.2019.106035

Clarke, P. B., Lewis, T. F., Myers, J. E., Henson, R. A., & Hill, B. (2020). Wellness, emotion regulation, and relapse during substance use disorder treatment. *Journal of Counseling & Development, 98*(1), 17–28. https://doi.org/10.1002/jcad.12296

Dingle, G. A., Neves, D. D. C., Alhadad, S. S., & Hides, L. (2018). Individual and interpersonal emotion regulation among adults with substance use disorders and matched controls. *British Journal of Clinical Psychology, 57*(2), 186–202. https://doi.org/10.1111/bjc.12168

Fahmy, R., Wasfi, M., Mamdouh, R., Moussa, K., Wahba, A., Wittemann, M., Hirjak, D., Kubera, K. M., Wolf, N. D., Sambataro, F., & Wolf, R. C. (2018). Mindfulness-based interventions modulate structural network strength in patients with opioid dependence. *Addictive Behaviors, 82*, 50–56. https://doi.org/10.1016/j.addbeh.2018.02.013

Fingerette, H. (1988). *Heavy drinking: The myth of alcoholism as a disease.* University of California Press.

Grant, L. P., Haughton, B., & Sachan, D. S. (2004). Nutrition education is positively associated with substance abuse treatment program outcomes. *Journal of the American Dietetic Association, 104*(4), 604–610. https://doi.org/10.1016/j.jada.2004.01.008

Jellinek, E. M. (1960). *The disease concept of alcoholism.* Hillhouse Press.

Jeynes, K. D., & Gibson, E. L. (2017). The importance of nutrition in aiding recovery from substance use disorders: A review. *Drug and Alcohol Dependence, 179,* 229–239. https://doi.org/10.1016/j.drugalcdep.2017.07.006

Kang, D., Fairbairn, C. E., & Ariss, T. A. (2019). A meta-analysis of the effect of substance use interventions on emotion outcomes. *Journal of Consulting and Clinical Psychology, 87*(12), 1106. https://doi.org/10.1037/ccp0000450

Kaskutas, L. A., Borkman, T. J., Laudet, A., Ritter, L. A., Witbrodt, J., Subbaraman, M. S., Stunz, A., & Bond, J. (2014). Elements that define recovery: The experiential perspective. *Journal of Studies on Alcohol and Drugs, 75*(6), 999–1010. https://doi.org/10.15288/jsad.2014.75.999

Kelly, J. F., & Eddie, D. (2020). The role of spirituality and religiousness in aiding recovery from alcohol and other drug problems: An investigation in a national US sample. *Psychology of Religion and Spirituality, 12*(1), 116–123. https://doi.org/10.1037/rel0000295

Kim, J. S., Brook, J., & Akin, B. A. (2018). Solution-focused brief therapy with substance-using individuals: A randomized controlled trial study. *Research on Social Work Practice, 28*(4), 452–462. https://doi.org/10.1177/1049731516650517

LeTendre, M. L., & Reed, M. B. (2017). The effect of adverse childhood experience on clinical diagnosis of a substance use disorder: Results of a nationally representative study. *Substance Use & Misuse, 52*(6), 689–697. https://doi.org/10.1080/10826084.2016.1253746

Lewis, T. F. (2014). *Substance abuse and dependence treatment: Practical application of counseling theory.* Pearson Education, Inc.

Luke, C. (2017, September 27). *Addiction as a relational disorder: A neuro-informed treatment perspective.* NAADAC recorded webinar. Retrieved from https://www.naadac.org/addiction-as-relational-disorder-webinar

Lydon-Staley, D. M., Cleveland, H. H., Huhn, A. S., Cleveland, M. J., Harris, J., Stankoski, D., Deneke, E., Meyer, R. E., & Bunce, S. C. (2017). Daily sleep quality affects drug craving, partially through indirect associations with positive affect, in patients in treatment for nonmedical use of prescription drugs. *Addictive Behaviors, 65*, 275–282. https://doi.org/10.1016/j.addbeh.2016.08.026

Marlatt, G. A., Demming, B., & Reid, J. B. (1973). Loss of control drinking in alcoholics: An experimental analogue. *Journal of Abnormal Psychology, 81*, 233–241.

Marlatt, G. A., Parks, G. A., & Witkiewitz, K. (2002). Clinical guidelines for implementing relapse prevention therapy. Illinois Department of Human Services Office of Alcoholism and Substance Abuse.

Meyers, R. J., Villanueva, M., & Smith, J. E. (2005). The community reinforcement approach: History and new directions. *Journal of Cognitive Psychotherapy, 19*(3), 247–260. https://doi.org/10.1891/jcop.2005.19.3.247

Miller, W. R., Forcehimes, A. A., & Zweben, A. (2019). *Treating addiction: A guide for professionals.* Guilford Publications.

Miller, W. R., Rollnick, S., & Moyers, T. B. (1998). *Motivational interviewing: Professional training videotape series.* The University of New Mexico.

Myers, J. E., & Sweeney, T. J. (2005). Introduction to wellness theory. In J. E. Myers & T. J. Sweeney (Eds.), *Counseling for wellness: Theory, research, and practice* (pp. 7–14). American Counseling Association.

Perry, C. J., & Lawrence, A. J. (2017). Addiction, cognitive decline and therapy: Seeking ways to escape a vicious cycle. *Genes, Brain and Behavior, 16*(1), 205–218. https://doi.org/10.1111/gbb.12325

Rhee, T. G., & Rosenheck, R. A. (2019). Association of current and past opioid use disorders with health-related quality of life and employment among US adults. *Drug and Alcohol Dependence, 199*, 122–128. https://doi.org/10.1016/j.drugalcdep.2019.03.004

Sliedrecht, W., de Waart, R., Witkiewitz, K., & Roozen, H. G. (2019). Alcohol use disorder relapse factors: A systematic review. *Psychiatry Research, 278*, 97–115. https://doi.org/10.1016/j.psychres.2019.05.038

Substance Abuse and Mental Health Services Administration (SAMHSA) (2012). SAMHSA's working definition of recovery: 10 guiding principles of recovery. https://store.samhsa.gov/sites/default/files/d7/priv/pep12-recdef.pdf

Substance Abuse and Mental Health Services Administration. (2022). Key substance use and mental health indicators in the United States: Results from the 2021 National Survey on Drug Use and Health (HHS Publication No. PEP22-07-01-005, NSDUH Series H-57). Center for Behavioral Health Statistics and Quality, Substance Abuse and Mental Health Services Administration. https://www.samhsa.gov/data/report/2021-nsduh-annual-national-report

Thombs, D. L., & Osborn, C. J. (2019). *Introduction to addictive behaviors* (5th ed.). Guilford Press.

Timko, C., & DeBenedetti, A. (2007). A randomized controlled trial of intensive referral to 12 step self-help groups: One-year outcomes. *Drug and Alcohol Dependence, 90*(2–3), 270–279. https://doi.org/10.1016/j.drugalcdep.2007.04.007

Tracy, S. W., Kelly, J. F., & Moos, R. H. (2005). The influence of partner status, relationship quality and relationship stability on outcomes following intensive substance-use disorder treatment. *Journal of Studies on Alcohol, 66*(4), 497–505. https://doi.org/10.15288/jsa.2005.66.497

van Wormer, K. S., & Davis, D. R. (2003). *Addiction treatment: A strengths perspective*. Brooks/Cole.

Volkow, N. D., & Baler, R. D. (2014). Addiction science: Uncovering neurobiological complexity. *Neuropharmacology, 76*, 235–249. https://doi.org/10.1016/j.neuropharm.2013.05.007

Wang, D., Wang, Y., Wang, Y., Li, R., & Zhou, C. (2014). Impact of physical exercise on substance use disorders: A meta-analysis. *PLoS One, 9*(10), e110728. https://doi.org/10.1371/journal.pone.0110728

White, W. L. (2007). Addiction recovery: Its definition and conceptual boundaries. *Journal of Substance Abuse Treatment, 33*(3), 229–241. https://doi.org/10.1016/j.jsat.2007.04.015

CHAPTER 2

AN OVERVIEW OF WELLNESS COUNSELING AND WELLNESS-BASED ADDICTIONS COUNSELING

WELLNESS

Traditional mental health counseling, psychotherapy, and addiction counseling are steeped in the medical model of symptom identification, classification into disorders, and designing treatments specifically for symptom reduction. The strengths and positive qualities of the client, preventing the occurrence of mental health concerns, maximizing life balance and the parts that make one well are not always prioritized. However, wellness counseling represents a shift in approach to mental health. Wellness has impacted mental health and medical care discussions in significant ways by (a) highlighting the importance of prevention, (b) demonstrating that one can live life fully beyond having or not having a disease, and (c) illustrating that the physical dimension is but one part of health and wellness. Before discussing wellness counseling, specifically, we'll start by reviewing the work of John Travis, Regina Ryan, and Bill Hettler in conceptualizing wellness and designing wellness interventions in the health arena.

John Travis and Regina Ryan made seminal strides down each of these roads. They described that "wellness is a way of life – a lifestyle you design to achieve your highest potential for well-being" (Travis & Ryan, 1988, p. xiv). Further, they conceptualized wellness as a holistic and a lifelong pursuit that rests within the autonomy of the individual to pursue or not pursue. Despite striving for the heights of holistic wellness, the authors were clear to note that "acceptance" is a part of the wellness definition, recognizing the value of the dialectic of both endeavoring for increased wellness while honoring one's current wellness.

One of the most reproduced diagrams and concepts in health and wellness is Travis' (1972) depiction of disease, health, and wellness. The "Illness/Wellness Continuum" contains a mid-point which represents an individual having no medical problems yet having made no positive steps toward wellness (Travis & Ryan, 1988). The "illness" side of the continuum shows increasing health risk levels proceeding into identifiable symptoms, then affecting one's ability to function, and eventually ending in preventable early death. In contrast, the wellness portion of the model indicates steps toward wellness enhancement starting with understanding one's strengths and areas for improvement, learning about ways to increase wellness, and enacting wellness behaviors (Travis & Ryan, 1988). The authors clarify that one can be extremely high in wellness while living with medical conditions as the continuum is referring to disease from lack of nurturing one's wellness.

We wish to highlight one additional notion put forth by Travis and Ryan (1988) – the idea that wellness is like energy processes in physics in which wellness behaviors are converted to helpful products in one's life. When I took a wellness course from wellness pioneer Jane Myers, she talked about the concept of "garbage in and garbage out" in regard to nutrition. For instance, if one eats something nutritious, that food is converted into healthy byproducts for the body with effects that can include better mood and clearer cognitions. However, negative wellness behaviors can result in energy "blocks" or toxic energy that can affect multiple other aspects of one's wellness. Hence, Travis and Ryan (1988) are emphasizing that wellness is holistic or interconnected because one area of wellness can impact others.

DOI: 10.4324/9781003147954-2

Bill Hettler created the Six Dimensions of Wellness model that is known to many health-care professionals and is pivotal to the work of the National Wellness Institute (Hettler, 1976; National Wellness Institute, n. d.). Part of Hettler's innovation was to extend and operation-alize the components of wellness. His model consists of

- Occupational Wellness: aligning one's job with one's abilities and principles leading to a gratifying work life.
- Emotional Wellness: identifying, acknowledging, and voicing one's feelings.
- Spiritual Wellness: living life in a manner that is congruent with one's principles and what is most important to the person.
- Intellectual Wellness: participating in "problem-solving, creativity, and learning" that are cognitively invigorating.
- Social Wellness: fostering nourishing connections with others and the environment.
- Physical Wellness: attending to exercise, nutrition, and other efforts to increase the health of one's body (Hettler, 1976; National Wellness Institute, n. d.).

WELL-BEING

The field of psychology has contributed substantially to the wellness literature via positive psy-chology. "Positive psychology is the study of the conditions and processes that contribute to the flourishing or optimal functioning of people, groups, and institutions" (Gable & Haidt, 2005, p. 104). Those using positive psychology approaches seek to identify and promote strengths and positive qualities (Downey & Henderson, 2021; Gallagher, 2019). There are several concepts in the positive psychology literature including, subjective well-being, thriving, and hope. Thriving and hope will be elaborated upon in later chapters (Chapters 3 and 10, respectively). Here we'll expound upon well-being to illustrate its similarities and differences from wellness because its concepts are integrated into Wellness-Based Addictions Counseling (WBAC).

Subjective well-being is "a person's evaluation of [their] life …" and "… can be in terms of cognitive states such as satisfaction with one's marriage, work, and life, and it can be in terms of ongoing affect …" (Diener, Sapyta, & Suh, 1998, p. 34). Carol Ryff's model of psychological well-being includes autonomy, environmental mastery, personal growth, posi-tive relations with others, purpose in life, and self-acceptance (Ryff, 1989). Autonomy entails being impervious to peer influence and using one's internal guide to inform life choices (Ryff, 2014). Environmental mastery is the confidence and proficiency to change environments or adapt to one's environment. Personal growth is the perception of progress in one's life. Positive relations with others involve possessing relationship-building skills and experiencing contentment with one's social life. A person with purpose perceives life as meaningful and has a vision for their life. Self-acceptance is related to adopting a constructive view of all of one's "qualities" (Ryff, 2014). Hedonic well-being, an element not in Ryff's model, per-tains to experiencing pleasant emotions and reducing negative emotions (Diener et al., 1998; Joshanloo, 2016 as cited in Diener, Suh, Lucas, & Smith, 1999).

WELLNESS COUNSELING

Myers, Sweeney, and Witmer (2000) defined wellness "… as a way of life oriented toward optimal health and well-being in which body, mind, and spirit are integrated by the individual to live more fully within the human and natural community" (p. 252). Their Wheel of Wellness (WoW) model (Figure 2.1) in counseling is unique when compared to well-being in setting spirituality and self-direction as signature life tasks at the center of the model. The spirituality circle lies within self-direction as the two go hand in hand: a sense of meaning and purpose and that one can experience fulfillment from engaging with something greater than ourselves facilitates self-direction (Myers & Sweeney, 2005b; Myers et al., 2000). Self-direction underscores "intentionality" or the ability to successfully navigate the challenges and objectives of one's day (Myers & Sweeney, 2005b, p. 20). Intentionality is a necessary piece of the wellness puzzle as one cannot productively engage in wellness behaviors in its absence (Myers & Sweeney, 2006).

Work and leisure, friendship, and love are also life tasks in the WoW model. Sense of worth, sense of control, realistic beliefs, emotional awareness and coping, problem-solving and creativity, sense of humor, nutrition, exercise, self-care, stress management, gender identity, and cultural identity were the subtasks ("spokes") linked with self-direction. According to WoW, wellness is a comprehensive construct that draws upon environmental factors that

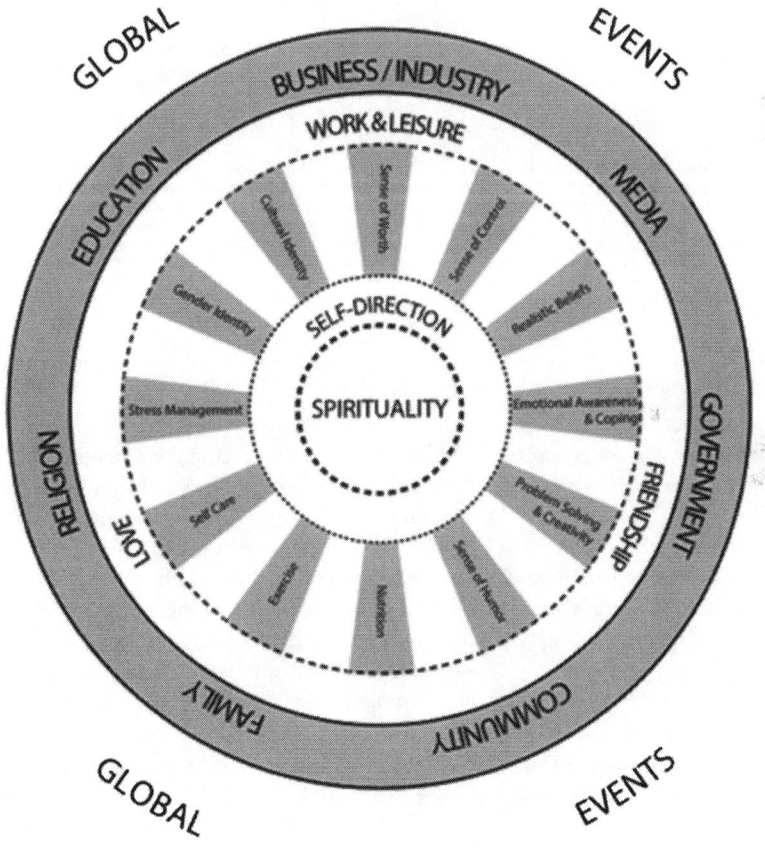

© J. M. Witmer, T. J. Sweeney, & J. E. Myers, 1996, reprinted with permission

Figure 2.1 Wheel of Wellness Model.

THE INDIVISIBLE SELF:
An Evidence-Based Model Of Wellness

CONTEXTS:

Local (safety)
Family
Neighborhood
Community

Institutional (policies & laws)
Education
Religion
Government
Business/Industry

Global (world events)
Politics
Culture
Global Events
Environment
Media

Chronometrical (lifespan)
Perpetual
Positive
Purposeful

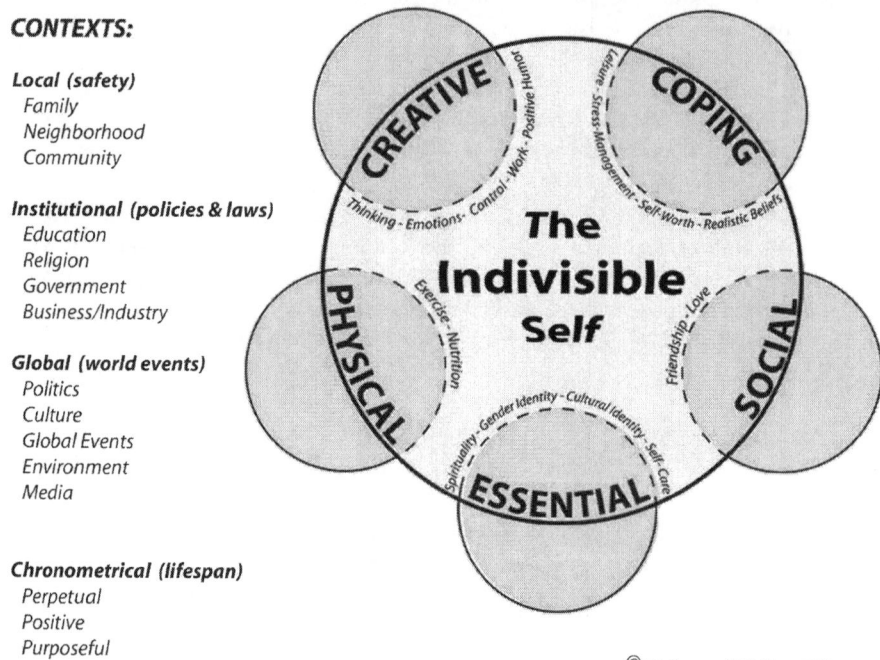

© T. J. Sweeney & J. E. Myers, 2003.

Figure 2.2 Indivisible Self Model of Wellness.

can influence one's wellness including family, religion, education, business/industry, media, government, community, and global events (Myers et al., 2000).

Analyses of the Five Factor Wellness Inventory (5F-Wel) were used to determine if the WoW framework most accurately represented the wellness data; the outcome was an update of the model from the Five Factor Model of Wellness to the Indivisible Self Model of Wellness (IS-Wel; Myers & Sweeney, 2004) pictured in Figure 2.2. Analyses indicated that wellness was most accurately understood when not divided into tasks or subtasks. This amendment signifies that wellness is holistic (Myers & Sweeney, 2004, 2005a,b, 2008). The component variables that did emerge were labeled the Creative Self (thinking, emotions, control, work, and positive humor), Coping Self (leisure, stress management, self-worth, and realistic beliefs), Social Self (friendship and love), Essential Self (spirituality, gender identity, cultural identity, and self-care), and Physical Self (exercise and nutrition) (Myers & Sweeney, 2004).

Myers and Sweeney went on to describe the process of wellness counseling in works like the *Wellness and Habit Change Workbook* (Myers & Sweeney, 2006) and *Counseling for Wellness: Theory, Research, and Practice* (Myers & Sweeney, 2005a). Wellness counseling involves the following:

- Providing information on the dimensions of wellness.
- Evaluating the client's wellness.
- Assessing the client's stage of change related to each wellness dimension.

- Identifying wellness goals, based in part on motivation to change for a given wellness dimension.
- Building the wellness goals into a wellness plan which contains facets that increase the likelihood of success such as the client's wellness strengths.
- Selecting and implementing wellness-enhancing techniques to assist the client in initiating and maintaining change (Myers & Sweeney, 2006).

These processes are also reflected in the counselor wellness competencies which include wellness assessment and wellness-based goal setting and plans (Gibson et al., 2021).

Wellness-based counseling has been applied or proposed with multiple client populations and presenting concerns. Below are a few examples:

- The IS-Wel model and affirmative therapy were used to ground assessment and treatment planning with adolescents who identified as LGBTGEQIAP+ (McKinney, Desposito, & Yoon, 2020).
- The WoW model tasks and subtasks provided the session themes and subject matter for a cancer survivor support group for women (Shannonhouse et al., 2014).
- Hartwig and Myers (2003) described implementing the WoW model for counseling with justice-involved adolescent females.
- The five second-order wellness factors of the IS-Wel model shaped the themes and subject matter for group counseling that targeted bolstering self-esteem in youth (Mills & McBride, 2016).
- Wellness counseling via the IS-Wel model was put forth as an approach for family caregivers of individuals with neurocognitive disorders (e.g. Alzheimer's disease) that includes bolstering the caregiver-care receiver relationship (Clarke, Adams, Wilkerson, & Shaw, 2016).

My (Phil) colleagues and I sought to contribute to the wellness counseling literature by synthesizing the numerous wellness factors into five domains and using terminology for each dimension that might be more accessible (mind, body, spirit, emotion, and connection wellness) (Ohrt, Clarke & Conley, 2019). From a clinical perspective, the five-domain wellness approach leaves room for the client to infuse their conceptualization and definitions of wellness. Throughout this book, we have made sure to discuss different assessment tools and resources to help you evaluate client wellness across these dimensions. Moreover, there are additional sub-components of these dimensions to examine regarding the addictive use of substances. We'll begin to survey the landscape of WBAC in the following sections.

WELLNESS-BASED ADDICTIONS COUNSELING

WBAC is a holistic and strength-based approach for counseling individuals with substance use disorders (SUDs). It is one of the first addictions interventions to be grounded in a wellness model, rather than wellness serving as an adjunct to treatment. It is important to describe how clinicians using WBAC conceptualize addiction and recovery. In this chapter, we will walk through the unique perspective of WBAC including how addiction and recovery are defined, conceptualized, and addressed in counseling. The key tenets of WBAC will be outlined. Additionally, we will elaborate on how WBAC fits into the SUDs treatment landscape so that you can begin to identify how this approach can be utilized in the settings at which you serve your clientele.

Addiction, according to WBAC, is defined as *compulsive engagement with substances or behaviors caused by diminished dimension-specific and overall wellness*. Recovery is defined as *a non-compulsive relationship with a substance or behavior that results when the effects of attending to one's holistic wellness outweigh those of compulsive engagement in the behavior. Moreover, recovery is the elimination or healthy integration of substance use or behaviors into a wellness-focused life*. In WBAC, decreased substance use is a byproduct of increased wellness. Therefore, holistic wellness is the centerpiece of addiction treatment. WBAC is a longitudinal, lifestyle approach that helps clients build a whole, fulfilling life and pursue their foundational and personal growth aims. Wellness is an equally important goal as the management of one's substance use. This is a shift in how SUDs treatment is typically provided. WBAC clinicians encourage clients to affirm themselves for wellness improvements as they would for a negative drug test or picking up a chip denoting one year of abstinence at an Alcoholics Anonymous (AA) meeting. In WBAC, figurative chips are imbued into sessions for positive steps attempted or accomplished.

WBAC interventions are a combination of approaches for increasing dimension-specific and holistic wellness and recovery skills integrated within a wellness framework. Some clients make substance use changes before making any substantive wellness improvements. For other clients, advancements in wellness precede reduction or abstinence from substance use. Whichever path is followed, the word "recovery" can include increased wellness, decreased substance use, or both. WBAC is another step forward in the clinical community moving toward a broader understanding of addiction and recovery, seeing recovery as more than simply someone abstaining or mitigating use. We believe that WBAC sends a powerful message to clients that can increase their motivation to change; that non-use or reduced use is but a part of a larger picture of your recovery process.

This perspective on recovery builds upon what researchers like William Miller and Stephen Rollnick (developers of Motivational Interviewing) have established; that most clients experience some level of ambivalence about change. When the clinician can widen the possibilities for change, adopting a holistic view, the risk of the client getting stuck in a place of ambivalence decreases. For clients who believe that quitting substance use is just a part of a bigger picture, clinicians can more thoughtfully address other aspects of recovery, such as wellness-based living, with a more invested client. Authors such as David Burns (1999) have discussed motivation as additive. Positive action steps further one's motivation to take additional action steps. Similarly, wellness scholars propose that positive steps taken in one area of wellness can produce wellness benefits in other wellness dimensions (e.g. Myers & Sweeney, 2005a). Hence, we believe that WBAC is not limited to helping clients stop or reduce substance use. Rather, the approach empowers clients to also plant seeds for taking care of themselves and living well. Let us further discuss the definitions and philosophies of WBAC.

In WBAC, we define wellness as *actively seeking life balance through identifying and engaging one's mental, emotional, physical, spiritual, developmental, cultural, and contextual strengths, needs and goals*. This is a definition you should share and explore with your clients, highlighting that wellness is about their involvement and empowerment. Convey that wellness contains multiple dimensions and hence relates to multiple aspects of their life. Confer with the client that they have ownership in discerning the areas of wellness that they wish to bolster. Emphasize that wellness is more about balance than perfection/flawlessness. In other words, the client should not expect each area of wellness to be equally fulfilled or "100%" fulfilled. Rather, wellness necessitates developing their ideal balance across the dimensions that enables them to achieve their wellness and substance use goals (Ohrt et al., 2019).

We have continued to revise the five-domain model by including development, culture, and contextual wellness as conceptual second-order factors. We also employ the word

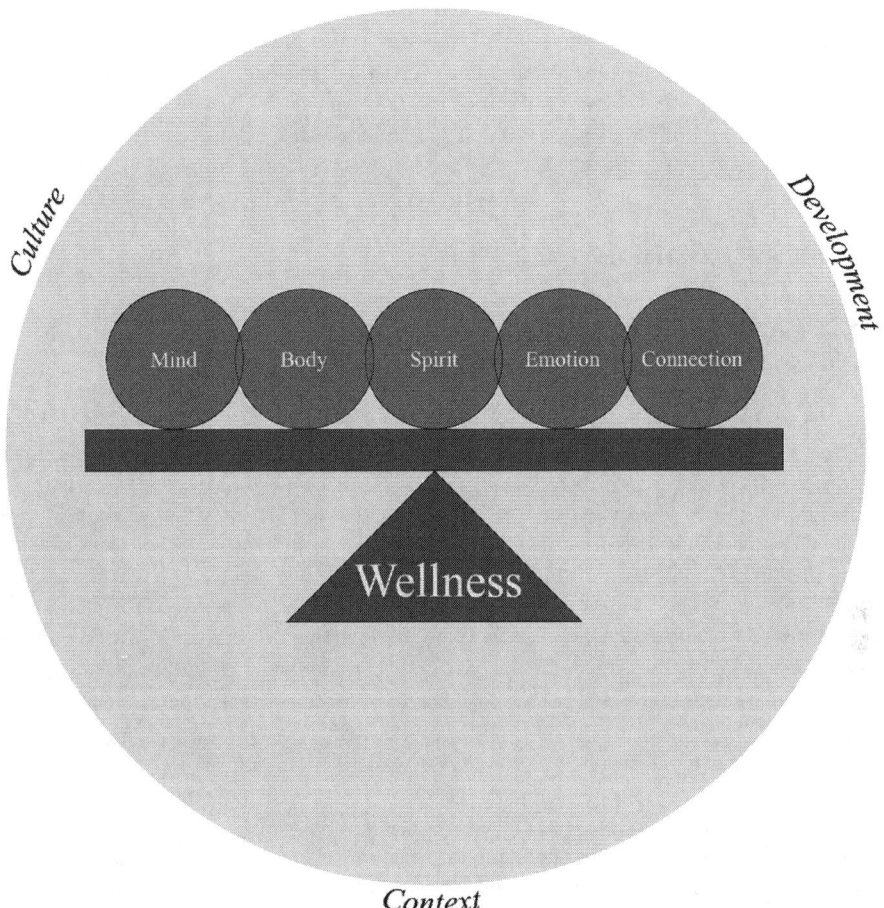

Figure 2.3 Five-Dimension Model of Wellness-Based Addictions Counseling. Adapted from the Five-Domain Model of Wellness (Ohrt et al., 2019).

"dimension" instead of "domain" to denote wellness as a flexible construct with depth and possibility. In Figure 2.3, we seek to visually depict the concept of lifestyle balance to reinforce our position that addictive behavior is the result of lifestyle imbalance which is further advanced by the addictive behavior itself. One of the goals of this model is to allow you to have conversations about balance with your clients, even inviting them to draw or share how much the scales are tipped for them currently and what that means for their holistic recovery.

The Wellness-Substance Use Relationship

Substance misuse and wellness have a reciprocal impact on each other. In other words, when a person ingests a substance compulsively or problematically, any single dimension of their wellness can be affected. Because the dimensions of wellness are interconnected, the effects in this one area can roll over into multiple wellness dimensions and result in decreased wellness overall. For example, the 24-year-old who binge drinks alcohol and is a daily cannabis user on top of taking psychotropic medication will likely experience negative impacts on her wellness. On the flip side, it is lower wellness that may fuel her substance use. Consider a person who lost his service industry job due to COVID-19 and feels a dearth of direction in his life (spiritual wellness) which substance use helps cover up. Additionally, this person is sheltered-in-place with apartment mates that frequently use substances (connection and contextual wellness). A *wellness-substance use cycle* is perpetuated and intensifies in which the wellness deficits get worse due to the substance use and the substance use is exacerbated by wellness challenges. Relapse, which may be a consequence of the wellness-substance use relationship, will be explored in depth in Chapter 4.

WBAC is Strengths-Based and Client-Centered

WBAC principles hold that one can be in recovery without complete abstinence from a substance. The writers of the *Diagnostic and Statistical Manual of Mental Disorders* (DSM-5; APA, 2022) have recognized that two people can have a cannabis use disorder, but this same disorder can vary widely in the number of symptoms and life disruptions that occur from that use. WBAC clinicians invite their clients to *share and develop their own personal model of addiction based on the dimensions of holistic wellness*. Clients are presented with the dimensions of wellness and asked to identify wellness struggles and dimensions of lower wellness that they believe factor into their substance use. Clients also process how their substance use either enhances or detracts from their wellness. Lastly, clients explore their strengths across the wellness dimensions and engrave these into the wellness plan (treatment plan) as skills and resources.

Strengths and solutions are a primary vehicle for improving wellness and substance use outcomes. Treatment as usual risks getting bogged down in the clinician being attentive to deficits in the client. Clinicians can become hyper-vigilant for manipulation or lying on the part of the client. Additionally, the remnants of the moral model stigma that individuals with SUDs are somehow lower in integrity still exist (Giordano, Stare, & Clarke, 2015). Treatment can also narrow-mindedly focus on correcting how the client responds to situations and internal impulses. WBAC clinicians conduct a deep dive into the client's positive qualities, unique coping skills, and resources and use these assets to derive progress. Take a moment and reflect on the many unique pathways to recovery you have witnessed in your tenure as a clinician. There is no way for you to prescribe exactly what would be best for every client. Hence, relying on what has worked for them in the past and drawing out positive qualities and resources that only that client may possess put you and the client at a therapeutic advantage. We will explore incorporating strengths within WBAC in greater depth in Chapter 5.

WBAC Guidelines

Ohrt et al. (2019) proposed "principles of wellness counseling" that we have synthesized and adapted for WBAC below. These guidelines hold the fundamental procedural and therapeutic elements of WBAC and can be referred to throughout your work with clients to assist you in upholding them.

- *Assess the client across the multiple wellness dimensions, ensuring that assessments of individual dimensions are related back to their relationship with the remaining dimensions.*
- *Assess the client's strengths during the evaluation process and throughout WBAC.*
- *Evaluate the client's substance use and explore the relationship between wellness and their use.*

- *Wellness plans should situate substance use in a manner that aligns with the client's goals. In other words, wellness plans allow for substance use goals to not be the primary objective or priority of the wellness plan.*
- *Wellness plans allow for abstinence and harm reduction substance use goals.*
- *Review client progress regularly during WBAC*
- *Frequently discuss the impact of interventions on the client's substance use goals and wellness.*
- *Seek opportunities to utilize and build upon client strengths throughout WBAC.*
- *Utilize a prolapse approach throughout WBAC: challenges experienced by the client are chances for new learning and growth (Marlatt, 1985).*

What about Maslow?

WBAC entails that holistic wellness is at the heart of addiction and recovery. Mental health and addictions professionals have asked questions such as, "how does wellness counseling work for my homeless client? Wouldn't a wellness focus be contraindicated for someone low in resources whose essential needs are not being met?" A myth and stereotype about wellness interventions is that they apply primarily to the "worried well"; in other words, clients whose fundamental needs are met and are not experiencing symptoms of an MHD or SUD. To these concerns, we respond that wellness is for all individuals and communities. Attending to the client's needs (whether obtaining employment, food, housing, medication adherence, childcare, etc.) nestles squarely within the realm of WBAC. This approach is first and foremost about meeting clients where they are, honoring what they identify will make them well, and then addressing how their substance use fits into the picture. In this way, WBAC is like interventions for individuals with multiple life challenges such as motivational harm reduction for clients with co-occurring disorders (Denning & Little, 2012; Mueser, Noordsy, Drake, & Fox, 2003). The difference is that wellness theory grounds our interactions with clients, providing a scaffolding for them to intentionally grow in nurturing these different aspects of themselves. The WBAC clinician asks the client struggling with homelessness, joblessness, or food insecurity to prioritize goals, however small, and how accomplishing them could benefit their overall wellness.

How Do WBAC and the Brain Science on Addiction Co-Exist?

Another question that arises for clinicians and clients alike is, "if addiction and relapse are related to low wellness, what about those whose genetics increase their risk to become addicted or whose brain processes result in craving and addictive use of substances?" WBAC is inclusive of research suggesting the significant involvement of brain processes in addiction. Remember that holistic wellness involves multiple aspects of the individual including their brain and mental processes. If a client experiences a relapse that could be explained by hijacked brain theory in which a person's behavior was influenced at the brain level with a desire to offset dopamine depletion or an individual's brain chemistry reacts more strongly than someone else's to exposure to a certain substance (Volkow, Koob, & McLellan, 2016), WBAC clinicians embrace this. These occurrences or possibilities are housed within the mental and physical components of wellness. Further, genes do not guarantee that one will become addicted. Genetics, depending on the substance, may only contribute about 30% to addictive behavior, whereas environmental can contribute upward to 50% or more, suggesting that lifestyle factors, such as wellness, can potentially have a powerful impact (Polk, 2015).

A client in a WBAC session who is de-constructing a recent relapse may describe how it originated cognitively with craving thoughts and likely being automatically triggered at the brain level from something he saw when going for a walk (mental/physical wellness). He might also describe viscerally experiencing the craving (physical wellness). However, what is sometimes missing with a sole emphasis on the disease/medical model is how the substance use impacts the client therein. The client describing the recent relapse with a clinician using WBAC would then process how the relapse affected different aspects of their wellness. Perhaps their substance use was wellness-enhancing in the short term in a few areas. But perhaps there also was a hangover (physical wellness), guilt (emotional wellness), the stress of telling their sponsor and partner about the relapse (emotional wellness), and the strain on the relationship with the partner from the relapse (connection wellness). The WBAC clinician can then discuss general wellness skills or wellness-based relapse prevention skills to assist the person. These include understanding what might be currently going on in the person's brain and body given the relapse and applying wellness-informed approaches to navigate these areas.

Co-Occurring Disorders

The wellness, recovery, and relapse definitions hold true for clients with co-occurring disorders. There are several hypotheses about how or why co-occurring disorders come about. Some researchers hypothesize that the mental health issue(s) arise first and that the individual then uses substances to manage the mental health symptoms (Miller, Forcehimes, & Zweben, 2019). Some believe that the SUD arrives first and can physiologically and/or psychologically activate the MHD. Other scholars believe there is a single cause that precipitates/influences the development of both the SUD and MHD (Miller et al., 2019).

It is possible that these different pathways are all true and that one theory accounts for the experience of one individual and another theory explains the manifestation/origin of another person's co-occurring disorder. Regardless, if one scrutinizes these theories, wellness is involved in each of them. As we discussed in Chapter 1, we believe that the development of the SUD and/or MHD sets off a cascade of negative effects across the individual's life that run into most or all aspects of the wellness including mind, body, spirit, emotion, and connection.

A powerful aspect of WBAC is that a wellness approach can help address both the MHD and SUD in an integrated way since wellness is a core factor implicated in both issues. Wellness is a useful platform for helping clients understand how their co-occurring disorders unfolded. These insights hold potential to be therapeutically normalizing, resulting in increased motivation and decreased shame. Integrated care or having the same treatment team providing services for both the MHD and SUD simultaneously is recommended for clients with co-occurring disorders. These approaches allow the MHP to employ interventions that help clients develop skills for addressing both issues. WBAC also offers this benefit in that when clients learn wellness information and skills that are helpful in managing both disorders, they can actively apply wellness-informed skills for preventing relapse in their MHD and SUD.

WBAC in Abstinence-Based Treatment Programs

WBAC has its roots in harm reduction perspectives and that a client's experience with addictive use is a journey with its own unique path. For some clients, a fulfilling path can still include substance use, and for others, this is not preferable or possible. We believe one of the great benefits of WBAC is its facilitation of intrinsic motivation as clients discern how substance use fits in with a life well lived. However, some clients are mandated through the criminal justice system or the structure of a treatment program to seek and maintain abstinence. This abstinence is typically tracked via drug testing.

WBAC can still be effective under abstinence-only treatment conditions and maintain its basic principles. Abstinence is still the client's choice. Clinicians using WBAC emphasize to clients that no one can technically force them to use or not use substances. Not even the justice system. A client can choose to relapse and break the terms of parole. A client can choose to relapse and lose custody or visitation with their children. A client can choose to relapse and be kicked out of their halfway house. A client can choose to relapse and be kicked out of their treatment program. Hence, WBAC clinicians reinforce client autonomy and will then build wellness principles and practices in and around that aim. Wellness clinicians use abstinence-required scenarios as an opportunity to underscore that clients can also choose to use in the future once their treatment program or period of probation, etc. ends. That even if they are not invested in abstinence in the long term, now is an opportunity to experiment with abstinence. The clinician stresses that given their abstinence, the client has the chance to develop strong wellness practices that will serve them. The client has the chance to see, with clear eyes, what life is like when focusing on wellness and not using substances.

CONSIDERATIONS FOR IMPLEMENTING WBAC

WBAC consists of formulating an overall treatment plan, centered upon a wellness plan and relapse prevention plan. The wellness plan is created during the first session and the relapse prevention plan is generated during the initial sessions. There are five dimensions of wellness along with development, cultural, and contextual factors. If you are leading addictions groups, you can devote learning modules to each of the five dimensions and the three cross-cutting factors (what are these factors?). When working with individual clients, the clinician may use relapse prevention and the client's wellness goal areas as the hub of the session plan. This includes providing psychoeducation, identifying, and practicing techniques specific to relapse prevention and the wellness dimensions the client seeks to address. However, the other wellness dimensions are consistently discussed because the client examines the impact of wellness and substance use changes on different dimensions of wellness. Further, as WBAC progresses, the client may benefit from in-depth discussions of all the wellness dimensions to (a) account for clients shifting their goals to new wellness dimensions over time and (b) to preserve a holistic perspective on the counseling process.

CLIENT EXAMPLE – ERIC

Throughout the book, a "running case study" of a fictional client is used to illustrate WBAC approaches. Eric is a fictional client based on multiple clients and insights that we have had in our clinical, supervision, and research experiences related to addiction. No client names or identifying information are included in this book. Below we describe the background, family history, and substance use history of Eric, who is coming to counseling due to increasing substance use problems and family-related issues. In many of the upcoming chapters, you will see examples of how wellness-based principles apply to this client. As you read about Eric, practice conceptualizing his presenting concerns through a wellness lens. Based on what you know thus far, how might WBAC inform your work with Eric?

Client Background

The client, Eric, is a 35-year-old biracial male (Caucasian and African American) who came to counseling at the insistence of his wife who recently informed him that she would end the marriage and seek primary custody of their daughter if he did not get help for his drinking. Additionally, his long-time friend (a physician) joined his wife and brother in an informal intervention, strongly recommending he attend treatment for his alcohol use. The relationship between Eric and his wife, Kelly, of ten years had become increasingly conflicted with both parties verbalizing threats of divorce. Eric and Kelly met while pursuing their associate's degrees and have remained together since then. They have a ten-year-old daughter, Lia. After their daughter was born, Kelly became pregnant on three more occasions but had a miscarriage with each of these children.

Eric and Kelly are currently experiencing financial stress. Eric, who had earned his associate's degree in business administration after high school, had bounced from job to job since completing his degree. He worked for years for a landscaping company, eventually landing a management role. Several years ago, he left that company for a sales representative position, and was ultimately fired. He currently holds an entry-level sales position for a technology company. During the pandemic, Kelly lost her job, and Eric's job was the sole source of income. Kelly obtained new employment also in a sales role. Eric's father has lived with he and Kelly for the past two years given multiple medical conditions (strokes that have affected his gait, fine motor skills, and resulted in mild cognitive impairment) that render independent living difficult. Their marriage is currently under duress. Two years ago, Kelly admitted to having an "emotional affair" with a long-time friend that she had grown up with. Kelly ended communication with this person after this admission occurred.

Family History

Eric is the middle child of three siblings. There was a lot of tension in his home growing up with a negative emotional tone much of the time. Stressors resulted from financial problems. Eric reports that he grew up in a lower middle-class household and that all his needs were provided for in terms of food and housing, but that his parents argued and "stressed" about money and finances consistently. Eric recalls feeling a special bond with his mother who, based upon his description, may have struggled with recurrent depression and anxiety and, during stretches of time, only left the house to go to work and complete essential tasks for the family (e.g., grocery shopping and depositing money at the bank). His mother did consume alcohol, but not frequently or to the point of intoxication, nor was he aware of drug use. Eric notes that his father worked 60 or more hours per week as an electrician and was not highly involved with him and his siblings while they were growing up. He describes that his father rarely drank and did not use any drugs. Eric believes his father probably had extramarital affairs based on his mother's comments, and his father regularly stayed out after work without his mother. He recalls often fearing that his parents would get divorced and split up the family. Eric does report some positive memories with both of his parents.

Substance Use History

Eric first consumed alcohol as a sophomore in high school on one or two occasions (once at a family gathering and once at a party with high school friends). He consumed alcohol at several parties during his junior year of high school but did not on a regular basis. He consumed alcohol and cannabis nearly every weekend of his senior year. Several friends he made in high school, college, and through his work in landscaping used alcohol and other drugs frequently. He reports in his 20s, consuming alcohol four to five days per week in the amount of four or more drinks per drinking day and on weekends typically consuming at least eight to ten drinks or more. When he met Kelly in his mid-20s, she also consumed alcohol approximately four days per week. Kelly (age 36) has not consumed alcohol for the past five years and had cut down substantially leading up to that. Eric cut down on his drinking several times in the past. He reduced his drinking ten years ago coinciding with Kelly's decision to reduce her drinking. Kelly expressed her concerns about their drinking and him receiving a DUI when he drove himself and Kelly home from a party and was pulled over for swerving. Eric reports his blood alcohol content was .14. Eric decreased his alcohol consumption to three to four days per week (limiting himself to no more than two drinks per day during the week and four to five drinks per day on weekends). Motivated by the birth of their daughter, he had decreased his drinking further to no more than two to three drinks every two to three days per week. However, in subsequent years, his alcohol use has increased, and he currently reports consuming alcohol at the frequency and quantity he did in his mid-20s. He typically begins consuming alcohol in the early evenings after work and starting early in the afternoons on weekends.

CONCLUSION

In this chapter, we presented an overview of wellness counseling and WBAC. Understanding the origins of wellness counseling will enable you to implement the approach with greater intentionality. Hettler's six-dimension model, the Wow model, the IS-Wel model, and the five-dimension model of WBAC can all be valuable in counseling clients with addictions. We also shared the philosophy and guidelines that shape WBAC. Lastly, we introduced Eric, a fictional client whose life experiences and WBAC experiences are incorporated in multiple chapters to demonstrate WBAC skills. Eric's introduction offered an opportunity to practice clinical thinking with a wellness mindset. The effective wellness clinician invites wellness and the whole client into each part of the counseling process. This will become increasingly clear as you venture further into the book, starting with the next chapter on evaluation which details the transformative role of wellness in assessment and treatment planning.

REFERENCES

American Psychiatric Association (2022). *Diagnostic and statistical manual of mental disorders* (5th ed., text rev.).

Burns, D. D. (1999). *The feeling good handbook*. First WholeCare.

Clarke, P. B., Adams, J. K., Wilkerson, J. R., & Shaw, E. G. (2016). Wellness-based counseling for caregivers of persons with dementia. *Journal of Mental Health Counseling, 38*(3), 263–277. https://doi.org/10.17744/mehc.38.3.06

Denning, P., & Little, J. (2012). *Practicing harm reduction psychotherapy: An alternative approach to addictions.* Guilford Press.

Diener, E., Sapyta, J. J., & Suh, E. (1998). Subjective well-being is essential to well being. *Psychological Inquiry, 9*(1), 33–37. https://doi.org/10.1207/s15327965pli0901_3

Diener, E., Suh, E. M., Lucas, R. E., & Smith, H. L. (1999). Subjective well-being: Three decades of progress. *Psychological Bulletin, 125*(2), 276–302. https://doi.org/10.1037/0033-2909.125.2.276

Downey, C. A., & Henderson, R. E. (2021). Speculation, conceptualization, or evidence? A history of positive psychology. In C. R. Snyder, S. J. Lopez, L. M. Edwards, & S. C. Marques (Eds.), *The oxford handbook of positive psychology* (3rd ed., pp. 8–17). Oxford University Press.

Gable, S. L., & Haidt, J. (2005). What (and why) is positive psychology? *Review of General Psychology, 9*(2), 103–110. https://doi.org/10.1037/1089-2680.9.2.103

Gallagher, M. W. (2019). Introduction to positive psychological assessment. In M. W. Gallagher & S. J. Lopez (Eds.), *Positive psychological assessment: A handbook of models and measures* (pp. 3–9). American Psychological Association. https://doi.org/10.1037/0000138-001

Gibson, D. M., Pence, C., Kennedy, S. D., Gerlach, J., Degges-White, S., & Watson, J. (2021). Development of the counselor wellness competencies. *Journal of Counselor Leadership and Advocacy, 8*(2), 130–145. https://doi.org/10.1080/2326716X.2021.1925997

Giordano, A. L., Stare, B. G., & Clarke, P. B. (2015). Overcoming obstacles to empathy: The use of experiential learning in addictions counseling courses. *Journal of Creativity in Mental Health, 10*(1), 100–113. https://doi.org/10.1080/15401383.2014.947011

Hartwig, H. J., & Myers, J. E. (2003). A different approach: Applying a wellness paradigm to adolescent female delinquents and offenders. *Journal of Mental Health Counseling, 25*(1), 57–75. https://doi.org/10.17744/mehc.25.1.kg4jy38q13xmfklb

Hettler, B. (1976). *Six dimensions of wellness.* National Wellness Institute. https://nationalwellness.org/about-nwi/

Joshanloo, M. (2016). Revisiting the empirical distinction between hedonic and eudaimonic aspects of well-being using exploratory structural equation modeling. *Journal of Happiness Studies, 17,* 2023–2036. https://doi.org/10.1007/s10902-015-9683-z

Marlatt, G. A. (1985). Relapse prevention: Theoretical rationale and overview of the model. In G. A. Marlatt & J. R. Gordon (Eds.), *Relapse prevention: Maintenance strategies in the treatment of addictive behaviors* (pp. 3–70). Guilford Press.

McKinney, R., Desposito, M., & Yoon, E. (2020). Promoting identity wellness in LGBTGEQIAP+ adolescents through affirmative therapy. *Journal of LGBT Issues in Counseling, 14*(3), 176–190. https://doi.org/10.1080/15538605.2020.1790464

Miller, W. R., Forcehimes, A. A., & Zweben, A. (2019). *Treating addiction: A guide for professionals* (2nd ed.). Guilford Press.

Miller, W. R., & Rollnick, S. (2013). *Motivational interviewing: Helping people change* (3rd ed.). Guilford Press.

Mills, B., & McBride, D. L. (2016). Increasing adolescent self-esteem: Group strategies to address wellness and process. *Georgia School Counselors Association Journal, 23,* 58–67.

Mueser, K. T., Noordsy, D. L., Drake, R. E., & Fox, L. (2003). *Integrated treatment for dual disorders: A guide to effective practice.* Guilford Press.

Myers, J. E., & Sweeney, T. J. (2004). The indivisible self: An evidence-based model of wellness. *Journal of Individual Psychology, 60*(3), 234–245.

Myers, J. E., & Sweeney, T. J. (2005a). *Counseling for wellness: Theory, research, and practice.* American Counseling Association.

Myers, J. E., & Sweeney, T. J. (2005b). The wheel of wellness. In J. E. Myers & T. J. Sweeney (Eds.), *Counseling for wellness: Theory, research, and practice* (pp. 15–28). American Counseling Association.

Myers, J. E., & Sweeney, T. J. (2006). *The wellness and habit change workbook.* Author.

Myers, J. E., & Sweeney, T. J. (2008). Wellness counseling: The evidence base for practice. *Journal of Counseling & Development, 86*(4), 482–493. https://doi.org/10.1002/j.1556-6678.2008.tb00536.x

Myers, J. E., Sweeney, T. J., & Witmer, J. M. (2000). The wheel of wellness counseling for wellness: A holistic model for treatment planning. *Journal of Counseling & Development, 78*(3), 251–266. https://doi.org/10.1002/j.1556-6676.2000.tb01906.x

National Wellness Institute (n.d.). *The six dimensions of wellness model.* Retrieved from https://cdn.ymaws.com/members.nationalwellness.org/resource/resmgr/pdfs/sixdimensinsfactsheet.pdf

Ohrt, J. H., Clarke, P. B., & Conley, A. H. (2019). *Wellness counseling: A holistic approach to prevention and intervention.* American Counseling Association.

Polk, T. A. (2015). *The addictive brain.* The Teaching Company.

Ryff, C. D. (1989). Happiness is everything, or is it? Explorations on the meaning of psychological well-being. *Journal of Personality and Social Psychology, 57*(6), 1069–1081. https://doi.org/10.1037/0022-3514.57.6.1069

Ryff, C. D. (2014). Psychological well-being revisited: Advances in the science and practice of eudaimonia. *Psychotherapy and Psychosomatics, 83*(1), 10–28. https://doi.org/10.1159/000353263

Shannonhouse, L., Myers, J., Barden, S., Clarke, P., Weimann, R., Forti, A., Moore-Painter, T., Knutson, T., & Porter, M. (2014). Finding your new normal: Outcomes of a wellness oriented psychoeducational support group for cancer survivors. *The Journal for Specialists in Group Work, 39*(1), 3–28. https://doi.org/10.1080/01933922.2013.863257

Travis, J. W., & Ryan, R. S. (1988). *The wellness workbook* (2nd ed.). Ten Speed Press.

Volkow, N. D., Koob, G. F., & McLellan, A. T. (2016). Neurobiologic advances from the brain disease model of addiction. *New England Journal of Medicine, 374*(4), 363–371.

CHAPTER 3

WELLNESS-BASED EVALUATION: SCREENING, ASSESSMENT, DIAGNOSIS, AND TREATMENT PLANNING

INTRODUCTION

When clients enter counseling, they most likely engage in an evaluation process where the clinician gathers relevant background information, inquires about current symptoms, and, if warranted, administers questionnaires. From this information, the clinician makes several decisions that significantly impact the direction of counseling. A thorough evaluation can be a clinician's best friend: it sets the tone for the clinical relationship, offers opportunity for client feedback, and provides information that could be critical to successful counseling. Wellness-Based Addictions Counseling (WBAC) evaluation begins with the assumption that substance use assessment is part of an overall wellness evaluation. This is because substance use is a part of the overall wellness picture and not representative of the whole person.

Substance use disorder (SUD) evaluation involves learning about the person's use *and* their context. We would argue that a well-conducted evaluation is even more important with issues related to substance use. The overall approach to wellness evaluation involves reducing a resistance dynamic, building motivation for improving wellness, making positive changes to substance use behavior, and gathering resources to assist the client in implementing changes. WBAC does this by pairing the substance use evaluation interview and formal assessments with wellness and strengths inventories. The clinician can then use wellness as a launching pad for the client to take an honest look at their substance use and how it fits within their life. Examination of the client's substance use can then be brought in through the side door of the platform that wellness provides. The evaluation culminates in the creation of a wellness plan that outlines the client's goals, action steps, treatment approaches to be used, and strengths and resources to draw upon.

In this chapter, we discuss the general process of clinical evaluation and its components: screening, assessment, diagnosis, and treatment planning. Using this discussion as a foundation, we then examine how wellness principles can be integrated into the substance use evaluation process. Wellness principles infused within the clinical evaluation help clients focus on positives and strengths from the start. Motivational interviewing (MI) principles, a natural fit with wellness, comprise a key component of WBAC assessment interventions. We conclude the chapter by exploring the components of a wellness-based treatment plan and case example. The client in the case example will be followed from the evaluation through the intervention process. This fictitious client is based on a compilation of clients with whom the authors have worked.

EVALUATION

Clinical evaluation is an umbrella term that encompasses *essential* activities designed to help clinicians figure out what is going on with the client. Although clients share information about their struggles from the start, additional information gathering is often necessary to get a complete picture. A thorough clinical evaluation can help clinicians assess the magnitude of

DOI: 10.4324/9781003147954-3

substance use problems (e.g., experimentation versus daily and problematic use), determine the fallout from problematic use, and identify contextual factors that partially maintain the addiction. Evaluations can help determine motivation, stage of change, degree of resistance, strengths, and other factors thought to be important for successful outcomes.

The evaluation for substance use concerns is the point of entry for real therapeutic value to commence. Some clients have been to treatment for SUDs previously, and many clients expect to be questioned about the problematic nature of their substance use and even their character. However, the WBAC clinician opens the process by informing the client of the following:

> We'll be exploring your holistic wellness. This includes learning more about your strengths, how well you feel in different areas of your life across mind, body, and spirit, and the behaviors you engage in that contribute to your well-being. Substance use is a part of your current wellness story and is a primary reason why you and I will be meeting, so the relationship between your substance use and wellness will be a part of this discussion.

Now, screening related to wellness and substance use problems, the first component of clinical evaluation, can effectively begin.

Screening

Screening allows clinicians to rule out the possibility of a SUD. It entails a broad, initial inquiry to find evidence of a substance use issue should one exist. Screening procedures are often brief in nature and can be informal or formal. SUD screening and assessment can garner significant resistance dynamics between the clinician and client for many reasons; one of which is that the client feels as if they are being picked apart and dissected by the clinician who is looking for things that are wrong with them (Doweiko, 2019). Hence, setting a positive tone starting early can pay dividends in rapport building and having a productive evaluation experience (Miller, Forcehimes, & Zweben, 2019).

In WBAC, the purpose of screening is twofold: to learn about the client's wellness and to learn about substance use. The client's substance use is a part of their wellness and thus becomes a natural extension of the dialog. To facilitate this, we start by conducting a wellness screening which involves first asking the client how they define wellness for themselves. This will provide you with valuable information about what wellness means to the client and their level of awareness about their own wellness behavior.

The clinician then presents the five-dimensional wellness model or a wellness model of their choice and processes the model's standard definitions of each wellness dimension. The client is invited to add to or take away any of these dimensions and to revise any wellness definitions. This ensures we are working within the client's unique perspective on wellness. Once each dimension is de-constructed, the wellness screening can proceed further. This entails the clinician asking the client to rate their level of wellness in each dimension and overall using a one to five or one to ten scale. "Level of wellness" can be operationalized as satisfaction with one's wellness, the extent to which one attends to that dimension of wellness, and/or the client's perception of how well they are in each dimension.

A visual alternative for initiating wellness screening is the wellness pie activity (Clarke & Scholl, 2022; Myers, Clarke, Brown, & Champion, 2012; Ohrt, Clarke, & Conley, 2019). It entails the clinician presenting a paper with a circle that spans the page. The clinician then directs the client to draw each slice of the pie to a size that corresponds with their level of wellness in that dimension. If mental wellness is their highest wellness dimension, for example, then that should be the largest slice of pie. Instead of drawing the pie, clients can elect to write a percentage that equates to their level of wellness for each dimension such that all the dimensions in total add to 100. As you review each dimension after the client has completed the activity, be sure to prompt the client to explain their rating. Clinicians then de-brief the wellness self-rating process by incorporating the following questions and prompts:

- What stood out to you the most from exploring your dimension and overall wellness?
- What surprised you now that you have rated your wellness?
- Talk about the reasons behind the rating you assigned for each dimension.
- What have you been doing that has resulted in _____ being one of your stronger wellness dimensions?
- What are some of the causes of _____ dimension being lower than other wellness dimensions?

The clinician then hearkens back to substance use being a part of wellness (Myers et al., 2012). The clinician should describe that substance use may have short- and long-term wellness costs and benefits and inquires accordingly,

- In what ways has your substance use affected your wellness?
- In what ways have areas of lower wellness affected your substance use?
- In what ways does substance use increase your wellness?
- What aspect(s) of your wellness are most negatively impacted by your substance use?

To concretize the discussion, the clinician can ask for examples of times when their substance use affected them in that area or when lack of attending to their wellness in a certain dimension influenced their substance use. For instance, a client may identify being hungover and not thinking clearly at work the next day (mental wellness).

Wellness screening in WBAC also includes observing the client and denoting indicators that further assessment is needed. The clinician should attend to these indicators in their conceptualization, diagnosis, and treatment with the client. These indicators include physiological (e.g., having family history of SUD, injection marks along the arms, physical signs of intoxication), psychological (e.g., depression, anxiety, and excessive mood swings), and behavioral (legal problems, occupational problems, and financial problems).

Methods of screening can be both informal and formal. For example, informal screening occurs during a mental status exam (MSE), where clinicians assess a client's mental state by observing affect, thought patterns, speech, appearance, and risk of self-harm. Most MSEs conducted by clinicians are purely observational; after an initial intake interview, the clinician will complete an MSE form followed by a brief mental status report. However, in some hospital settings, the MSE is a more formal procedure (e.g., having the client count backward from 100 to 7 and remembering three words that were said five minutes earlier). Formal screening usually involves one or more brief screening instruments that typically take ten minutes or less to complete. We briefly review three of these below: the Substance Abuse Subtle Screening Inventory – 4 (SASSI-4), the Michigan Alcoholism Screening Test (MAST), and the CAGE.

A popular screening tool used within the SUD treatment community is the SASSI-4 (Miller, 1985). The SASSI-4 takes about 10–15 minutes to complete, is easy to score, and is relatively accurate at predicting the presence of a SUD (e.g., higher in sensitivity; Stevens & Smith, 2013). In addition to assessing the intensity of drinking and/or drug use, the SASSI queries clients about the more "subtle" aspects of substance use behavior that, at first glance, would appear to be unrelated (e.g., questions about having memory issues or frequently feeling angry). Indeed, the strength of the SASSI is in its ability to look beyond obvious substance use signs and consider other behaviors that are correlated with problematic use.

Another screening instrument is the MAST. The MAST, created in 1971 by M. L. Selzer, is one of the most researched alcoholism screening instruments and, as with the SASSI, has a remarkably high sensitivity rate for correctly identifying alcoholism (Stevens & Smith, 2013). The MAST includes 25 items, is easy to score, and takes five to ten minutes to complete. It has been administered to both adolescents and adults and has a wide applicability across many populations (Stevens & Smith). A short version (SMAST) consists of 13 of the original 25 items.

The CAGE screening assessment entails variations on four questions: (a) Has anyone ever recommended that you cut back or stop drinking? Have you ever felt annoyed or angry if someone comments on your drinking? Have there been times when you have felt guilty about or regretted things that have occurred because of drinking? Have you ever used alcohol to help you get started in the morning to steady your nerves [Eye-opener]? Two or more positive responses indicate the presence of a severe alcohol use disorder with 90% accuracy (Stevens & Smith, 2013). The CAGE is a remarkably simple and accurate screening tool. It can easily be incorporated into any intake assessment, even if the focus of one's practice is not on substance use.

To broaden its applicability, Brown, Leonard, Saunders, and Papasouliotis (1998) modified the CAGE by creating the CAGE-AID and adding "drug use" in addition to alcohol use within the four original CAGE questions (e.g., has anyone ever recommended that you cut back or stop drinking *or drug use*? The CAGE-AID has been found to have sufficient reliability and validity among Northern Plain American Indians (Leonardson et al., 2005), in detecting SUDs among adolescents in Norway (Couwenbergh, van der Gaag, Koeter, de Ruiter, & van den Brink, 2009), and shows greater sensitivity than the CAGE for identifying primary care patients with alcohol and drug use disorders (Brown & Rounds, 1995). The advantage of the CAGE-AID is that clinicians can conjointly screen for alcohol and drug use problems. It holds promise as an effective clinical tool toward this goal (Brown & Rounds, 1995).

Screening for SUDs is designed to be overinclusive (Miller, Forcehimes, & Zweben, 2011), assessing for the possible presence of a substance use issue. If a client shows signs of problematic use through the screening process, a more thorough inquiry is warranted. Assessment is the next step in the evaluation process and includes a deeper analysis that can shed additional light on the occurrence of problematic use.

Interview

WBAC assessment for substance use problems can take several forms, including clinical interviews, semi-structured interviews, the use of wellness and substance use assessment instruments, or some combination. Screening questions, such as the CAGE or CAGE-AID, also can be infused within clinical interviews. Thus, the line between screening and assessment is sometimes blurred as the clinician gathers data. Doweiko (2009) proposed that the clinical interview is one of the best methods for addiction assessment. Based on the clinical interview, the clinician usually has enough information to inform a diagnosis and treatment plan (Lewis, 2014).

The clinical interview is a semi-structured process in which the clinician probes for indicators and correlates that might suggest a substance use problem. The clinical interview is contextualized within the client's holistic wellness. Hence, questions and prompts about the client's wellness, strengths, and resources are part of the interview. Questions are formulated around quantity and frequency (i.e., intensity) of use, perceived benefit of using, what role substance use plays in the client's life, family history of use, and consequences of use. Lewis (2014) outlined seven key components of a clinical interview, along with sample questions, focused on substance use. We have integrated wellness questions and prompts into these components and have added an additional item about trauma.

1. *Referral source.* Who referred you? Self? Others? Why were you referred?

2. *History of substance use and misuse/Periods of reduced use or abstinence that followed periods of problematic use.* When did your substance use begin? When did your use become problematic? What changes in your wellness have you noticed because of changes in your substance use? Tell me about times when you have reduced your substance use or quit using. What were your reasons for reducing or quitting? What impact did reducing or quitting have on your wellness? What did you do differently that helped you reduce or quit? What wellness behaviors, strengths, skills, and/or resources helped facilitate this reduced use or abstinence?

3. *Prior treatment history/Prior treatment insights.* Have you been to SUD treatment before? If so, what was that experience like? What was helpful and what was not helpful? List two to three things you learned about yourself, your substance use, and/or your wellness from your previous experience(s) in treatment.

4. *Current life functioning.* What current challenges are you facing in regard to your daily functioning whether mental, emotional, physical, spiritual, or social? Note: The clinician should explore any areas of concern or red flags related to substance use. What aspects of your wellness are strongest/most helpful in your daily functioning?

5. *Family history of substance use.* Do you recall or know of substance use problems within your family? If so, how has this affected you or your family's wellness? Who in your life – whether blood relatives or friends/significant others – have been or could be supportive in you reaching the goals you set in counseling?

6. *Consequences of substance use.* What have been the specific consequences of your substance use? How have these consequences affected you across the dimensions of wellness? How, if at all, has the impact of your substance use on your wellness changed over time?

7. *General personal history.* Many elements of the client's personal history may have been covered up to this point in the clinical interview. However, components of work history, legal history, relationship history, and emotional functioning may need clarification and/or further exploration.

8. *Trauma history.* Have you experienced one or more traumas that impact your wellness and substance use? If so, in what ways has the trauma affected your wellness and substance use?

There are many other areas one can cover using the clinical interview, depending on the agency, client issues, and clinician preference. The beauty of the clinical interview is that, as Juhnke (2002) noted, it humanizes the process. Its flexibility allows clinicians to build rapport, which can enhance motivation and encourage sharing. The clinician can pursue specific questions in more depth or back off if information is not relevant. The clinician can be more in tune with nonverbal information, such as emotional reactions, which may lead to additional insight and information.

Substance Use Assessment Instruments

Substance use instruments can be an excellent way for clinicians to assess the extent of use, experiences and characteristics that may underlie use, and other external correlates of use (e.g., presence of family violence). These methods are more structured than the clinical interview; clients typically complete them via paper and pencil or online administration. Although instruments are thought to be objective, the clinician still has responsibility in interpreting the findings and using them to inform a diagnosis and/or treatment plan. The strength of using instruments is that they can reveal aspects of substance use that might be out of the client's awareness. Personality assessments, for example, can uncover underlying tendencies and characteristics that may either drive or exacerbate a substance use problem. A client whose score is elevated on a depression scale may alert the clinician that negative mood may be an underlying cause of addiction (or vice versa). This information enriches the clinical picture and allows for a more expanded treatment plan.

To provide an in-depth review of substance use instruments is beyond the scope of this chapter. However, there is a bevy of information online where clinicians can explore possibilities, objective measurements, and the psychometric integrity of potential instruments (e.g., the reliability and validity of an instrument) for their SUD practice. The U.S. government publishes extensive assessment resources open to the public. For example, the National Institute on Drug Abuse (NIDA) publishes *the Screening and Assessment Tools Chart* (https://www. drugabuse.gov/nidamed-medical-health-professionals/screening-tools-prevention; NIDA, 2019) complete with access to several high-quality screening and assessment instruments. Many of these tools can be accessed on the NIDA website or corresponding links. Additionally, NIDA publishes content on the description and psychometric properties of these instruments. Another excellent resource is the *Substance Use Screening and Assessment Instruments Database*, created by the Alcohol and Drug Abuse Institute Library (ADAI Library) at the University of Washington (https://tinyurl.com/2p8vc8b7; ADAI, 2010). The database is a compendium of substance use assessment instruments, both in the public dimension as well as copyrighted. Search results provide author information, instrument descriptions, psychometric properties, relevant articles and links, how to locate the instrument, and whether it is in the public dimension (Lewis, 2014). Instruments in the database range from assessing the use of specific drugs (e.g., cocaine) and drug classes (e.g., amphetamines) as well general substance use.

In the substance use screening and assessment portion of the evaluation, the MI style of elicit-provide-elicit is utilized (Miller & Rollnick, 2013). The clinician queries the client about what they think the screening and assessment tools revealed about their wellness and their substance use. This communicates the importance of the client's perspective and increases client openness to the evaluation results. When the clinician "provides" the results and interpretation of the evaluation, the client is then re-enlisted by not only processing their thoughts on the results but also inviting the client to identify screening and assessment items that stood out to them and that most strongly reflect substance use concerns. No substance use assessment should be used in isolation as this would omit key aspects of the whole person that relates to their substance use and overall goals for wellness and mental health. The clinical interview and substance use assessment instruments should be linked to the client's wellness. The clinician and client thus examine the relationship between these flagged responses and the client's wellness and vice versa (Clarke, Adams, Wilkerson, & Shaw, 2016).

Wellness Assessment Instruments

Holistic wellness is difficult to measure, and the lack of these measures may be a result of that (Ohrt et al., 2019). For those practicing wellness counseling, the Five Factor Wellness Inventory (Myers & Sweeney, 2014) is one of those few such measures. It assesses the respondent's engagement in wellness behaviors and perception of one's levels of wellness across dimensions. The strengths of this measure lie in its thoroughness, examination of behaviors rather than solely one's satisfaction with wellness, and positive psychometric outcomes (Shannonhouse, Erford, Gibson, O'Hara, & Fullen, 2020). It also assesses overlooked aspects of wellness such as humor, self-worth, and gender and cultural identity (Myers, Luecht, & Sweeney, 2004).

The Perceived Wellness Survey (Adams, Bezner, & Steinhardt, 1997) also takes a holistic approach to wellness assessing for psychological (positive outlook), emotional (self-efficacy and self-worth), social (social support), physical (perceptions and outlook on physical health), spiritual (meaning and purpose), and intellectual ("mental stimulation") health and wellness. The view on wellness presented in this measure is based on how well one believes oneself to be across these dimensions.

Well-being and quality-of-life measures tend to assess factors related to wellness. For example, Ryff's (1989) well-being model comprised self-acceptance, positive relations with others, autonomy, environmental mastery, purpose in life, and personal growth (p. 1072). Several well-being measures address one or more of these elements such as the Mental Health Continuum-Short Form (Lamers, Westerhof, Bohlmeijer, Klooster, & Keyes, 2011), the Brief Inventory of Thriving, and the Comprehensive Inventory of Thriving (Su, Tay, & Diener, 2014). The conceptualization of the variable, quality of life, ranges from "happiness" to one's "living conditions" (Barcaccia et al., 2013). The World Health Organization's QoL Brief scale incorporates physical, psychological, social, environmental, and spiritual (2004). The clinician should thus be intentional in identifying what they want to learn about their client.

Finally, provided that the clinician is intentional, a piecemeal approach to holistic wellness assessment can be acceptable. For instance, the clinician may elect to utilize separate measures to represent each dimension of wellness. Each chapter on the different dimensions will include assessments that address each respective dimension.

Recovery capital assessments offer a means for evaluating client strengths specific to their substance use. You'll recall that recovery capitals are the resources that enable the addicted individual to productively address their substance use concerns. Those include physical financial, social, human (abilities, health, education, and other facets), and cultural (values align with a culture of recovery and lifestyle not involving the addictive use of substances; Cloud & Granfield, 2008). The Recovery Capital Scale (White, 2009; White & Cloud, 2008) will inform clinicians and clients on the recovery capital dimensions, and White noted that it can be helpful in determining the client's level of care. For instance, a physical (financial) item states "I have the financial resources to provide for myself and my family". A human capital item states "I live in an environment free from alcohol and other drugs".

White and Cloud (2008) present a structure for goal setting based on the survey results involving identifying lower scores. We recommend that clinicians also identify their higher scores and discuss ways to mobilize the recovery capital to achieve their substance use goals. The Brief Assessment of Recovery Capital (BARC-10) (Vilsaint et al., 2017) is an empirically validated scale that measures ten factors from the Assessment of Recovery Capital (Groshkova, Best, & White, 2012) and consists of items that link elements of wellness to recovery (Vilsaint et al., 2017). For example, one item states "There are more important things to me in life than using substances" (Vilsaint et al., 2017, p. 74).

The therapeutic magic of the formal wellness assessment is in the added perspective of their results. The screening prompts and questions listed above can be used to process formal wellness assessments. Clinicians and clients also now have specific items as a launching point from which to explore further. This exploration is distilled into meaningful content by the client noting the most vital strengths and resources that were unearthed via the screening, interview, and assessment. The clinician can facilitate this unearthing of strengths by simply having the client list them on a paper or a dry-erase board. These strengths and resources will be incorporated into treatment planning and the wellness plan (see Handout 3.1).

SUD Diagnosis

After a positive screen and assessment, the next step in clinical evaluation is making a diagnosis. Clinicians consider the client data and determine if there is a match between signs and symptoms to established criteria outlined in the *Diagnostic and Statistical Manual of Mental Disorders* (currently in its fifth edition, text revision, DSM-5; APA, 2022). If clients meet the criteria threshold for a disorder, a diagnosis is made. All addictive disorders outlined in the DSM-5 include substance-induced disorders and SUDs. Substance-induced disorders refer to substance-related syndromes that manifest from recent ingestion of a substance (intoxication) or recent cessation of a substance (withdrawal). SUDs refer to substance-specific problems related to the intensity (i.e., quantity and frequency) of use.[1]

To be diagnosed with a SUD, a client must have, "A problematic pattern of alcohol (or any other substance) use leading to clinically significant impairment or distress, as manifested by at least two of the following [11 criteria], within a 12-month period" (APA, 2022, p. 583). In other words, for at least a year, the client must experience significant life disruption due to substance use. Specific diagnoses are made according to the class of substance from which a client is struggling (e.g., alcohol use disorder, cannabis use disorder, and stimulant use disorder). The DSM-5 lists ten classifications of substances based on how they affect the brain and nervous system (e.g., alcohol and stimulants). Table 3.1 outlines the 11 criteria in the DSM as well as the ten drug classifications.

The clinician must also assess for co-occurring disorders and/or trauma. If these factors are identified, they are examined through a wellness lens. The clinician explores the relationship among the client's trauma and mental health symptoms, substance use, and wellness. Following are some prompts and questions to assess these relationships.

- How does the presence of trauma/mental health symptoms and substance use affect your wellness? What areas of wellness are most affected?
- What symptoms have the biggest impact on your wellness?
- In what ways has lower wellness in certain dimensions affected your trauma/mental health symptoms?

Table 3.1 Classifications of Substances and Diagnostic Criteria (Adapted) for Substance Use Disorders[a] in DSM-5

Drug Classifications within the DSM	
Alcohol	Inhalants
Stimulants[b]	Tobacco
Caffeine[c]	Opioids
Cannabis	Sedatives, hypnotics, or anxiolytics
Hallucinogens	Other
Phencyclidine	
Other hallucinogens	

Diagnostic criteria for SUDs

A maladaptive pattern of substance use leading to clinically significant impairment or distress, as manifested by two (or more) of the following, within a 12-month period

1. Substance is often taken in larger amounts or over a longer period than was intended.
2. There is a persistent desire or unsuccessful efforts to cut down or control substance use.
3. A great deal of time is spent in activities necessary to obtain/use/recover from its effects.
4. Craving or a strong desire or urge to use a specific substance.
5. Recurrent substance use resulting in a failure to fulfill major role obligations at work, school, or home (repeated absences, poor work performance, suspensions, or expulsions).
6. Continued substance use despite having persistent or recurrent social or interpersonal problems caused or exacerbated by the effects of the substance (arguments and physical fights).
7. Important social, occupational, or recreational activities are given up or reduced.
8. Recurrent substance use in situations in which it is physically hazardous (e.g., driving).
9. The substance use is continued despite knowledge of having a persistent or recurrent physical or psychological problem that is likely to have been caused or exacerbated by the substance.
10. Tolerance
11. Withdrawal

Based on American Psychiatric Association (2013). *Diagnostic and Statistical Manual, Fifth Edition* (DSM-5). Washington, DC: American Psychiatric Association (APA).
[a]The generic criteria listed in this table are applicable across the 13 classifications of substances. Specific diagnoses are made depending on the substance from which the client struggles.
[b]Includes amphetamines and cocaine.
[c]There is no SUD for caffeine.

- What areas of wellness are most helpful in addressing your trauma/mental health symptoms?
- Reflect on a time when you felt you have had success in managing your trauma symptoms/co-occurring disorder. What aspects of your wellness were most helpful?

Lutz (2013) noted that clinicians incorporating a solution-focused perspective in assessing trauma can inquire about (a) "How did you cope with these situations?", (b) "Supposing 10 is you are satisfied with how you are coping and 1 is the opposite, where would you say you are now?", (c) "What makes it not lower?", and (d) "What would it take to raise it by one point?" (p. 140). Further, the Substance Abuse and Mental Health Services Administration (SAMHSA) assembled a list of trauma measures in their *Treatment Improvement Protocol 57: Trauma-Informed Care in Behavioral Health Services* (SAMHSA, 2014).

Do a Client Map

In WBAC, treatment plans need to be comprehensive, flexible, and open to providing a wellness-based vision for the client's recovery. One model that meets these requirements and is used in conjunction with the wellness plan is Reichenberg and Seligman's (2016) Client Map. Considering important treatment factors such as objectives of treatment, clinician characteristics, assessments, interventions, and prognosis, the Client Map is comprehensive and easy to use, and allows for creativity in the treatment planning process. The Client Map is a clinical conceptualization based on 12 key factors, spelling the mnemonic DO A CLIENT MAP. The Client Map is appropriate for any disorder group in the DSM, including substance-related disorders and co-occurring disorders. Its flexibility also allows for the inclusion of the wellness plan which contains wellness-based goals and interventions. Each letter representing one of the 12 key factors is briefly described below.

Diagnosis. The first step in the treatment plan. All disorders, including non-substance-related, are listed in order of clinical importance.

Objectives/goals. Objectives/goals refer to what the client will accomplish in counseling. The process should be collaborative, and objectives should be written in a clear and measurable way (Reichenberg & Seligman, 2016).

Assessments. List all relevant screening and assessment interviews, tools, inventories, scales, tests, journals, or checklists you plan to use. Medical status assessments can be listed, although make sure to confirm from a medical specialist (or that one is needed). Incorporate a balance of symptom-based and wellness and strength-based measures.

Clinician characteristics. List clinician characteristics that may be important to successful counseling, depending on the client and presenting issue. Relevant to both wellness and addictions counseling would be characteristics such as empathy, collaborativeness, and compassion. Demographic characteristics, experience, and professional expertise also can be listed here, although these items may or may not be important to the client (Reichenberg & Seligman, 2016).

Location. Note treatment setting most appropriate for the client. Options include withdrawal management, residential, inpatient, half-way house, intensive outpatient, and outpatient (Lewis, 2014). Discussion on actualizing the wellness plan in the context of the treatment location should occur.

Interventions. Interventions include how the clinician will intervene to help the client accomplish their objectives/goals. Ideally, both theoretical and technique-based applications are offered in this section. Consider interventions that address motivation, substance use, and wellness issues.

Emphasis. Different emphases include directiveness (directive vs. non-directive), structure (structured vs. non-structure), support (supportive vs. encouraging more individuality), confrontation (confrontational vs. non-confrontational), and exploration (exploration vs.

behavioral; Reichenberg & Seligman, 2016). These will vary depending on the client and the severity of substance use. For example, some clients might respond well to structure and support, whereas others may respond better to non-structure and exploration. In general, clients struggling with addiction usually require more structure and support upfront and, when their recovery strengthens, flourish with less direction and more flexibility. Emphasis on wellness issues should be evident throughout treatment.

Number. List how many people will participate in counseling and what mode of counseling will be used. Options include individual counseling, family counseling, couples counseling, group counseling, or some combination. All modes can be used in addictions counseling.

Timing. Note the frequency and length of counseling. Frequency refers to how often you will meet with your client(s), such as once a week. Length of counseling refers to the duration of care (e.g., 12 months) and length of counseling sessions (e.g., 50 minutes). If the client is in more than one mode of counseling, list frequency and length for each mode (e.g., once a week, 50-minute individual sessions; once a week, 90-minute sessions for the group).

Medication. List all relevant medications the client is currently taking. Consultation with a medical specialist may be warranted to receive accurate information.

Adjunct services. These services can play a major role in recovery. The most common example would be Alcoholics Anonymous (AA) and other 12-step mutual support groups. Other examples might be community organizations, volunteering programs, and animal-assisted therapy for addicted individuals. Community and individual wellness programs, groups, and activities can be considered as well. List all relevant adjunct services in which the client participates. Like the Interventions segment of the Client Map, the wellness model can help the client and clinician co-create these options.

Prognosis/possibilities. Consult screening and assessment results, diagnosis, and consultations to arrive at a prognosis. Many factors can play into a prognosis, although two critical factors include the severity of the diagnosis/disorder and motivation to make changes (Reichenberg & Seligman, 2016). What is the likelihood that the client will reach their objectives/goals? Although somewhat subjective, use clinical intuition, assessments, and other data as the basis of your prognosis. In general, words to describe prognosis include *excellent*, *very good*, *good*, *fair*, and *poor*. Reasons for your prognosis can be briefly summarized. Although not a formal part of the Client Map, the clinician should also log client possibilities and strengths. These include reasons the client might be successful in reaching their treatment goals, even if their prognosis is less favorable/guarded/less promising. Identifying client strengths fits squarely within the WBAC protocol for treatment and counseling. In essence, the clinician can help the client identify strengths and explore ways that these can be incorporated into the wellness and recovery plan.

Treatment planning serves several important functions. First, it can help the clinician and client track clinical progress by determining to what extent goals have been met (Reichenberg & Seligman, 2016). Second, it can be referred to when counseling gets off track, thus providing structure and focus. Relatedly, a thorough treatment plan facilitates accountability for both the client and the clinician. For example, is the client following through on assigned tasks? Is the clinician incorporating interventions agreed to in the plan? We advocate that clients and clinicians co-construct the treatment plan, with significant client input as to goals, interventions, and types of counseling. In our experience, a collaborative, well-conceived treatment plan increases the odds for successful counseling.

We have reviewed five key components of clinical evaluation: screening, clinical interview, assessment, diagnosis, and treatment plan. In the next section, we will describe the wellness plan, which is formulated during treatment planning. It is a comprehensive document that outlines the direction of counseling moving forward.

WELLNESS PLAN

In WBAC, a wellness plan is created as part of the treatment plan. The wellness plan is the client-facing document that contains the goals, subgoals, action steps, strengths/resources, and how they can be utilized toward goal attainment and wellness. The wellness plan also highlights the substance use benefits of goal pursuit and achievement, and wellness and substance use consequences of not changing. Goal setting is one of the first steps in building the wellness plan and necessitates prompting the client to identify the wellness areas they would like to improve upon by the end of counseling. Another option is to inquire what facets of wellness the client wants to give more attention.

The wellness goals are operationalized by using scaling questions from the wellness screening and assessment. For example, if a client who sets a mental wellness goal scored themselves at a three out of ten on mental wellness, the clinician requests that the client identify what their mental wellness self-score would be at the completion of counseling if they had accomplished their goal (Guterman, 2013; Lutz, 2013). The client is asked to elaborate on what they would observe that would indicate a successful counseling outcome or what they would notice that would let them know they had reached their goal of a six out of ten on mental wellness, for example (O'Hanlon, O'Hanlon & Weiner-Davis, 2003). Ensure that the client reports on measurable/observable wellness behaviors, thoughts, and/or feelings and a time frame for completion. The outcomes of this process can yield both the goals and action steps.

The goal is the vision for what the client wants to be different and the clinician can safeguard that the goal is measurable by incorporating the phrase "as evidenced by". The content that follows "as evidenced by" is considered a subgoal or extension of the original goal. The action steps can be separated out from the goal as these are reflective of the thoughts, feelings, behaviors, and beyond that will enable accomplishment of the goal. Below is an example that illustrates and differentiates goals from action steps.

- **Goal 1:** Increase mental wellness from a three to a six out of ten as evidenced by
    - **Subgoal:** Identifying at least one hobby that is mentally stimulating.
        - **Action Step 1:** Make a list of mentally stimulating hobbies within the next two weeks.
        - **Action Step 2:** Try out at least two of those activities on more than one occasion over the next two to four weeks.
        - **Action Step 3:** Select 1 of those hobbies and commit to doing it at least once per week.
    - **Subgoal:** Exploring opportunities to broaden work possibilities that would be more mentally challenging.
        - **Action Step 1:** Consult with at least two colleagues who have gotten their master's degree in my field of interest to learn about pros and cons and recommended schools within the next month.
        - **Action Step 2:** Conduct a web search of multiple regional programs and learn about coursework, cost, timeline to degree completion, etc. within the next month.

    ○   **Action Step 3:** Explore other job opportunities via web search and possibilities for advancement at current job via consulting with at least two colleagues.

The clinician now shifts to facilitate the client's examination of their substance use as part of the wellness goals. "What role would your substance use play in achieving this wellness goal?" Other questions could include the following:

What would your substance use look like if you reached your wellness goal?

If you make no changes to your substance use, what is the likelihood that you can attain your wellness goal?

How would your relationship with your substance use change if your wellness improved in the goal area you have identified?

What effects might you notice on this wellness area if you made constructive changes to your substance use?

These same questions can be posed for each wellness goal area noted by the client. When it comes to change goals, it also is important to assess the client's importance, confidence, and readiness to make changes (whether wellness, substance use, or both) (Miller & Rollnick, 2013). To achieve this, importance, confidence, and readiness ruler questions from MI are utilized. For example, the clinician inquires about how important it is for the client to fully abstain from their substance use, reduce their substance use, or explore making changes to their substance use on a 1–10 scale with 1 representing "not at all important" and 10 representing "extremely important" (Miller & Rollnick, 2013). This scaling question structure is also used to determine the client's level of confidence and readiness to change. Formal measures of motivation for change can be incorporated such as the Readiness to Change questionnaire (Heather & Rollnick, 1993), Change Questionnaire (Miller & Johnson, 2008), or the Problem-Recognition Questionnaire (Cady, Winters, Jordan, Solberg, & Stinchfield, 1996). The importance, confidence, and readiness questions can also be directed at the client's wellness goals (Myers & Sweeney, 2006).

If through the above process, the client does not value examining or addressing their substance use, the focus can be on wellness-specific goals. The clinician listens for new insights that may arise for the client related to their substance use as they pursue their wellness goals and periodically inquires about how their wellness goal progress or lack thereof has affected their thoughts, feelings, and behaviors related to substance use. If the client falls into the category of seeking an abstinence goal (on their own volition or a requirement of treatment), a harm reduction goal (on their own volition or a requirement of treatment), or is willing to reflect on their substance use, the clinician should delve into generating substance use specific goals in addition to the wellness goals.

Alternatively, if changing one's substance use felt like a better fit for the client within an existing wellness goal, a substance use subgoal is added to the wellness goal. For instance, in the mental wellness example above, the client decides that heavy cannabis use on weekends and the occasional weekday lead to mental fogginess and dulling of their mental processes the next day. This client's harm-reduction-related subgoal entails limiting their cannabis use to no more than one joint in total between Friday and Sunday and eliminating weekday cannabis use. Action steps would then flush out the changes needed to accomplish this.

Harm Reduction

Clients interested in pursuing harm reduction should be informed about the benefits and potentially serious consequences of this recovery pathway. The clinician is obliged to share that harm reduction is not advisable if any of the following is true for the client (note: this is not an exhaustive list) (Tatarsky & Kellogg, 2012; Tatarsky & Marlatt, 2010):

- Client is physiologically dependent on the substance (in other words, face high likelihood of withdrawal symptoms upon reducing use).
- Client who has incurred severe consequences from their use (e.g. hospitalization, domestic violence, and incarceration)
- Substance(s) used by client possess powerful addictive properties that reduce the likelihood of effectively reducing use (e.g. opiates, amphetamines, and sedatives
- Client has a moderate or severe SUD.
- Client has a co-occurring mental health disorder, in particular, if they have any history of crises such as suicidal ideation, homicidal ideation, violence, or impulse control concerns that are associated with their substance use.
- Client has a co-occurring behavioral addiction(s).
- Client has a co-occurring medical condition(s) that has or could be negatively affected by substance use.
- Client has attempted harm reduction previously and was not able to maintain the harm reduction goal.

Clients who incorporate harm reduction goals or subgoals for their substance use should create an ideal use plan as part of their wellness plan (Tatarsky, 2007). The components of this can include setting a limit on total quantity of consumption per week or month, number of using days per week, maximum quantity of use in a given day, when use can and cannot occur, etc. (NIAAA, n.d.; Tatarsky & Kellogg, 2012). For drug use, clinician and client should discuss ways to reduce risk regarding administration of the drug (Kilmer et al., 2012). Clinician and client track the effectiveness of the plan (NIAAA, n.d.; Tatarsky & Kellogg, 2012; Tatarsky & Marlatt, 2010), for instance, the extent to which the client adheres to the ideal use plan versus breaks the boundaries they have set.

The wellness structure allows the clinician to constantly refer the client back to the impact of the ideal use plan (or breaching that plan) on their dimensions of wellness. This eases the shift in treatment goals should the client elect to transition to abstinence and increases client self-efficacy in cases of success with the ideal use plan. Further, upon realizing the benefits of decreased substance consumption through examining its relationship with their wellness, clients may terminate their substance use (Tatarsky & Kellogg, 2012). The key is for the clinician to create the conditions for informed choice on the part of the client; maintaining their autonomy to determine their wellness path and the role of substance use in that journey (Denning & Little, 2012).

Substance-Specific Goals

Similar goal-setting questions are used for the substance-specific goals. Additionally, the clinician discusses the impact of substance use goal attainment on each wellness goal area and overall wellness. For example, "If you were able to reduce your alcohol use to once per month, what would you be doing, thinking, or feeling differently that would have a positive result on your wellness?" or "If you were to stop drinking, what wellness areas would be most impacted and in what way?"

If the goals, subgoals, or action steps are still unclear, solution-focused exception questions can be utilized. In WBAC, this involves requesting the client to "Tell me about a time in your life when you were more satisfied with your wellness in this area. What were you doing, thinking, feeling, differently at that time that resulted in your wellness being higher then?" Follow-up questions can insert substance use into the discussion such as "In what ways was your substance use different during this time of higher wellness? What impact did this different level of substance use have on your wellness?" To situate the exception on the substance use, the clinician inquires,

> Tell me about a time when you were able to successfully reduce or abstain from use (even if only for a few days). What were you doing, thinking, feeling differently that helped you change your substance use? What impact did reducing or abstaining from substance use have on your wellness at that time?

Addressing Strengths in the Wellness Plan

The clinician reviews the client's strengths, exceptions, resources, and stronger wellness areas and invites the client to make a list of these and how they can be implemented toward achieving their wellness plan goals. See the sample wellness plan in Handout 3.1 which includes an example of a resource list. You'll notice multiple additional components to the wellness plan. The wellness vision grounds the client in the rationale and motivation for seeking wellness changes and beginning to cultivate what they want those changes to entail. The wellness plan prompts the client to reflect and document the relationship between their wellness and substance use. Solution-focused questions and concepts are incorporated such as the failed solutions (identifying what has not worked in the past to address the presenting concern in order to avoid similar pitfalls) and the exception question to explore what has worked previously (O'Connell, 2012; O'Hanlon, et al., 2003). An exercise like "Flagging the Minefield" (Erford, 2020) is included in which the client, as the expert of challenges they could encounter in achieving their goals, anticipates what could get in their way. Ideally, the client can then more quickly identify and navigate around those obstacles should they arise, and these barriers can also be further explored during counseling.

Handout 3.1 Wellness Plan

Wellness Vision: What lets you know that you have not reached the level of wellness and life balance that you desire? What does balance in your life/holistic wellness look like for you and mean to you? What would you notice that would let you know that your life had reached higher levels of wellness?

The wellness dimensions most negatively affected by the concerns for which I am seeking help/my substance use are _____ _____.

When _____ wellness dimen- sions are out of balance, the concerns for which I am seeking help/my substance use becomes more concerning or stressful to me in the following ways:

Below is a list of solutions I have attempted in order to address the concerns for which I am seeking help/my substance use that have not been helpful in the short and/or long term:

-
-
-
-
-
-

My areas of highest and lowest wellness are _____.

Goal 1:

- Subgoal:

  - Action Steps:

Goal 2:

- Subgoal:

  - Action Steps:

Goal 3:

• Subgoal:

    • Action Steps:

In the past, attending to _____
wellness dimensions has helped me make positive changes to my
substance use. The positive impact on my substance use resulting from attending to these wellness dimensions includes:

In the table below, list the strengths and resources that you
possess and how they can be utilized toward achieving your
wellness plan goals.

Strength/Resource	Strength/Resource Implementation

Knowing obstacles you have faced in the past, if you were to predict what could get in the way of you achieving your wellness goals, what would those obstacles be? What ideas do you have for ways to navigate them? In what ways could your strengths/resources be helpful?

Obstacle	Potential Solution

We strongly recommend that the client keep a wellness journal during the treatment process (see Handout 3.2). The purpose of the wellness journal (titled "Weekly Wellness Journey") document is threefold: (a) Assessing weekly progress, (b) strength and growth building, and (c) increasing motivation. Clients can record progress, challenges, and how to address them, deepening their insight into the wellness-substance use relationship, and noting new strengths and resources. The client's regular review of progress serves to increase motivation for goal attainment which is an important factor in clients remaining in treatment and actualizing changes to their substance use (Groshkova, 2010).

Handout 3.2 Weekly Wellness Journey

List one wellness goal/substance use success from the past week. How did this success impact other dimensions of your wellness?

What evidence of wellness/substance use improvement did you notice from this week? What other dimensions of wellness were affected by these improvements? What does seeing this improvement mean to you?

Have you become aware of any new strengths or resources over the past week?

What challenges did you experience this week? What insights can you take away from these challenges that may help you going forward?

What wellness challenges do you foresee in the coming week? How might you overcome those challenges?

What are the one or two most important things you can do over the next several days to nurture/sustain your wellness and/or take positive steps toward your wellness/substance use goals?

ERIC'S WELLNESS SCREENING AND ASSESSMENT

The evaluation and treatment planning process consisted of eliciting Eric's wellness and substance use history, substance use and wellness screening, and formal assessment followed by identifying treatment goals and filling out the wellness plan. During wellness screening, he rated his mental wellness highest (seven out of ten), then spiritual wellness (six out of ten), cultural wellness (four out of ten), physical, emotional and contextual wellness (three out of ten), and connection wellness lowest (two out of ten). Eric declined to rate his developmental wellness noting he would like to attend more sessions and get a clearer grasp on the concept before self-assessing. The clinician had an inkling that incorporating wellness into the substance evaluation and treatment planning already had a therapeutic affect as it changed the tone of the session and affect of the client from one of defensiveness and seriousness to more pleasant and reflective. The clinician also gained a fuller picture of the client through learning about his strengths and wellness dimensions.

The results of the World Health Organization Brief scale (2004) reinforced these ratings and were a point of departure for further discussion. The clinician invited Eric to provide context for his wellness ratings and responses to the outcomes of the WHO. He disclosed that his mental wellness was highest because he feels mentally engaged in his new job and has to learn new information consistently to succeed. He also builds furniture occasionally which contributed to this score. He rated spiritual wellness higher than other dimensions because through his job and parenting his daughter, he derives meaning. Playing sports and building furniture also stimulate/generate spiritual wellness for Eric.

Based on a recent physical, Eric's physician stated he was pre-diabetic and pre-hypertensive and that he needed to watch his weight and diet resulting in his low physical wellness rating. Eric reported emotional wellness challenges due to stress management. He stated, "I have a hard time changing my mindset from work stress to being present at home and also I'll just worry about things like money and I literally can't stop myself". Contextual wellness was lower for the client due to the disorganization in scheduling and his home often being in disarray. The client stated he rated his cultural wellness lower because of fear he had been hired because he was a person of color, lack of racial/ethnic diversity of employees at work, and microaggressions he had experienced there. Additionally, Eric felt he was not doing a good job of imparting information and conveying appreciation for their cultural heritage to his daughter.

The clinician directed the client to also share about his wellness strengths, even in the areas he rated as lower. This seemed to carry therapeutic value since the client struggled to do this. Eric eventually shared about pride in his biracial heritage noting "his culture has always made him feel special, deep down" (cultural wellness). He talked about the close bond he felt with his daughter and positive experiences they had (connection wellness). He gave himself credit for still obtaining physical activity occasionally (physical wellness). Further, Eric revealed that he could see that he possesses some level of inner strength (mental and emotional wellness) to endure stressors at home and the shame of being confronted about his drinking and yet staying open to attending counseling.

Impact of Substance Use

Eric's gradual increase in alcohol has coincided with the miscarriages Kelly had in Eric and Kelly's efforts to grow their family. Additionally, years ago, Eric took a risk to leave the land-scaping company he had been with for many years for a chance at a higher salary in a sales position. However, he was eventually fired as he failed to progress in his sales production (in part due to starting work late from being hungover on days he was permitted to work remotely). Eric's father coming to live with him added a significant stressor. Specifically, it seemed to intensify feelings of confusion as his relationship with his father was not close while he was growing up. He felt torn as he did not want his father in assisted living, yet he experienced resentment toward him for his upbringing. Further complicating matters, his father's personality had seemed to soften as he aged, possibly related to the vascular issues he had experienced.

Several incidents of concern have accumulated concerning his wife and others in his life. Two years ago, Eric picked up their daughter and drove her while intoxicated on at least two occasions and his father on other occasions. Kelly was not aware of the first time, but upon the second time when she identified this, she made an ultimatum that she would divorce him and seek custody of their daughter if he did this again. Eric agreed that she could take his keys once he arrived home from work if he was going to consume any alcohol.

In another set of incidents, Eric had gotten a ride to his daughter's dance performance and was intoxicated upon arrival. This also occurred at her soccer game. Again, Kelly set a rule that if he had consumed any alcohol, he was not to attend her events. Eric complied with this. On several occasions when he was intoxicated, Eric became verbally abusive to his spouse. Their daughter had not witnessed these occurrences. For example, he would become incensed at times, when she commented on his irresponsibility (needing to step up at work because they needed the money and spend more time with their daughter) and questioning if he talked to other women when out with colleagues. He expressed that his wife would say negative things about him to his daughter, effectively turning her against him at times.

Eric described these incidents of yelling as unusual for him, as he is normally a relatively calm person. These verbal altercations scared her because he seemed very different from the normally calm person he was when not consuming alcohol. Eric would often become tearful in sessions when talking about his daughter. He felt like a failure as a father. Kelly stated that Eric can be a loving father, but she and her daughter felt like they were "walking on eggshells" when he was drinking, and that Eric's anger seems to increase when drinking. Eric presented in counseling as a soft-spoken person with a gentle demeanor but, in his narrative and Kelly's perspective, alcohol seemed to be the single common factor when he had angry outbursts.

Relationship between Eric's Wellness and Substance Use

Eric and the clinician began drawing connections between the client's wellness and substance use. The client commented that he tended to hold in his feelings until they exploded out of him (emotional wellness) which may explain the incidents of yelling. He also remarked that he felt ashamed (emotional wellness) about the drinking and driving and that his wife had to monitor his driving as if he were a child. The clinician knew this likely affected his drinking and well-being. Eric stated that talking aloud and ranking his wellness dimensions helped him more fully see the negative impact his drinking was having on his connection wellness.

SUBSTANCE USE EVALUATION AND DIAGNOSIS

The substance use evaluation included administering the Alcohol Use Disorders Identification Test (AUDIT; Babor, Higgins-Biddle, Saunders, & Monteiro, 2001) and a clinical interview. Eric was oriented to time, person, place, and situation. His speech, dress, and appearance were unremarkable. He had not consumed alcohol for nearly two days, knowing his initial counseling appointment was approaching. The Clinical Institute for Withdrawal Assessment for Alcohol, revised (CIWA-AR; Sullivan, Sykora, Schneiderman, Naranjo, & Sellers, 1989) protocol was administered to assess for alcohol withdrawal risk, and the client did not report or exhibit withdrawal symptoms via the CIWA-AR and overall clinical assessment. His judgment without alcohol in his system seemed normal, although his intake history, and information from Kelly, shows multiple instances of poor judgment when under the influence. Thinking is neither obsessive nor peculiar. He has been emotional in several sessions, especially when he talks about his daughter. He denies having suicidal or homicidal ideation. Despite having a slender frame in college and young adulthood, he begrudgingly noted he has gained a lot of weight in the past few months. His energy levels seem low, and he acknowledges that his diet has "gone to pot". He reports waking up in tears in the days after his first sessions because he feels he has let his family and himself down.

Based on Eric's description of the presenting issues, the clinician proceeded to complete the following DSM 5 diagnosis:

F10.20 Alcohol use disorder, severe
World Health Organization Disability Assessment Schedule 2.0 (WHODAS 2.0) – overall scale average – 3.5 (moderate to severe)
Other clinical observations: pre-diabetic; pre-hypertensive

Eric met the criteria for an alcohol use disorder, with severe intensity, as he met 9 out of 11 criteria. Alcohol seems to be the organizing factor around his difficulties. From the WHO-DAS 2.0 assessment, Eric is experiencing moderate-to-severe difficulty in his life. Additional information seemed pertinent to his case. Based on a recent physical, Eric's physician stated he was pre-diabetic and pre-hypertensive and that he needed to watch his weight and diet. His physical health has denigrated over the past year, and he was functioning sub-optimally. In the upcoming chapters, we will continue to explore Eric's wellness through the lens of each respective wellness component: mind, body, spirit, emotion, and connection.

The Start of Eric's Goal-Setting Process

With a clearer view of his wellness and the role of his drinking, Eric felt more affirmed in abstaining from alcohol while he was in treatment. Eric identified this would quickly benefit his relationships at home and already had by him coming to counseling (connection wellness), that he would likely feel better physically (physical wellness), reduce the risk of emotional outbursts (emotional wellness), and enable him to be more organized and present at home which could improve contextual wellness. Eric hypothesized that building upon his interest in increasing physical and leisure activity which facilitates both physical and spiritual wellness for him, engaging in family counseling (connection wellness) would also be helpful. Related to contextual and emotional wellness, he desired to maintain an active wellness journal and to use this as a space to share freely about his thoughts and feelings. He also planned to brainstorm ways with Kelly and the therapist to improve scheduling and organization in their home.

CONCLUSION

The evaluation is your opportunity to set the tone for the wellness counseling. Marrying wellness, substance use, and mental health evaluation tools conveys a meta-message of holism and provides a more accurate view of the client's life and goals. The client begins to learn more about the wellness perspective that will be utilized during this time as well.

The goal of the wellness plan and WBAC is to help the client maximize their wellness via goal pursuit. The wellness plan and activities assist the clinician in funneling the wellness discussion into practical goals and should be reviewed consistently as it increases client confidence and awareness of the wellness-substance-use relationship. The versatility of the wellness plan helps the clinician meet clients where they are as the client determines where and how substance use is situated in their plan.

You may be wondering about the feasibility of utilizing this approach given the time limitations where you provide addiction services. Here are a few keys:

- Use a brief wellness inventory rather than a longer one.
- Make sure to include at least one wellness goal in your treatment plan.
- Ascertain at least a few client strengths and resources.
- Filter your discussion of substance use through a wellness lens, helping the client make connections between their use and wellness and vice versa.

NOTE

1   For our purposes, we will only be covering substance use disorders in this chapter. Substance-induced disorders are more likely to be seen in hospital and emergency settings and require medical supervision and care. Thus, these diagnoses would rarely be seen (although not impossible) in non-medical residential or outpatient settings.

REFERENCES

Adams, T., Bezner, J., & Steinhardt, M. (1997). The conceptualization and measurement of perceived wellness: Integrating balance across and within dimensions. *American Journal of Health Promotion, 11*(3), 208–218. https://doi.org/10.4278/0890-1171-11.3.208

American Psychiatric Association. (2022). *Diagnostic and statistical manual of mentaldisorders* (5th ed., text rev.). American Psychiatric Association.

Babor, T. F., Higgins-Biddle, J. C., Saunders, J. B., & Monteiro, M. G. (2001). *AUDIT: Thealcohol use disorders identification test: Guidelines for use in primary health care* (2nd ed). World Health Organization. Retrieved from https://apps.who.int/iris/handle/10665/67205

Barcaccia, B., Esposito, G., Matarese, M., Bertolaso, M., Elvira, M., & De Marinis, M. G. (2013). Defining quality of life: A wild-goose chase? *Europe's Journal of Psychology, 9*(1), 185–203. https://doi.org/10.5964/ejop.v9i1.484

Brown, R. L., Leonard, T., Saunders, L. A., & Papasouliotis, O. (1998). The prevalence and detection of substance use disorder among inpatients ages 18–49: An opportunity for prevention. *Preventative Medicine, 27*, 101–110.

Brown, R. L., & Rounds, L. A. (1995). Conjoint screening questionnaires for alcohol and other drug abuse: criterion validity in a primary care practice. *Wisconsin Medical Journal, 94*, 135–140.

Cady, M. E., Winters, K. C., Jordan, D. A., Solberg, K. B., & Stinchfield, R. D. (1996). Motivation to change as a predictor of treatment outcome for adolescent substance abusers. *Journal of Child & Adolescent Substance Abuse, 5*(1), 73–91. https://doi.org/10.1300/J029v05n01_04

Clarke, P. B., Adams, J. K., Wilkerson, J. R., & Shaw, E. G. (2016). Wellness-based counseling for caregivers of persons with dementia. *Journal of Mental Health Counseling, 38*(3), 263–277. https://doi.org/10.17744/mehc.38.3.06

Clarke, P. B., & Scholl, M. B. (2022). Integrating the models of addiction into humanistic counseling for individuals with substance use disorders. *The Journal of Humanistic Counseling, 61*(1), 2–17. https://doi.org/10.1002/johc.12171

Cloud, W., & Granfield, R. (2008). Conceptualizing recovery capital: Expansion of a theoretical construct. *Substance Use & Misuse, 43*(12–13), 1971–1986.

Couwenbergh, C, van der Gaag, R. J., Koeter, M., de Ruiter, C., & van den Brink, W. (2009). Screening for substance abuse among adolescents: Validity of the CAGE-AID in youth mental health care *Substance Use & Misuse, 44*, 823–834.

Denning, P., & Little, J. (2012). *Practicing harm reduction psychotherapy: An alternative approach to addictions*. Guilford Press.

Doweiko, H. E. (2009). *Concepts of chemical dependency*. Brooks/Cole.

Doweiko, H. E. (2019). *Concepts of chemical dependency* (10th ed.). Cengage.

Erford, B. T. (2020). *45 techniques every counselor should know* (3rd ed.). Pearson.

Groshkova, T. (2010). Motivation in substance misuse treatment. *Addiction Research & Theory, 18*(5), 494–510. https://doi.org/10.3109/16066350903362875

Groshkova, T., Best, D., White, W. (2012). The assessment of recovery capital: Properties and psychometrics of a measure of addiction and recovery strengths. *Drug and Alcohol Review, 32*, 187–194.

Guterman, J. T. (2013). *Mastering the art of solution-focused counseling* (2nd ed.). American Counseling Association.

Heather, N., & Rollnick, S. (1993). *Readiness to change questionnaire: User's manual (revised version).* National Drug and Alcohol Research Centre.

Juhnke, G. A. (2002). *Substance abuse assessment and diagnosis.* Brunner-Routledge.

Kilmer, Ja. R., Cronce, J.M., Hunt, S. B., Lew, C. M. (2012). Reducing harm associated with illicit drug use: Opiates, amphetamines, cocaine, steroids, and other substances. In G. Allen Marlatt, Mary E. Larimer, & Katie Witkiewitz, (Eds.) *Harm Reduction: Pragmatic strategies for managing high-risk behaviors* (2nd ed., pp. 170–200). The Guilford Press.

Lamers, S. M. A., Westerhof, G. J., Bohlmeijer, E. T., ten Klooster, P. M., & Keyes, C. L. M. (2011). Evaluating the psychometric properties of the mental health continuum-short form (MHC-SF). *Journal of Clinical Psychology, 67*(1), 99–110. https://doi.org/10.1002/jclp.20741

Leonardson, G. R., Kemper, E., Ness, F. K., Koplin, B. A., Daniels, M. C., & Leonardson, G. A. (2005). Validity and reliability of the audit and CAGE-AID in Northern Plains American Indians. *Psychological Reports, 97*, 161–166.

Lewis, T. F. (2023). *Substance abuse and addiction treatment: Practical application of counseling theory.* Cognella.

Lutz, A. B. (2013). *Learning solution-focused therapy: An illustrated guide.* American Psychiatric Publishing.

Miller, G. (1985). *The substance abuse subtle screening inventory.* SASSI Institute.

Miller, W. R., Forcehimes, A. A., & Zweben, A. (2011). *Treating addiction: A guide for professionals.* Guilford Press.

Miller, W. R., Forcehimes, A. A., & Zweben, A. (2019). *Treating addiction: A guide for professionals* (2nd ed.). Guilford Press.

Miller, W. R., & Johnson, W. R. (2008). A natural language screening measure for motivation to change. *Addictive Behaviors, 33*(9), 1177–1182. https://doi.org/10.1016/j.addbeh.2008.04.018

Miller, W. R., & Rollnick, S. (2013). *Motivational interviewing: Helping people change* (3rd ed.). Guilford Press.

Myers, J. E., Clarke, P. B., Brown, J. B., & Champion, D. A. (2012). Wellness: Theory, research, and applications for counselors. In M. B. Scholl, A. S. McGowan, & J. T. Hansen (Eds.), *Humanistic perspectives on contemporary counseling issues* (pp. 17–44). Routledge.

Myers, J. E., Luecht, R. M., & Sweeney, T. J. (2004). The factor structure of wellness: Reexamining theoretical and empirical models underlying the wellness evaluation of lifestyle (WEL) and the five-factor wel. *Measurement and Evaluation in Counseling and Development, 36*(4), 194–208. https://doi.org/10.1080/07481756.2004.11909742

Myers, J. E., & Sweeney, T. J. (2006). *The wellness and habit change workbook.* Author.

Myers, J. E., & Sweeney, T. J. (2014). *Five factor wellness inventory.* Mind Garden.

National Institute on Alcohol Abuse and Alcoholism, National Institutes of Health, U.S. Department of Health and Human Services (n.d.). *Rethinking drinking: Alcohol and your health.* Retrieved March 21, 2023, from https://www.rethinkingdrinking.niaaa.nih.gov/

O'Connell, B. (2012). *Solution-focused therapy* (3rd ed.). Sage.

O'Hanlon, B., O'Hanlon, W. H., & Weiner-Davis, M. (2003). *In search of solutions: A new direction in psychotherapy.* W. W. Norton & Company.

Ohrt, J. H., Clarke, P. B., & Conley, A. H. (2019). *Wellness counseling: A holistic approach to prevention and intervention.* American Counseling Association.

Reichenberg, L. W., & Seligman, L. (2016). *Selecting effective treatments: A comprehensive, systematic guide to treating mental disorders* (5th ed.). Wiley.

Ryff, C. D. (1989). Happiness is everything, or is it? Explorations on the meaning of psychological well-being. *Journal of Personality and Social Psychology, 57*(6), 1069–1081. https://doi.org/10.1037/0022-3514.57.6.1069

Shannonhouse, L., Erford, B., Gibson, D., O'Hara, C., & Fullen, M. C. (2020). Psychometric synthesis of the five factor wellness inventory. *Journal of Counseling & Development, 98*(1), 94–106. https://doi.org/10.1002/jcad.12303

Stevens, P., & Smith, R. L. (2013). *Substance abuse counseling: Theory and practice* (5th ed.). Pearson.

Su, R., Tay, L., & Diener, E. (2014). The development and validation of the Comprehensive Inventory of Thriving (CIT) and the Brief Inventory of Thriving (BIT). *Applied Psychology: Health and Well-Being, 6*(3), 251–279. https://doi.org/10.1111/aphw.12027

Substance Abuse and Mental Health Services Administration (2014). *Trauma-informed care in behavioral health services.* Treatment improvement protocol (TIP) series 57. HHS Publication No. (SMA) 13-4801. Substance Abuse and Mental Health Services Administration.

Sullivan, J. T., Sykora, K., Schneiderman, J., Naranjo, C. A., & Sellers, E. M. (1989). Assessment of alcohol withdrawal: The revised clinical institute withdrawal assessment for alcohol scale (CIWA-Ar). *British Journal of Addiction, 84*(11), 1353–1357. https://doi.org/10.1111/j.1360-0443.1989.tb00737.x

Tatarsky, A. (2007). *Harm reduction psychotherapy: A new treatment for drug and alcohol problems.* Jason Aronson/Rowman and Littlefield.

Tatarsky, A., & Kellogg, S. (2012). Harm reduction psychotherapy. In G. A. Marlatt, M. E. Larimer, & K. Witkiewitz (Eds.), *Harm reduction: Pragmatic strategies for managing high-risk behaviors* (pp. 36–60). The Guilford Press.

Tatarsky, A., & Marlatt, G. A. (2010). State of the art in harm reduction psychotherapy: An emerging treatment for substance misuse. *Journal of Clinical Psychology, 66*(2), 117–122. https://doi.org/10.1002/jclp.20672

Vilsaint, C. L., Kelly, J. F., Bergman, B. G., Groshkova, T., Best, D., & White, W. (2017). Development and validation of a Brief Assessment of Recovery Capital (BARC-10) for alcohol and drug use disorder. *Drug and Alcohol Dependence, 177*, 71–76. https://doi.org/10.1016/j.drugalcdep.2017.03.022

White, W. (2009). Recovery capital scale. Posted at www.williamwhitepapers.com

White, W. & Cloud, W. (2008). Recovery capital: A primer for addictions professionals. *Counselor, 9*(5), 22–27.

World Health Organization. (2004). *The World Health Organization quality of life (WHOQOL) BREF, 2012 revision.* World Health Organization. Retrieved from https://apps.who.int/iris/handle/10665/77773

CHAPTER 4

HOLISTIC RELAPSE PREVENTION

INTRODUCTION

A primary role of substance use counseling is to help clients prevent relapse or manage a relapse if one occurs so that it does not get out of control. As such, relapse prevention (RP) is an essential component of any addictions counseling process. It is one thing to stop using substances and quite another to prevent the return of problematic use. Different strategies are needed to prevent or manage relapse. The WBAC approach uses traditional RP models and key wellness principles to help clients identify relapse triggers and wellness strategies for how to best manage these triggers. In this chapter, we first define relapse, discuss key terms, and show how relapse fits into the broader experience of recovery. Next, we briefly review Marlatt's (1985) Covert Antecedents Model. This model provides a foundation from which to build wellness-based interventions within WBAC. In the second half of the chapter, we focus on these wellness-based interventions and conclude with a brief case study to demonstrate key principles.

WHAT IS A RELAPSE?

Before we dive into the concept of relapse, let's define some terminology. A *lapse* is a return to use after a committed period of abstinence. Lapses tend to be minor and do not involve returning to pre-treatment levels of use (Marlatt, 1985). An example of a lapse might be a person who is trying to abstain from alcohol but has a glass of beer at a party; shortly thereafter, they recommit to abstinence and avoid "falling off the proverbial wagon". For reasons explained below, lapses are often seen as myths according to more traditional treatment perspectives (such as proponents of the disease model of addiction; Thombs, 2006). A *relapse* is the return to uncontrolled pre-treatment levels of substance use after a period of abstinence or sobriety. Relapse in one's co-occurring disorder can also involve an increase in mental disorder symptoms reaching a level that impacts the person's daily functioning or precipitate a substance use relapse (Doweiko, 2019; Miller, Forcehimes, & Zweben, 2019). As you proceed through the chapter, relapse can refer to substance use or co-occurring disorders. A relapse is more serious than a lapse, although if a lapse is not addressed, it can lead to a full-blown relapse. Making attributions of self-blame, having a strong self-image as a hard-working person in recovery, and experiencing a strong abstinence violation effect (AVE) all increase the odds of a slip turning into a relapse (Thombs, 2006). The AVE involves emotional reactions to a lapse such as anxiety, guilt, embarrassment, and shame that increase the likelihood of a relapse (Thombs & Osborn, 2019). The thinking goes something like this: [after a lapse] "I can't believe I screwed up. I'm so stupid. What a loser. I might as well go all the way because it doesn't matter anymore!" (Thombs & Osborn, 2019).

Relapse has been conceptualized in one of two ways. First is the traditional view, which states that either a person is ill and has symptoms or is well and does not (Lewis, 2014). The traditional view holds that a person is either abstinent or using, there is no "in-between".

DOI: 10.4324/9781003147954-4

Relapse Based on the Process View

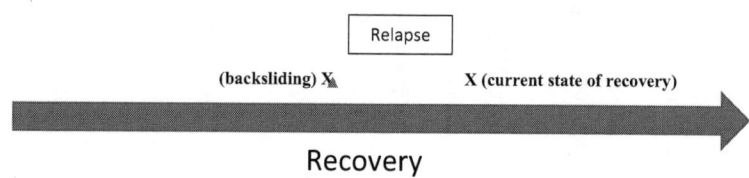

Figure 4.1 Relapse Based on the Process View.

As you can see, the word "either" is important in the traditional view, making this a very black-and-white perspective. The second conceptualization is the process view. Here relapse is seen as a backsliding or worsening of substance use during the recovery process. Rather than an either-or concept, relapse is considered part of the process of change and allows the client to learn new skills to help her down the road. Consider Figure 4.1. Think of an arrow on this page pointing to the right. This arrow represents one's recovery process. A relapse in the process view means that the person moved backward on the arrow but did not completely fall. They can pick themselves up, dust themselves off, and recommit to their recovery trajectory.

At the risk of overgeneralizing, strict adherents to the traditional view do not believe in "backsliding"; either you are drinking, or you are not. This is one reason why Alcoholics Anonymous (AA) exclusively advocates for abstinence from alcohol. The only requirement to join AA is to have a desire to *stop* drinking (rather than cutting back or engaging in controlled drinking). Unfortunately, this rigid posture can contribute to the very behavior it is trying to prevent – more relapse. The guilt and shame that one feels after a relapse is partially created by the rigidity of the traditional view.

The process view of relapse was, at first, scorned by proponents of the traditional view. After all, if a person returns to use, however small, it is a slippery slope to full-blown relapse. In addition, conceptualizing a slip as a "mistake" may not convey the seriousness of the drug use problem. Slipping a little bit here and there may be seen as ok once and awhile – what is the big deal if the person quickly gets back on track? The danger of this pattern is that many lapses can and do lead to relapse. This perspective is rooted in the long-held belief that those struggling with alcohol or drug addiction lose control once the substance enters their system. One drink, let alone a sip, can easily turn into ten. However, this loss of control hypothesis has not held up to scientific scrutiny. Intentions to drink and other cognitive, behavioral, and social mechanisms play a significant role in returning to drinking (Thombs & Osborn, 2019).

So, which is the correct conceptualization? Well, both viewpoints have merit. The traditional view removes any ambiguity on what constitutes addiction and recovery. The only goal for SUD treatment is abstinence. However, the traditional view of relapse is largely grounded in the disease model of addiction, which surprisingly has little to say about coping and skills needed to prevent or manage relapse (Thombs & Osborn, 2019). It is unrealistic to assume that, despite good intentions, clients will keep to their abstinent commitment 100% of the time and never slip. Consequently, we argue that the process view is more in line with WBAC. From the wellness perspective, clients can learn valuable lessons from the inevitable adversity and environmental temptations that arise during recovery. Further, a dichotomous view of relapse diverges from WBAC which is a harm reduction approach that can also be used with clients who wish to pursue abstinence. Helping clients reconceptualize a slip not as falling off the wagon but as a backsliding event where they can quickly get back on track has tremendous value. It counteracts the AVE, a major player in pushing one from slip to relapse, and helps clients refocus on infusing wellness behaviors as part of their recovery.

THE COVERT ANTECEDENTS MODEL OF RELAPSE

The Covert Antecedents theoretical model illustrates that relapse is a process rather than an event (Marlatt, 1985). Further, the model indicates that lifestyle imbalance or stress resulting from a lopsided ratio of daily stressors to pleasures in one's life can spark cravings followed by relapse. This is because the stress yields a thirst for addictive avenues for self-care or a "desire for indulgence or immediate gratification", according to Marlatt (1985, p. 48). To add to this, WBAC follows that when one or more dimensions and/or one's overall wellness is at a deficit, one seeks to fill those gaps with substances or engaging addictively in a behavior. WBAC draws upon Kasl's notion that the urge to use substances is not a bad thing; rather it is a signal that one has a need that has been unmet and substance use occurs as an attempt to meet that need (1992). If the client can (a) identify that there is a wellness need, (b) recognize what that need might be, and (c) implement wellness skills and resources to meet that need, their risk of relapse may decrease.

Research supports the idea of a wellness-relapse connection. A review of 321 alcohol use disorder studies uncovered evidence of a link between biological, psychological, social, and spiritual variables and relapse (Sliedrecht, Waart, Witkiewitz, & Roozen, 2019). For example, from a biological or physical wellness lens, study participants who were physically healthier were less likely to relapse. From a psychological lens (mental wellness and emotional wellness), participants with a co-occurring mental health disorder or who had experienced trauma relapsed with greater frequency. Individuals reporting more social support whether via intimate partnership or others (connection wellness) were less likely to relapse. Finally, spiritual wellness was supported as a relapse factor in 13 studies (Sliedrecht et al., 2019). Although wellness is not always directly named, decreased wellness as a setup for relapse is implied in widely used behavioral interventions such as Dialectical Behavior Therapy's (DBT) behavioral chain analysis (Linehan, 2015).

The wellness challenges that precipitate urges to use substances may stem from aspects of wellness not being attended to for long periods of time or lower wellness due to obstacles a person has faced to improve a specific wellness dimension. The urge to use can also be the consequence of a need that arises in the moment or low wellness on a given day(s). In either instance, there is typically a spark that triggers the relapse. The relapse taxonomy used in RP and cognitive-behavioral RP approaches encompasses several dimensions of the wellness spectrum. The taxonomy assists the client in pinpointing "high risk situations" that can cause a relapse (Marlatt, 1985). The situations are dichotomized into social (interpersonal determinants) and within-person (intrapersonal) scenarios or triggers. Social triggers are those arising from tension with others, peer pressure to use, and fostering pleasant feelings while with others. Within-person triggers arise from cravings, negative feelings, aversive physical experiences, the intention to foster pleasant feelings, and the intention to prove one's ability to abstain in the face of relapse cues (Marlatt, 1985).

The taxonomy is integrated into WBAC as it is evidence-based (Donovan & Witkiewitz, 2012) and recognizes connection, emotion, physical, and cognitive wellness. However, WBAC uses the five-dimensional wellness framework to help clients identify relapse risks. This is because there are a myriad of relapse precipitants not covered by the taxonomy and RP approaches in general such as cultural and spiritual factors (Williams & Gorski, 2007).

Additionally, there are relapse processes across connection, emotion, physical, and cognitive wellness other than the ones accounted for by the taxonomy.

RELAPSE AND WELLNESS RECOVERY

A discussion of relapse and RP would not be complete without considering its role in the recovery process. Recovery can be defined as a period of deliberate and intentional non-use of substances (Lewis, 2014). Many make the mistake of assuming that recovery is simply the cessation of use; in reality, it involves efforts to abstain or reduce *and* incorporate new and positive behaviors to live a more productive and healthy life. Recovery has an identified beginning point but no firmly established endpoint (Lewis, 2014). It is often difficult, challenging, and life-long. At the same time, it can be an exhilarating process as clients learn new ways to be in the world, slowly regain their lives, and repair damaged relationships. We would add that within a recovery based on wellness, the client learns to embrace the wellness factors as a roadmap to a more preferred life.

RP in WBAC starts with a foundation of facilitating a deeper awareness of the wellness-substance use connection in the client's life. Self-monitoring is used to enhance the client's awareness of their relapse triggers in each wellness dimension and what underlies them. These two components fall within what Prochaska and DiClemente (1983) term "consciousness raising" because the client learns more about their substance use issues and what causes them. WBAC practitioners mine the client's experiences of lapses, relapses, close calls to relapse, past treatment, and RP successes to add and reinforce information and skills for the client. All the above processes are compiled into a relapse resource toolbox for the client to incorporate. Let's start by discussing the RP process that illuminates the wellness-substance use relationship.

THE STEPS OF RELAPSE PREVENTION IN WBAC

Several WBAC RP techniques will be presented below. The RP process should begin once a treatment plan is in place. The wellness story, in the next section, launches client and counselor into exploring the context for the causes of relapse and approaches to preventing it. Self-monitoring is assigned to the client early in counseling to obtain a sharper view of relapse triggers, as one does in RP (Marlatt & Witkiewitz, 2005). Then the client participates in matching relapse triggers with wellness coping skills. Strength-building via ascertaining positive qualities, wellness strengths, and skills that have helped the client increase wellness and address substance use in the past are also layered into the coping skills of this plan. The RP process also includes ways the clinician can respond if a client relapses.

THE WELLNESS STORY

Marlatt, Parks, and Witkiewitz (2002) included autobiography as a component of assessment and intervention in their RP approach. An integral part of WBAC is for the client to form connections between their wellness and substance use. The autobiography method used by Marlatt et al. (2002) and others is one avenue toward achieving this. It should be presented as homework to the client to be discussed in the first two to three sessions (Note: If the client is not able to complete on their own, this can be worked on during the session). The client is asked to write their wellness story and the role of substance use needs to be a part of the narrative. Responses to the following questions guide the wellness story:

- What was your wellness like in your youth (you can decide which age in your youth you'd like to discuss)? Did your life/wellness feel in balance or out of balance? What memories do you have that provide insight into your wellness as a youth? What were your higher areas of wellness and lower areas of wellness?

- How has your wellness changed over the past five to ten years? In what ways has it improved? In what ways has it declined? Provide a specific example or two to illustrate this. What factored into these changes? How has your substance use changed over the past five to ten years? What factored into these changes?

- Write about a time in your life when your wellness was at its peak? What was going on in your life at the time/what did your life look like at the time? What were you doing at the time that contributed to this higher level of wellness? What was your substance use like at the time in terms of frequency, quantity, and stress/problems resulting from use?

- Write about a time in your life when your wellness was at its lowest. What was going on in your life at the time/what did your life look like at the time? What do you believe factored into this period of lower wellness? What was your substance use like at the time in terms of frequency, quantity, and stress/problems resulting from use?

- Give examples of times in your life when your substance use positively affected your wellness?

- Give examples from times in your life when your substance use negatively affected your wellness?

- What do you envision your life will look like (including your substance use) if you successfully achieve your wellness goals?

Each question provides the client an opportunity to pause and reflect about their wellness at different points in their life. This reflection is paired with additional prompts that facilitate clients identifying elements associated with higher or lower wellness throughout their life including substance use. The wellness story encourages clients to focus on specific experiences that highlight these connections. The clinician's job is then to elicit the client's appraisals about the pathways to wellness and the role of substance use in progressing down that path. Ideally, the client will walk away from this debriefing with additional ideas for ways to increase their wellness and an understanding of the implications of substance use on wellness and vice versa.

In the next section, we'll talk about self-monitoring which can be initiated alongside the wellness story process. Self-monitoring enables the client to drill down further from the wellness-substance use relationship to variables that precipitate relapse.

SELF-MONITORING

WBAC also adapts self-monitoring from RP (e.g., Marlatt et al., 2002), using these techniques to help clients learn about their in-the-moment wellness needs, ongoing wellness needs, and how they are associated with cravings and relapse. To that end, clients are first provided with psychoeducation about cravings. This entails sharing definitions of craving and then inviting the client to define what craving looks like for them. Craving is "an intense desire or urge for the drug" or addictive behavior that can be experienced across the wellness dimensions (APA, 2022, "SUD Diagnostic Features," para. 3)." For instance, spiritual cravings may be represented by a sense of a void needing to be filled, feeling spiritually conflicted (e.g., "the enemy is on my one shoulder telling me to use and an ally is on the other shoulder saying not to use"). The clinician can ask the client questions like, (a) What lets you know you are experiencing a craving?, (b) What are you experiencing mentally, emotionally, physically, and spiritually when you are having an urge to use?, (c) What behaviors do you engage in that let you know you are having an urge to use?, and (d) What physical sensations do you experience when you have an urge to use? (Carroll, 1998).

To self-monitor, clients are asked to track their daily cravings over a span of one to two weeks (see Handout 4.1). On the handout, clients identify the type of craving (was it experienced in mind, body, spirit, emotionally, or across multiple dimensions), its level of intensity, and the time of day the craving occurred. Clients must also answer an essential question on the self-monitoring form – "What were you wanting in that moment? What were you wanting the substance to do for you?" Maslow's Hierarchy of Needs (1943) is a starting point for identifying what the client was wanting in the moment of craving. Maslow's hierarchy includes physiological, safety, love and belonging, esteem, and self-transcendence needs (Koltko-Rivera, 2006; Maslow, 1943).

Handout 4.1 Self-Monitoring Handout

Type (Mind, Body, Spirit, Emotion, Connection)	Intensity (1–10)	Day/Time	Need (Phys, Safety, Love/Belong, Esteem, Transcend/Feel Good)

Type (Mind, Body, Spirit, Emotion, Connection)	Intensity (1-10)	Day/Time	Need (Phys, Safety, Love/Belong, Esteem, Transcend/Feel Good)

Physiological examples of cravings are clearer. However, the other needs may be less clear. Cravings related to physical safety can include using substances to cope with physical pain or withdrawal symptoms whereas emotional safety cravings can pertain to trauma triggers or problems managing emotional activation. Cravings generated from love and belonging needs may involve feelings of loneliness, alienation, boredom, emotional pain from ruptured relationships, or stressors with a close friend. Esteem craving can come from feelings of disappointment, discouragement or failure, and negative comments from others. Self-transcendence urges entail a desire to consume substances to enhance creativity or one's experiences, reduce boredom, and increase personal growth and discovery.

Self-monitoring can be an effective way to learn about acute wellness-related relapse triggers and how unmet wellness needs result in relapse. Reviewing the client's previous relapses fills in the relapse picture for additional types and incidents of relapse linked to wellness (Marlatt, 1985).

WELLNESS-BASED RELAPSE TRIGGERS

The five-dimensional wellness model presented in this book (as well as other wellness models) in conjunction with Marlatt's (1985) relapse taxonomy can facilitate the client's identification of relapse triggers. A trigger is when the desire to enhance one's wellness, cope with wellness deficits, or cope with isolated incidents that decrease one's wellness results in cravings, a near relapse, or actual relapse. Triggers are warning signs that a relapse may be impending unless action is taken. The clinician can provide the client with a copy of the wellness model and invite them to reflect upon, "what warning signs in this dimension let me know that I might be at risk of relapsing?" If clients struggle to respond to this prompt, the clinician can ask about what was occurring for them in the hours or days leading up to a prior relapse or close call in their different wellness dimensions. The clinician can also offer examples of wellness-based relapse red flags including several from the "high risk situations" of the relapse taxonomy (Marlatt, 1985). For instance:

- What mental wellness triggers or challenges to your mental wellness were you experiencing leading up to your relapse (e.g., job or school concerns, boredom, mental health symptoms, and cravings)?
- What physical wellness triggers or challenges to your physical wellness were you experiencing leading up to your relapse/close call (e.g., physical cravings, pain,

sleep concerns, energy levels [too low or high], pain/discomfort or other health problems, and cravings)?

- What spiritual wellness triggers or challenges were you experiencing leading up to your relapse/close call (e.g., lack of meaning and purpose, struggles related to religious beliefs or practices, and cravings)?

- What emotion wellness triggers or challenges were you experiencing leading up to your relapse/close call (e.g., stress, grief and loss, mental health symptoms, emotion regulation challenges, cravings, "enhancement of positive emotional state", and "coping with negative emotional states") (Marlatt, 1985, p. 80)?

- What connection wellness triggers or challenges were you experiencing leading up to your relapse/close call (e.g., social pressure, interpersonal conflict, and enhancement of positive emotional states [Marlatt, 1985, p. 81])?

- What triggers or challenges related to culture, context, or development were you experiencing leading up to your relapse/close call (e.g., microaggressions, financial stress, and absence of meaning in retirement)?

The self-monitoring activity from the previous section will give clients a head start in identifying some of these relapse triggers. However, systematically going through the wellness dimensions using the prompts above will provide additional relapse precipitants that may have gone unnoticed or may not have occurred during the self-monitoring period.

RP RESOURCES

Concurrent to clarifying relapse triggers is discovering and reinforcing RP skills, strengths, and resources. The goal of the relapse resource process is to make the wellness skills, strengths, and resources that have protected the client from relapse more salient and accessible to the client. One starting point is to go through each of the cravings and triggers flagged by the client and identify ways to cope with or circumvent them. These solutions are generally derived in three ways: (a) brainstorming new ideas with the clinician, (b) identifying what has worked in previous situations when the client was exposed to the trigger and was able to abstain or adhere to their harm reduction plan, and (c) drilling down into specific resources or skills from the client's wellness strengths that could be used in high-risk situations. Handouts 4.4 and 4.5 may help you and your client organize their needs, triggers, skills, and resources so that the client can easily refer to this information outside of the session. Handouts 4.2 and 4.3 contain the results from Eric's engagement in this work.

Strengths-Building Using Lapses, Close Calls, Past Treatment, and Past Successes

Clients possess a wealth of information that can help prevent future relapses via their experiences of lapses, relapse close calls, past substance use successes, and past treatment. What if as clinicians we are missing an opportunity to support and expedite this learning and growth process by not devoting time to exploring periods of abstinence or harm reduction success that happened between treatment or before the person sought treatment? Do we allot sufficient time to de-constructing what the client learned about wellness and RP from their previous times in treatment? A thoughtful investigation of these incidents enables the

Handout 4.2 Sample Needs and Relapse Prevention Resources Handout

Needs	Skills/Resources
Physiological • Forgetting to eat • Forgetting to drink water • Sleep	• Set alarm reminder to drink water • Set alarm reminder for snacks and meals • Pack lunch to take to work • Use cue of loss of focus or alcohol craving as a re-minder to eat food or drink non-alcoholic drink • Need more resources to help with sleep*
Safety (emotional) • Criticism from spouse • Father's gestures of kindness that make me feel confused	• Use grounding activities practiced during session • Tell Kelly how I feel/ask for support • Call one of the three friends I stay in touch with (resets me emotionally, reminds me I'm OK)
Love and Belonging • Distance and conflict with Kelly • Conflict with Lia • Perceived lack of be-longing at work • Loneliness/Isolated	• Call one of the three friends I stay in touch with (resets me emotionally, reminds me I'm OK) • Use communication skills from family sessions • Talk with Kelly about my feelings • Practice acceptance (of the situation) if Lia responds in a way I do not like and self-talk reminder that she loves me despite certain in-the-moment responses
Esteem • Receiving feedback at work	**Do something that reminds me of my strengths** • Get a small task done at work • Think about a goal I have made progress on • Work on furniture project • Tennis, walk, or soccer

Needs	Skills/Resources
Self-Actualization **Feelings of failure as** • Employee • Marriage • Father • Son • Drinking	• Examine my self-talk – challenge my self-talk if it is not helpful. • Identify a strength in the aspect in which I feel like a failure • Do one small thing to better myself in the area in which I feel like a failure (e.g., do one small thing to help out with care for Dad or Lia, make a kind comment to Kelly that will make her feel good) **Do something that reminds me of my strengths** • Get a small task done at work • Think about a goal I have made progress on • Work on furniture project • Tennis, walk, or soccer
Self-Transcendence • Desire to escape • Helps with ideas • Helps me see possibility for self-actualization	• Sit with the feeling **Find another way to reach that feeling** • Sports • Furniture project • Art project

Handout 4.3 Sample Wellness Triggers and Relapse Prevention Skills Handout

Wellness Triggers and Relapse Prevention
Mental Wellness Triggers/Relapse Prevention Skills and Resources

- Trigger: self-talk statements, e.g., "one drink will not be a big deal", "you don't have a drinking problem", "I need a drink right now because I can't deal with _____".
- Skills/Resources: constructive self-talk: "you have more important things in your life than risking what you care about for one drink", "your drinking has become a problem", "you have dealt with high stress before without a drink and you can now".

Physical Wellness Triggers/Relapse Prevention Skills and Resources

- Trigger: feeling worn down physically/lack of sleep over several days.
- Skills/Resources: self-care via earlier bedtime and reduced screen time in bed (seven hours of sleep minimum).

Spiritual Wellness Triggers/Relapse Prevention Skills and Resources

- Trigger: feeling bored or isolated. Strings of thoughts about wasted years of life.
- Skills/Resources: engaging in activities (hobby) or with daughter. Calling a friend or recovery peer. Walk.

Emotional Wellness Triggers/Relapse Prevention Skills and Resources

- Trigger: stress (sources – work, financial, disorganization at home, and relationships at home).
- Skills/Resources: identify the stressful thought/feeling. What's one small step I can take toward fixing the problem? If not fixable, challenge stress thoughts with helpful thoughts. Do something to get your mind off of it. Talk to someone.

Connection Wellness Triggers/Relapse Prevention Skills and Resources

- Trigger: arguments/conflict/stress with Kelly, Lia, or Dad
- Skills/Resources: take a time out if I need it. Do something different to calm down. Don't talk to them if I notice the volume of my voice raising. Challenge self-talk that "I need a drink" to deal with stress to "I can deal with this". Notice my stress level before talking to them. Look at my thoughts – remember that my recovery is a change for them and things can get better.

client to crystallize strengths and insights that can be incorporated into their RP and wellness plans (Marlatt et al., 2002).

To unlock the wellness-recovery-enhancing potential of strengths building, we recommend exploring the following with clients: think about a time when you were abstinent or reached a harm reduction goal for any length of time – (a) what two or three skills or lifestyle changes were most helpful in achieving this?, (b) name and describe at least two to three strengths that you possess that enabled you to achieve this, (c) describe something you learned about your substance use from this experience, (d) describe something you learned about your wellness and/or the relationship between your wellness and substance use from this experience, and (e) describe something you learned about yourself from this experience? After processing the client's response to these prompts, the clinician transitions into the next steps by identifying (a) what principles, skills, insights, and/or strengths from this reflective exercise will be particularly helpful in their recovery at this time, and (b) how they can be applied in the here and now to help them reach their wellness and substance use goals. This set of questions can also be utilized in exploring previous treatments. The clinician would instead inquire about the most beneficial skills or lifestyle changes garnered from past treatments, meetings, or other clinical activities. These outcomes can be added to the wellness and RP plans.

Relapse close calls are times when a client nearly relapsed but did not. Lapses, as noted previously, are a short resumption of substance use followed by a prompt return to abstinence or harm reduction plans (Marlatt & Witkiewitz, 2005). Close calls and lapses can be frequent for clients in the initial weeks and months of treatment. These experiences can be carefully examined so that strengths and RP skills can be extracted using the same question sequence from the paragraph above. The clinician asks the client to identify two or three specific examples from the past days or weeks in which they experienced a strong desire to use or believed they would relapse but did not. The clinician should then ask the client, "What did you do that helped you to not relapse in those moments?" For clients who have lapsed, the clinician queries, "How did you keep the lapse from becoming a relapse?" (Marlatt et al., 2002; Marlatt & Witkiewitz, 2005). Thoughts or behaviors that can be replicated in future challenging situations should be identified from the client's response. To take this a step further, the clinician also incorporates the solution-focused question, "What is it about you that helped you maintain abstinence/harm reduction in this situation?" (Lutz, 2013; Ratner, George, & Iveson, 2012). With this question, you are attempting to elicit specific strengths from the client. The clinician follows this up by processing how these strengths can be utilized in the current and other related scenarios.

RESPONDING TO RELAPSE AND CHANGES IN MOTIVATION

Prolapse is an RP concept (Marlatt et al., 2002) that reconceptualizes a relapse as a chance for new learning and growth by re-examining the steps and processes that led to the relapse occurring. With this new knowledge, the client will be better prepared to avoid future relapses. Situating a relapse as a prolapse in RP also has the effect of preventing decreased importance, confidence, and readiness for change which can result in further relapse (Marlatt et al., 2002; Miller & Rollnick, 2013). It is possible that the relapse reminds the client of the benefits of substance use, reducing the sense of the importance of abstinence or the harm reduction plan. Further, the client can experience disappointment and perceive that recovery is no longer worth the effort (Marlatt et al., 2002). Relapse can deliver a blow so powerful to the client's self-efficacy for wellness and substance use change that the importance of change and readiness to maintain changes also declines for the client (Miller & Rollnick, 2013). It is critical to honor the client's experience and validate their thoughts and feelings including if they are considering abandoning some of their wellness-substance use goals and plans. Again, the clinician should listen with non-judgment and avoid leaping into advice-giving. In our experience, clients usually get back on track with the right guidance, collaboration, and enhanced self-motivation.

The clinician and client seize the opportunity for learning by examining wellness-related relapse triggers:

- What deficits in wellness existed that day or in the days leading up to the relapse?
- What areas of your wellness have not been attended to recently?
- What experiences have you had recently that may have resulted in decreased wellness?
- In what ways has your life been out of balance, even if in a small way?

The clinician will want to help the client pinpoint the ways in which this lower wellness or wellness challenges may have sparked the relapse. Within this, it can be helpful to review the wellness concept of holism – that the wellness dimensions are interconnected thereby impacting each other (Myers & Sweeney, 2005). Extending this idea, the clinician confers with the client about the possibility of lower wellness in one dimension creating a negative snowball effect into other wellness dimensions, ultimately spilling over into a relapse. The self-monitoring form questions (specifically those using Maslow's Hierarchy of Needs [1943]) are also incorporated to isolate the needs the client had leading up to relapse. This can illuminate how they sought to meet these needs through substance use.

In addition to providing a listening ear, the WBAC clinician can use MI scaling questions (scale of 1–10) to assess the client's levels of importance of change and self-efficacy about change (Miller & Rollnick, 2013). Separate scales can be employed for wellness and substance use. In exploring the client's response, the clinician should inquire how, if at all, the relapse had affected their rating. To build importance and self-efficacy, there is value in examining the strides the client has made in their wellness-substance use goals. The clinician assists the client in taking time to consider improvements in their substance use and wellness across dimensions, noting even the smallest of positive changes. The impact of these wellness and substance use gains on the client's life and holistic well-being are explored to elevate the importance of change. The clinician then funnels the conversation into further MI-solution-focused processing to increase self-efficacy, including the question, "what do these examples of improvement suggest to you about your ability to make changes to your wellness and substance use?" (Lutz, 2013; Miller & Rollnick, 2013; Ratner et al., 2012). It is tempting for clients who relapse to spiral into a negative mindset where they focus only on their "mistake", neglecting all of the positive steps they have taken in their recovery. The clinician's task is to gently remind the client of all the progress they have made.

Dedicate an extended amount of time to ascertaining how the client was able to decelerate or stop the lapse or relapse (Marlatt, 1985; Marlatt et al., 2002; Marlatt & Witkiewitz, 2005). Strengths and valuable insights lie within your client's ability to resume change during challenging times. The clinician's job is to find out the strengths and dimensions of wellness the client drew upon that enabled them to accomplish this. These conversations can reduce some of the injury to the client's importance, confidence, and readiness for change.

Clinicians must find a way to make the advantages of wellness pursuit and substance use goals salient in response to relapse or decreased motivation. One method is the benefits activity in which the client aggregates the positive aspects of wellness and recovery growth. The first part of this activity involves the client listing their reasons for pursuing their wellness and substance use goals. Underneath this, there is space for the client to keep a running list of all benefits that they notice have resulted from their seeking their wellness and substance use goals. The wellness model frames this inventory, reminding the client to attend to benefits across the wellness dimensions. With each advantage listed, the client has the option to elaborate on what it means to them.

To preserve the importance of change for the client, you can also ask them to reflect on the implications of no longer pursuing the wellness-substance use plan over the next year (or five years) (Miller & Rollnick, 2013). Invite the client to contemplate what their wellness and substance use might be like at different points in their future should they choose not to address what they had outlined in their wellness-substance use plan. What would be the positive and negative impacts on their wellness and substance use over time? This combines two MI techniques called the looking forward question and aspects of the decisional balance (Miller & Rollnick, 2013).

Another facet of prolapse in WBAC involves deriving added motivation and insight toward one's substance use and wellness goals via exploring the consequences of a relapse. This technique must be utilized with caution because of the risk of exacerbating painful emotions such as guilt, and thus activating the AVE, which is antithetical to recovery. The clinician must frame the discussion as one to increase insight into the relationship between the client's substance use and wellness. The client is informed that engaging in this reflective work can widen their window of understanding. Client and clinician then look at the wellness model being used and identify which dimensions of wellness have been affected by the relapse and in what ways.

The above process leads to another critical juncture: determining how to address the wellness "injuries" inflicted by the relapse. This is a point where rallying the client's wellness strengths and priorities can be impactful. The clinician invites the client to identify their stronger wellness dimensions and brainstorm specific ways they can be facilitative. Additionally, the clinician can incorporate a solution-focused coping question and find out wellness facets that have helped them successfully cope with major stressors and or past relapses. Example insights from this process could be that prayer or meditation (spiritual wellness), exercise (physical wellness), or connecting with their sponsor (connection wellness) may be grounding, growth-inducing, and prevent further relapse.

CLIENT EXAMPLE

Eric noticed how his clinician spent time in a session exploring what he had learned and how he had grown from his wellness challenges and substance use problems prior to counseling. He began to realize that there was wisdom in his experiences that could promote success with his wellness plan. Eric shared a few key insights:

Eric also had relapsed on alcohol for two days after about two months of counseling. His wife, daughter, and father were away for the weekend and he stopped by the liquor store after work on Friday, consuming alcohol Friday evening and much of Saturday. He was feeling dejected and angry with himself when his counseling session began on Tuesday. The WBAC clinician met Eric where he was emotionally and processed what he was experiencing. Later in the session, the clinician began to shift into rebuilding Eric's motivation and increasing insight that could prevent relapse in the future.

> CLINICIAN: Eric – I know this two-day relapse has thrown you for a loop. I really want to credit you with your ability to stop drinking after two days and to continue attending counseling. How were you able to do that? [Affirming the client and eliciting strengths the client used to stop the relapse].

ERIC: I didn't want my family to think I had given up and was going to go back to drinking how I had been. And I knew I didn't want to be hungover for work Monday. And I feel like if I kept drinking, it would be hard to stop. But also, something didn't feel right when I was drinking. I knew that I was working on other things in my life.

CLINICIAN: Your family – connection wellness is a powerful motivator for you as is the contextual and mental wellness from your job. And sticking to your wellness plan is important to you. It sounds like your wellness goals took priority over drinking. Let's talk about ways you can hold onto these insights during times when you experience craving. [Reflection highlighting the wellness dimensions noted by the client and encouraging brainstorming into applying client strengths].

THE WBAC CLINICIAN PROCESSED INSIGHTS ABOUT WHAT TRIGGERED THE RELAPSE.

CLINICIAN: Let's pretend we can rewind the tape of your life back to the days leading up to the start of the slip or that very day. What warning signs can you identify across the wellness dimensions that the risk of a slip was going on? [Initiating process of learning from the relapse].

ERIC: Oh man. Dad's health has continued to go downhill. I just have to keep doing more and more to take care of him at home. Then my wife keeps bringing up the conversation of needing to find a nursing home for him. So we've been arguing.

CLINICIAN: You have faced some emotional wellness challenges with stress from caring for your dad and connection wellness challenges with Kelly. What else? [Reflection highlighting the wellness dimensions noted by the client].

THE CLINICIAN ALSO ENGAGED ERIC IN THE BENEFITS ACTIVITY.

CLINICIAN: I know that you have been feeling down since the slip with alcohol. During these times, it can be difficult to connect with your motivation, progress, and goals. So I want to be intentional about making those connections. What are your reasons for pursuing abstinence and your wellness goals?

ERIC: I want my daughter and wife and even my dad to be proud of me. I want Lia to look back and know I was a valuable part of her life. I want to be a great husband to Kelly. That's what she deserves. And I want balance and to find more enjoyment in life.

CLINICIAN: Your relationships with family are at the center of your goals. You want to make time for what's most important regarding nurturing yourself and those relationships. What progress and benefits have you noticed from pursuing abstinence and wellness over the past two months? [Reflection highlighting the importance of the client's wellness goals and open-ended question exploring wellness progress and benefits].

ERIC: Several things. My relationships with my family have all improved. I make time for myself. My stress levels have come down a lot.

CLINICIAN: What do these things mean to you? [Open-ended question exploring progress and benefits in more depth].

ERIC (TEARFUL): I can't remember feeling so good, so hopeful. I messed up with drinking the other day, but I'm going to get back to my plan.

CLINICIAN: You can see your wellness vision coming to fruition. Having a slip with drinking won't deter you from your wellness goals. At the start of this session, you rated your confidence in abstaining from alcohol at a 4 or 5 and the importance of not drinking at a 7. What would you rate your importance and confidence right now?

[Reflection then scaling question to discern importance and confidence levels and impact of clinician response to client relapse].

ERIC: My importance is back to the highest level. My confidence is down a bit because of what happened, but it is a 7 right now.

CLINICIAN: As we always do, let's talk about some ways to keep the progress, benefits, and reasons for your wellness plan in the front of your mind as you continue your wellness journey. [Encouraging brainstorming into applying client strengths and insights].

CONCLUSION

Several important WBAC skills were illustrated in the case study with Eric. First, notice how the clinician used wellness language; labeling dimensions of wellness that arose from the client. The wellness framework provides a way for the client to make sense of their experiences. There also was an emphasis on learning from the relapse rather than judging the relapse. Moreover, the clinician invited the client to transform their insights into RP and wellness-enhancing skills that they can implement. The chapters on the wellness dimensions include additional ideas for how to accomplish this.

The subsequent chapters of the book dive deeper into the different wellness dimensions. In each of these chapters, you will learn more about dimension-specific relapse triggers and resources. You will also learn about how to support your clients whose treatment plans focus on certain wellness dimensions. Consider revisiting this relapse chapter again after completing some of the dimension chapters as you will be able to further apply this knowledge toward facilitating your clients' wellness and RP skills.

Handout 4.4 Blank Needs and Relapse Prevention Resources Handout

Needs	Skills/Resources
Physiological	
Safety (emotional)	
Love and Belonging	
Esteem	
Self-Actualization	
Self-Transcendence	

Handout 4.5 Blank Wellness Triggers and Relapse Prevention Handout

Wellness triggers and relapse prevention
Mental wellness triggers/relapse prevention skills and resources

- Trigger:
- Skills/resources:

Physical wellness triggers/relapse prevention skills and resources

- Trigger:
- Skills/resources:

Spiritual wellness triggers/relapse prevention skills and resources

- Trigger:
- Skills/resources:

Emotional wellness triggers/relapse prevention skills and resources

- Trigger:
- Skills/resources:

Connection wellness triggers/relapse prevention skills and resources

- Trigger:
- Skills/resources:

REFERENCES

American Psychiatric Association. (2022). *Diagnostic and statistical manual of mental disorders* (5th ed., text rev.). https://doi.org/10.1176/appi.books.9780890425787

Carroll, K. M. (1998). *A cognitive-behavioral approach: Treating cocaine addiction*. National Institute on Drug Abuse, NIH Publication Number 98-4308.

Donovan, D., & Witkiewitz, K. (2012). Relapse prevention: From radical idea to common practice. *Addiction Research & Theory, 20*(3), 204–217. https://doi.org/10.3109/16066359.2011.647133

Doweiko, H. E. (2019). *Concepts of chemical dependency* (10th ed.). Cengage.

Kasl, C. D. (1992). *Many roads, one journey: Moving beyond the 12 steps*. Harper Perennial.

Koltko-Rivera, M. E. (2006). Rediscovering the later version of Maslow's hierarchy of needs: Self-transcendence and opportunities for theory, research, and unification. *Review of General Psychology, 10*, 302–317.

Lewis, T. F. (2014). *Substance addiction: Practical application of counseling theory*. Pearson.

Linehan, M. M. (2015). *DBT skills training manual* (2nd ed.). Guilford Press.

Lutz, A. B. (2013). *Learning solution-focused therapy: An illustrated guide.* American Psychiatric Publishing.

Marlatt, G. A. (1985). Relapse prevention: Theoretical rationale and overview of the model. In G. A. Marlatt & J. R. Gordon (Eds.), *Relapse prevention: Maintenance strategies in the treatment of addictive behaviors* (pp. 3–70). Guilford Press.

Marlatt, G. A., Parks, G. A., & Witkiewitz, K. (2002) *Clinical guidelines for implementing relapse prevention therapy.* University of Washington.

Marlatt, G. A., & Witkiewitz, K. (2005). Relapse prevention for alcohol and drug problems. In G. A. Marlatt & D. M. Donovan (Eds.), *Relapse prevention: Maintenance strategies in the treatment of addictive behaviors* (pp. 1–44). The Guilford Press.

Maslow, A. H. (1943). A theory of human motivation. *Psychological Review, 50*(4), 370–396. https://doi.org/10.1037/h0054346

Miller, W. R., Forcehimes, A. A., & Zweben, A. (2019). *Treating addiction: A guide for professionals* (2nd ed.). Guilford Press.

Miller, W. R., & Rollnick, S. (2013). *Motivational interviewing: Helping people change* (3rd ed.). Guilford Press.

Myers, J. E., & Sweeney, T. J. (2005). Introduction to wellness theory. In J. E. Myers & T. J. Sweeney (Eds.), *Counseling for wellness: Theory, research, and practice* (pp. 7–14). American Counseling Association.

Prochaska, J. O., & DiClemente, C. C. (1983). Stages and processes of self-change of smoking: Toward an integrative model of change. *Journal of Consulting and Clinical Psychology, 51*(3), 390–395. https://doi.org/10.1037/0022-006X.51.3.390

Ratner, H., George, E., & Iveson, C. (2012). *Solution focused brief therapy: 100 key points and techniques.* Routledge.

Sliedrecht, W., de Waart, R., Witkiewitz, K., & Roozen, H. G. (2019). Alcohol use disorder relapse factors: A systematic review. *Psychiatry Research, 278*, 97–115. https://doi.org/10.1016/j.psychres.2019.05.038

Thombs, D. L. (2006). *Introduction to addictive behaviors* (3rd ed.). New York: Guilford.

Thombs, D. L. (2019). *Introduction to addictive behaviors* (5th ed.). New York: Guilford.

Williams, R., & Gorski, T. (2007). *Relapse prevention counseling for African Americans: A culturally specific model.* CENAPS/Herald Publishing House.

CHAPTER 5

STRENGTH AND SOLUTION-BUILDING

INTRODUCTION

In the world of substance use and addictions, it is easy to focus on what is wrong with the person who cannot stop using addictive substances. Society's perception is often aligned with problem-based or deficit-dominated stories about their lives. The "down and out drunk", being "strung out on drugs", or the "loser addict" are common reframes people use to refer to those struggling with substance addiction. Traditional substance use disorder (SUD) treatment approaches, either intentionally or unintentionally, promote this deficit model thinking: "You (the addict) are *flawed* and I (therapist) know how to *fix* you". We italicized the words flawed and fix because this approach assumes that clients have no inner resources, strengths, attributes, or even choices in their own recovery; they must be healed by a system that may not respect persons struggling with addictions. Undoubtedly, the life of an addicted person *is* filled with challenges and negative experiences. These deficits, problems, and diagnoses are worthy of exploration for the purposes of triage, assessment, and treatment. However, what is often overlooked are the strengths, possibilities, and resilience inherent in all clients. Strengths are important because they offer a platform to build upon for successful recovery. They offer hope. These strengths can be (a) personal qualities or character strengths, (b) areas in which the client is higher in wellness, or (c) resources external to the client. As such, assessing for and utilizing client strengths forms a major portion of WBAC.

Since the mid-1980s, strength-based approaches have offered an alternative to the prominent deficit-based model interpretations and interventions of addictive problems and issues. Although strength-based ideas have not permeated all traditional SUD programs, many of their ideas have been infused throughout the United States (e.g., harm reduction). In general, strength-based approaches focus on what is working in the client's life and build upon strengths, goals, and positive characteristics. Further, they can help clients identify what is *not* working and reduce or eliminate behaviors that are counterproductive or not preferred. In this chapter, we introduce the concept of strength-based therapy and review the philosophies and techniques of two primary strength-based counseling approaches: positive psychology and its related techniques and solution-focused therapy (SFT). After a review of each, we discuss how strength-based approaches in general integrate into WBAC. Special emphasis will be given to strength-based techniques and strategies to help addicted clients cultivate hope and envision positive change as they navigate the path to recovery.

STRENGTHS-BASED THERAPY

Proponents of strength-based counseling and therapy stress that even when an addicted person hits "rock bottom", she or he still has possibilities, resilience, and choices that encourage change (van Wormer & Davis, 2003). Strength-based approaches counter the common narrative that addicts are "lost causes", especially if they are in treatment for months (or even years). Single episodes of treatment are rarely effective for those struggling with addiction;

DOI: 10.4324/9781003147954-5

substance use disorders are chronic, relapsing problems that often require significant intervention over time (van Wormer & Davis, 2003). Rather than focusing exclusively on problems and limitations, strength-based practitioners keep an eye out for possibilities, positive goals, and inspiration. Common terms used in the strength-based movement include *empowerment, membership (belongingness), resilience, healing, wholeness, dialog, collaboration*, and finding ways to *trust* that the client will find their way (van Wormer & Davis, 2003).

A common theme in strength-based interventions is choice (van Wormer & Davis, 2003). Miller and Rollnick (2013) suggested that mental health professionals offer clients a *menu of options* from which the client can make choices about their own treatment and care. For example, addicted clients may choose from selected goals (harm reduction, controlled drinking, and complete abstinence), a list of treatment contexts and settings (inpatient, outpatient, individual, family, and mutual help groups), and treatment methods (relapse prevention, CBT group therapy, 12 steps, MI, and SFT). Clients who feel like they have some ownership in their care are generally more motivated with a sense of freedom and empowerment (Miller & Rollnick, 2013). In more traditional treatment approaches, choice is either non-existent or restricted. Clients tend to respond better when offered options rather than being told what to do (Miller & Rollnick, 2013).

In some situations, the clinician may not have much wiggle room related to client choice. For example, I (TFL) worked with a client diagnosed with severe alcohol use disorder. He had multiple physical problems related to years of heavy drinking with major life disruption, did not have much motivation to stop, and had a family history of alcohol dependence. This client was not a suitable candidate for harm reduction in the form of controlled drinking (Miller & Munoz, 2005). Due to numerous health concerns, there was only one treatment goal: to completely abstain from alcohol. However, even when there was only one choice for treatment, the client still had the autonomy to participate in that treatment. In addition, there were other aspects of his care, such as treatment setting and context, where choices were offered (e.g., choosing individual instead of group counseling). In strength-based treatment approaches, the clinician is always looking to enhance client autonomy by promoting choice, even if it might be restricted in some circumstances.

Strength-based therapy is about empowering clients by helping them uncover their own resources for change, such as motivation, persistence, resilience, and confidence. It is about finding and shining a bright light on strengths so that clients can take these and build their recovery. In the sections that follow, we highlight two common strength-based therapy approaches: the techniques of positive psychology and SFT. What these approaches have in common, like all strength-based approaches, includes respecting self-determination, being sensitive to the client's motivation to change, and focusing on both inter and intrapersonal skills and resources (van Wormer & Rae Davis, 2003).[1]

Positive Psychology

According to Peterson (2008), positive psychology is the scientific study of what makes life most worth living; it is the scientific study of human thoughts, feelings, and behaviors with a focus on strengths instead of limitations, wellness instead of disease, and building a life where one flourishes instead of "just getting by" (Peterson, 2008). Common elements associated with positive psychology include emotions (happiness, joy, inspiration, and love), characteristics and traits (gratitude, resilience, and compassion), and positive energy (optimism, life satisfaction, well-being, self-esteem, self-confidence, and hope). At first glance, one can see how these elements of positive psychology provide a counternarrative to the deficit-based treatment models that govern most drug-addicted individuals. Later in this chapter, we will discuss how infusing positive psychology into the treatment process fits squarely with the WBAC model.

Positive psychology emerged from the work of psychologist Martin Seligman, who initially studied the concept of "learned helplessness", a phenomenon that has been intricately linked with depression (Ackerman, 2020). Learned helplessness is the idea that humans, through cognitive mechanisms and other contingencies, can learn to feel powerless in their lives, believing they have no control. Learned helplessness has been found to have direct application to addictions (Wang, Zhang, & Zhang, 2017). The concept of relapse bears this out; addicted clients often find themselves solidly in recovery only to fall into a relapse. It is not uncommon for this cycle to repeat itself four, five, or six or more times until eventually the client maintains sobriety. Each time the client relapses, these "failures" engender discouragement and helplessness, leading to a pervasive sense of shame. Seligman's work on learned helplessness and its connection to depression led to treatment approaches that were focused more on resilience and learned optimism (Ackerman, 2020); if helplessness could be learned, then so could optimism.

The PERMA Model

The PERMA model was proposed by Seligman to provide depth to the concept of well-being (Ackerman, 2020). According to Seligman (2012), there are five key facets to well-being.

Positive emotions – Positive emotions such as joy and happiness are important components of well-being. To access these, clients are encouraged to engage in activities that provide or elicit these emotions and to stay in the present moment to savor these experiences. Importantly, positive emotions are necessary, but not sufficient, for healthy well-being. That is, it would be inappropriate (and ineffective) to tell clients to just do things to make one happier and everything will be ok. Authentic well-being includes positive emotions in context of the other aspects of the PERMA model.

Engagement – Engaging in activities in which one excels and enjoys is another important component of well-being. In this context, engagement means becoming totally absorbed in a healthy activity that provides meaning, pleasure, sense of fulfillment, etc. Whether at work or for leisure, it is difficult to imagine a strong sense of well-being if one is not engaged with life activities (Seligman, 2012).

Relationships (positive) – Not surprisingly, meaningful positive relationships strongly contribute to a sense of well-being. Our connections to other human beings help us flourish and provide opportunities that we simply would not have alone. One of the most common symptoms of the addictive process is *isolation*, where, metaphorically, the addiction does everything in its power to keep the individual isolated from others. In other words, the addiction wants the individual to develop a relationship with the drug, rather than with other human beings. A powerful antidote to this isolation is 12-step mutual help groups. The mutual support found in these groups can be a powerful way to counter isolation.

Meaning – A developed sense of well-being rests on having a purpose in life. One can be happy-go-lucky all day but without a sense of purpose and meaning, well-being is compromised. Dedicating oneself to larger causes, engaging in important work, or finding ways to help others are some common ways people find meaning. This aspect of well-being is enormously helpful when working with addictions. Assisting addicted clients to "get out of their own head" by focusing on larger causes, for example, can be a profound way to bolster the client's well-being and recovery process.

Accomplishment/achievement – When we achieve success, there is increased energy, positive feelings, and enhanced motivation to keep going. Success does not need to be monumental; even small, everyday successes can add up and contribute to well-being. Darren Hardy, a pioneer in the psychology of success movement, discussed in his book *The Compound Effect* (2012) how everyday successes are like small bricks that we add to building our metaphorical house. Brick by brick, we add positive habits, behaviors, and successes to our life. The consequences of these positive experiences become *compounded* over time, multiplying in ways that propel one toward a life worth living.

A common refrain in Alcoholics Anonymous (AA) circles is "one day at a time". This statement is a mantra that is repeated so that the prospect of giving up alcohol forever does not seem so daunting; taking "one day" to stop drinking instead of "the rest of my life" is manageable. However, we would argue there is another important element to this philosophy. Namely, that a day free from alcohol is a success, and as the compound effect predicts, small successes build upon each other until the benefits of living a wellness-based life are realized. Accomplishments and achievements, no matter the size, significantly contribute to well-being.

Positive Psychology Techniques

Positive psychology techniques are designed to focus on wellness and strengths, while still acknowledging the client's difficulties. They are intentional activities meant to promote both personal pleasure (hedonic) and contentment (eudaimonia) with life (Pawelski, 2020). By studying individuals with high levels of well-being, researchers have been able to identify those emotions, cognitions, and behaviors that lead to greater happiness and prosperity.

Pawelski (2020) broke down positive psychology interventions (PPIs) into their basic elements. The five elements include desired outcomes, target system, target change, active ingredient, and activity. *Desired outcomes* refer to the effect of the target change, such as greater contentment and enhanced purpose in life. *Target system* refers to the life component that changes, such as thinking, emotion, intention, or relationships. *Target change* refers to preferred changes within a domain, such as engaging with others more often, increasing self-confidence, and being a better _____ (insert "father", "spouse/partner", etc.). The *active ingredient* is what causes a change in the target system, such as stressing autonomy, offering a menu of options, or providing information with permission. Finally, *activity* includes the actions that will bring about the desired outcome, such as journaling, thinking a different way, or engaging in some physical activity. Pawelski further argued that each of these elements can be combined in imaginative ways to create innovative techniques consistent with positive psychology philosophy.

Applied to substance addictions, Pawelski's (2020) analysis can help MHPs design interventions aimed to help clients cut down use, abstain, or bolster recovery efforts. Taking each of the five elements discussed above, practitioners can map out an addictions-focused treatment plan that reflects the strengths-based perspective (generally) and positive psychology principles (specifically). Table 5.1 highlights an example of what this might look like with a client struggling with addiction.

Three PPIs are considered "iconic" in the field (Pawelski, 2020). They include *the three good things exercise, the gratitude visit*, and *using your signature strengths in new ways*. We briefly review each technique below, along with how they might apply in the case of clients struggling with substance addiction.

Table 5.1 Elements of PPIs Applied to a Client Struggling with Addiction

Desired Outcome	Target System	Target Change	Active Ingredient	Activity
Abstain from alcohol Repair/improve relationships Find purpose in life	Cognition and thinking Willpower Relationships	Increase motivation to change Strengthened refusal skills Better listening skills with spouse/partner Articulating one's purpose to others	Creating a change plan Overcoming fear of intimacy Goal setting Values clarification	Journaling Using 3 × 5 reminder cards Speaking clearly Exercise

THREE GOOD THINGS EXERCISE

In this exercise, the clinician encourages the client to write down three good things that happened each day and why they happened. The purpose of this technique is to help clients create a shift in mindset from negativity (something bad ALWAYS happens) to positivity (I am noticing good things happening now). However, this exercise is more than just writing down something positive that happens; it also entails helping the client identify *why* it happened. Inevitably, clients come to realize that positive things happen because of their own volition and behavior. Recorded over time, clients create their own record of success, which bolsters self-efficacy and counters more problematic self-narratives.

We can easily adopt this exercise in WBAC by asking the client to write down three good things that happened each day *related to their wellness and/or recovery*. Assume a client struggling with heroin addiction was asked to complete this exercise and, after a week, shared three good things that happened each day related to his recovery with his clinician (leaving 21 total items recorded). The conversation between the clinician and the client intentionally focused on positive wellness and recovery behaviors and how the client was able to make these events happen. Client strengths were emphasized, with encouragement from the clinician to fall back on these strengths in difficult times (e.g., when pressured by peers to use again). For example, the client might share how he attended Narcotics Anonymous every day during the past week and started a moderate exercise program. The clinician can then highlight perseverance and courage as strengths that allowed him to do this.

THE GRATITUDE VISIT

Expressing gratitude has been shown to be a powerful activity that can help improve mood, increase contentment, and promote well-being (Field, 2021). The gratitude visit (Seligman, Steen, Park, & Peterson, 2005) is a simple exercise where clients are asked to write a gratitude letter to someone who has helped them or has had a positive influence on them, but with whom they have not had a chance to thank. In the classic technique, the client reads the letter to the other person; however, there may be circumstances where that is not always possible. Alternative possibilities might include reading the letter using the empty chair technique, reading the letter to a therapy group but not sending it, or reading it back to the clinician.

This technique is different from step #8 within the AA 12 steps, where members are asked to "make amends" for wrongdoing. When making amends, clients are focused more on asking for forgiveness from those whom they have hurt because of their addictive behavior and consequences. The eighth step is designed to help clients get out of their own minds and recognize how they have hurt others. Expressing gratitude is not asking for forgiveness but rather giving thanks to someone who has helped them. Indeed, both making amends and expressing gratitude could be a powerful combination toward greater healing among those struggling with addiction.

In recovery, clients interact with many people who help them along their journey. Encouraging clients to acknowledge this help and actively show gratitude promotes positive feelings, reduces shame and guilt, and counters perceptions that all addicts are selfish. Making this a consistent practice would be an important adjunct to one's recovery plan.

USING YOUR SIGNATURE STRENGTHS IN NEW WAYS
In this exercise, clients are asked to identify their top five strengths and try to use them daily in new ways. For example, a client might identify trustworthiness as a strength and is encouraged to incorporate this into her wellness and recovery. She may be trustworthy to other people but not to herself. She could remember that an expanded definition of being trustworthy has to do with keeping promises to herself, such as following her relapse prevention plan if tempted to use again.

The framework of positive psychology focuses on client wellness and strengths, instead of deficits and disease. This is not to suggest that we should never focus on problems, symptoms, and the disease process of addiction. However, shifting attention to positive emotions, characteristics, and energy acknowledges a vast field of potential that is often ignored within traditional SUD treatment approaches.

Solutions-Focused Therapy

Solution-focused therapy (SFT) has gained recognition as a viable alternative to more traditional substance addiction treatment approaches (Lewis, 2023; Linton, 2005), and fits squarely within wellness-based addictions counseling. The strength-based orientation, with a focus on what is working instead of client deficits, has gained both national and international appeal in addressing substance use issues (McCullum, Trepper, & Smock, 2003; Smock et al., 2008). SFT clinicians hold unique views about the relationships between clients and their problems, how problems (and solutions) are generated, and how using language can shape a more positive experience in the counseling setting. In this section, we provide a brief overview of SFT counseling and how its methods may be utilized for substance addiction. We also explore some common SFT techniques that counselors can utilize when working with clients.

In SFT, clinicians monitor and conceptualize progress by starting with what the client wants. As clients increase their awareness of when they are getting what they want, they start to build a positive perspective of their lives. SFT clinicians challenge clients to identify times when the problem is *not* happening. This shift in focus may lead to insights into what they were doing, thinking, and feeling, and other factors that contribute to those positive moments. When clients identify the people, behaviors, feelings, and thoughts when things are going well (or going better), they set the path from which solutions can emerge.

SFT is about helping clients act. Rather than believing one must feel a certain way before positive change can happen, SFT clinicians focus on helping clients accomplish behavioral goals, engage in more preferred ways of living, and reinforce behaviors that are not associated with the problem. The emphasis on *doing* reflects the reciprocal nature of thoughts, feelings, and behaviors; that is, engaging in positive behaviors is likely to lead to more positive thoughts and emotions. SFT clinicians stress personal responsibility and redirect clients who want others to be responsible for their own change process (Lewis, 2018).

SFT with Addictions

It is a rare circumstance that clients struggling with addiction present to counseling with only one problem. Their narratives (i.e., life stories) are often *problem saturated*, meaning that client self-talk, communications from significant others, and (unfortunately) messages from the treatment community reinforce negative, stereotypical characteristics and traits of the addict. Addicted clients come to internalize these negative messages, realizing that not only do they have problems but also they *are* the problem! SFT clinicians strive to disentangle these stories from clients' sense of self by helping them shift perspective to moments when things are going in a more preferred way, goals are accomplished, and problems are not so dominant (Lewis, 2018).

Strategic Questioning: Setting Quality Goals in Addictions Counseling

A series of main questions guide the SFT counseling process. Key questions include,

    a.   What does the client want?

    b.   What has the client already done, if anything, to get what they want?

    c.   What can the client do to get more of what they want?

    d.   What are the client's counseling goals? (Allyn & Bacon Professional, 2001).

Although these questions provide the general framework from which SFT clinicians operate, we would like to focus on the fourth question because setting positive goals is foundational to SFT (as well as the wellness-based addictions counseling approach). Goals are co-constructed, must be relevant to the client, and manageable. Goals that come from someone else (e.g., counselor and family members) or that seem overwhelming to the client (e.g., ceasing all drug use immediately for the rest of one's life, confronting loved ones, and taking financial responsibility) will usually result in backsliding and little progress (Berg & Miller, 1992).

Berge and Miller (1992) provided some additional strategies regarding goal setting for clients struggling with alcohol addiction. For example, preliminary goals may not have anything to do with substance use (i.e., the literal ingestion of substances), although they may be related in some way. Prematurely focusing on substance use, especially for those in the *pre-contemplative* stage of change (i.e., clients who do not see a problem with their substance use and are resistant to change; Prochaska & DiClemente, 1992), may unintentionally push clients away (Berg & Miller, 1992). Clients may initially set goals related to the fallout of severe substance addiction such as wanting to improve relationships, work through the legal system, and secure employment. In our experience, when clients make the connection between mounting life problems and addiction, they are more amenable to taking a closer look at their problematic substance use. Berg and Miller (1992) called this strategy *finding the hidden customer* – helping the client with what they want, followed by opening conversations about drug use as the counseling relationship improves.

Goal setting in addictions counseling usually involves taking something away from the client's behavior (e.g., the drug use). Whereas this is an obvious area of focus, it also is important to help clients add something to their lives, so they are not left with a gaping hole in their day (Lewis, 2018). A question we like to ask our clients is, "what will you be doing *instead* of using?" In SFT, the purpose of quality goal setting is to help clients determine what is working, when the problem is not happening, and how they could do more of these behaviors (Lewis, 2018). Indeed, clients seem to respond better when they can imagine success and happiness rather than just avoiding drug use (Mott & Gysin, 2003). The wellness model is an excellent tool for brainstorming goals based on the SFT process. For example, the clinician can ask clients what is working and when the problem is not happening related to addiction as well as all domains of wellness, including body, mind, and emotions.

What might serve as a positive substitute for addictive behavior? As with all goal setting, this is determined in a co-constructive fashion, with the counselor and client identifying those activities that provide fulfillment and/or enjoyment. Importantly, counselors do not want to create another burden for the client by encouraging behaviors they think are beneficial but which the client does not find useful. As a common example, consider a counselor who strongly encourages exercise (weight training, cardio) as a positive substitute for drug use, but the client sees exercise as boring and has little motivation (Lewis, 2018). However, she may enjoy reading (joining a reading club), tai chi (a less boring form of exercise), or reconnecting with non-using friends. Gently encouraging substitute activities that are consistent with the client's interests, abilities, and lifestyle will help ease the burden when inevitable urges and cravings emerge.

Counseling goals help put the client in the right mindset toward change. However, to be most effective, goals should be perceived as challenging (Berg & Miller, 1992). Clients who accomplish challenging goals build momentum and confidence, setting the stage for additional goal setting and success (Lewis, 2018). In addition, *not* accomplishing a goal does not mean the client is a failure, only that more effort may be needed. SFT clinicians acknowledge the difficulty of goals, effort, and positive steps, however small, toward change (Berg & Miller, 1992).

Talking about Solutions

In SFT, conversations between counselor and client gently guide clients toward exploring solutions to problematic substance use, intentionally moving away from problem narratives to ones of opportunities, assets, and what is working (and not working). Many clients who come into counseling for substance-related reasons are already making changes. For example, Lewis (2018) noted that even before the first session, clients have most likely (a) attempted to cut back or stop drug use, (b) realized that their life is not where they want it to be, (c) have had some successes, even small, and (d) have been their own worst enemy when unable to stop. Although clients tend to overlook these small achievements, SFT clinicians intentionally point out and support clients in what they are already doing. Taken together, a–d above suggests that clients may have several strengths, including willpower, insight, persistence, and high expectations for self (Lewis). The astute clinician will not only focus on these strengths but also inquire how clients will continue to build on these to promote their own recovery (Lewis, 2023).

SFT Techniques

Below is a brief list of some of the more common SFT techniques which make significant use of strategic questioning (Linton, 2005).

EXCEPTIONS TO THE PROBLEM QUESTIONS

Human beings are naturally biased toward threats and negativity in what Hanson (2011) calls the negativity bias. Problems tend to become enormous roadblocks in life whereas successes tend to be overlooked. Counselors who ask exception to the problem questions counter the negativity bias by asking clients times when the problem is not happening. Positive client experiences without the problem happening become the basis for building a good life and creating solutions (Lewis, 2014; Linton, 2005; McCollum et al., 2003). If counselors can encourage clients to do more of what is working, they can escape the mindset that problems are intractable, create more space to try new behaviors, and begin to build the path to recovery.

Clients struggling with addiction may find it difficult to find exceptions to poor wellness narratives. In WBAC, clinicians can intentionally use this exercise to inquire and explore wellness exceptions. For example, questions such as, "What were some times in the last week that your overall wellness was high? What high wellness areas related to less substance use? What high wellness areas led to fewer consequences of use?" can start the process. Wellness exceptions can be explored across each domain so that several positive behaviors can be noted.

PRESUPPOSITION QUESTIONS

These questions presume that clients have made changes relatively soon. In SFT, language plays a major role in helping clients create a preferred way of living (Lewis, 2018). As such, SFT clinicians strategically ask about when in the future the problem is not happening and what the client will be doing when that happens. Here is an example: six months from now, *when you have completely stopped cocaine use*, what steps would you have taken to get there? How will you be living your life differently? The clinician is strategically presuming that cocaine use has stopped, thus instilling confidence (Lewis, 2018). Stage of change can be an important consideration when using this exercise. For example, clients in pre-contemplation (i.e., do not see their substance use as a problem despite numerous consequences) could focus on changes within wellness domains rather than substance use (focusing on substance use too early for clients in the pre-contemplative stage of change may engender resistance and discord). The clinician can then ask the client what substance use might look like if the client were to make these wellness-based changes. If the client can imagine positive changes in wellness, it is reasonable to assume that substance use would not be a part of the alternative narrative.

It is recommended that clinicians do not use unreasonable time frames for this question. For example, presuming that the client has stopped his addiction in two weeks is probably unreasonable, and projecting out five years from now is a horizon that is too distant. With presupposition questions, we like to use the six months to one-year time frame, which allows enough time for change to happen but does not look too far ahead to make the technique meaningless.

MIRACLE QUESTION

In this familiar SFT technique, counselors ask clients to imagine a miracle happening overnight in which the problem that brought them into counseling is solved (Berg & Miller, 1992). Because this happened while the client was sleeping, they did not know the miracle occurred. Once this brief setup is provided, the counselor asks any variation of the following question, "What do you think you will notice tomorrow morning that indicates to you that there has been a miracle overnight and the problem we have talked about is solved?" (Berg & Miller, 1992).

This question directs clients to prioritize behaviors, thoughts, and feelings that would be happening if they were experiencing wellness goal success related to their recovery from substance use. For example, a client might respond that her miracle would be that she wakes up from a satisfying seven-hour sleep, engages in meditation upon waking, and commits to an exercise program before heading to work. Getting up in the morning and calling a sponsor could be part of one's miracle. As with other SFT techniques, through this question, clients become active participants in building their own solutions.

MIRACLE DAY

Closely aligned with the miracle question is the *miracle day*. The clinician begins by asking clients how a day without the problem might unfold; that is, what would a *miracle* (i.e., problem-free) day look like in terms of thoughts, behaviors, emotions, relationships, communications, etc. (Lewis, 2018). Addicted clients usually come up with several ideas, such as not using substances, avoiding common triggers, or re-engaging in a long-lost hobby. The important point is to make sure the miracle day is co-constructed and defined with significant client input. Once defined, the clinician encourages the client to have one miracle day between the current session and the next session. When the client returns, the counselor reviews the miracle day, with emphasis on affirming strengths and positive experiences (Lewis, 2018).

This technique also can focus specifically on wellness, creating a *miracle wellness day* exercise. Here the miracle must be defined according to principles aligned with the domains of wellness, such as eating healthier (body), meditation (mind), or working through emotions (emotion). In debriefing the experience, the counselor can inquire how substance use fits or does not fit with this miracle wellness day.

If the miracle or miracle wellness day is a success, the assignment can expand from one to several days between sessions. As with other techniques, stacking up positive experiences, where the problem is not happening, encourages the client to build his own path forward in recovery. We have found the miracle day to be effective not just with addicted individuals but with couples and families as well.

SCALING QUESTIONS

Scaling questions are useful strategies to determine goal progress and levels of motivation to change. Used strategically, this technique can be a great way to explore what holds clients back from accomplishing goals, as well as what needs to happen for the client to meet the goal. Mott et al. (2003) noted that a typical scaling question asks clients where they fall on a scale of 1–10 related to their goal(s). Here is an example

On a scale of 1 to 10, with 1 being no progress on abstaining from alcohol and 10 being able to completely abstain, where would you rate yourself on this goal?

The technique continues with the follow-up question, "what makes your progress a [specific number] and not a [lower number]?" This follow-up is strategic; by asking about the current number and why it is not lower, the client naturally reports some success, otherwise there would be no initial number. In other words, there must be some progress associated with any number, even numbers considered low (i.e., below 5). Most clients will not be at a 10; however, even at a 3, 2, or 1, *some* progress is acknowledged!

Strength-based approaches, including positive psychology and SFT, remind clinicians to focus on wellness, strengths, what is working, and solutions. They counter interventions that solely focus on liabilities and deficits.

INTEGRATION OF STRENGTHS-BASED APPROACHES WITH WBAC

In WBAC, we advocate seeing clients as important allies in their own therapy and recovery. We do not discount the importance of diagnosis, deficits in behavioral skills, and comprehension of an underlying problem. However, the balance of intervention is focused on promoting wellness, building on strengths, and cultivating hope. It is our contention that these positive aspects are sorely missing within current SUD counseling practice. Strengths and a solutions focus are inherent to wellness counseling. In this section, we review methods for how to incorporate strength-based interventions and how they can be built into the WBAC to augment positive outcomes for clients.

Transforming Strengths into Recovery Strategies

Focusing on strengths creates a shift in thinking for clients, but how can strengths transform into effective recovery strategies for clients? Before we help clients transform strengths into positive action, we need to first identify them. There are two methods to do this: first, clinicians can simply ask clients about their strengths. Second, clinicians can point out strengths they notice by observing and working with the client. Whatever method is used, the next step is to acknowledge client strengths followed by intentionally affirming these inherent characteristics within the client. Affirmations, when done correctly, can be powerful statements that set the tone for a wellness-based perspective. Consider that some clients in the throes of an addiction or active recovery may not have heard much positive in their life. Indeed, when asked about their strengths, clients struggling with addiction may have difficulty coming up with any due to feelings of shame and guilt. Affirmation can be an effective strategy to counteract some of these intense feelings that can serve as roadblocks to recovery.

How to Affirm

Affirmations are statements that acknowledge positive characteristics and strengths within the client. The goal is to affirm *inherent* qualities, rather than behaviors. Once these positive inherent strengths and qualities are identified, the WBAC clinician makes an affirmative statement. Here is an example that a clinician might use:

Affirmation: You have a lot of resolve given what you have gone through and desire to stop using.

Affirmations seem to be more effective when using "you" statements rather than "I" statements (Rosengren, 2019). "I" statements tend to be more aligned with praise. Affirmation, however, is not the same as praise. Praising clients implies an unequal partnership and includes an element of judgment. Consider the affirmation example again, this time contrasted with a statement of praise:

Affirmation: You have a lot of resolve given what you have gone through and desire to stop using.

Praise: I think you have gone through a lot and I am pleased you want to stop using.

In the first example, the WBAC clinician is pointing out the strength of *resolve* that they observe within the client, as well as the *desire to stop using*. In the second example, the words "I think" and "I am pleased" are judgmental and imply an unequal therapeutic relationship: the client is there to please the therapist and, if that happens, the therapist will acknowledge this. The distinction between affirmation and praise is often subtle but important.

Affirmations (with "you" statements) directly convey what the WBAC clinician is observing and noticing about the client.

Affirmations always begin with identifying strengths, followed by a statement that acknowledges them. A helpful exercise for WBAC clinicians is to make a list of client strengths after a counseling session. For the next session, pick one or two of these strengths to affirm. Although the impact may be subtle, never underestimate the power of affirming. Remember that some clients struggling with addiction may be unaccustomed to hearing anything positive about themselves. Unfortunately, shame runs deep, which can sabotage recovery efforts. Affirmations can be a starting place to begin untangling the client from these emotional trappings. We have been astonished at how affirmations can brighten a client's mood. Simple, clear, and effective.

Once strengths have been uncovered and affirmed, WBAC practitioners encourage clients to find ways to utilize these strengths in their recovery effort. In our experience, common strengths we see among addicted clients include resolve, resilience, courage, motivation, caring, wanting to improve, and perseverance. Courage, for example, can be called upon when a client confronts an old using buddy who is pushing a return to drug use. The client's resolve can be reflected on 3×5 notecards that he carries with him for those times when he is in a tight situation. Caring can be encouraged when the client visits mutual help groups for support. Importantly, MHPs are encouraged to co-create with clients how to use strengths as part of one's recovery plan. As strengths are cultivated and utilized, more strength tends to emerge as the client builds a successful wellness-based recovery.

Identifying Wellness Factors

At the heart of strength-based approaches is determining what factors contribute to when the problem (in this case, addiction) is not happening and then building on these experiences to create more of them. The idea is that if clients can string enough small successes together, they build self-efficacy and momentum in their recovery. Over time, the benefits of living a life of wellness and abstinence or harm reduction are realized – healthier mind and body, happier relationships, and stronger connection to a sense of purpose.

What does it mean to say when the "problem is not happening?" There is no universal definition, although a helpful conceptualization would be that *any* improvement be construed as the problem "not happening". For example, a client may cut down on his drinking between sessions – the problem of alcohol use is still there to some extent, but it is better than before. Another might be that the client experienced a trigger yet was able to avoid relapse or break his harm reduction goals. We advocate celebrating all improvements, no matter how small. In WBAC, it is important that clinicians explore the wellness factors that led to these successes.

With strategic questioning, clients can gain insight into aspects of wellness that were prominent during times of sobriety, successful harm reduction, or effective recovery. Specifically, MHPs intentionally steer clients toward awareness of what they were doing, from a wellness perspective, during these more successful times. For example, assume a client reports that she had a rather good week by abstaining from cocaine use and resisting social pressure to use. The MHP can then explore this success by asking questions related to any of the wellness factors – mind, body, emotions, spirit, and connection. Table 5.2 provides a list of potential questions.

Table 5.2 Wellness-Based Questions to Use Following Client Successes within Addictions Treatment

Mind	Body	Emotions	Sprit	Connection
What types of thoughts were you having that helped you stop using this past week?	What role do you believe exercise had on your ability to resist relapse?	What did you notice about how you were feeling when you had that urge? After the urge passed?	Now that you have abstained for a while, what gives you a new sense of purpose?	Who has been in your corner to help you not use?
How did you use your mind to control those urges?	What did you notice about your physical self when you stopped using this week?	How were you able to keep your feelings in check when you decided to quit?	How has the AA philosophy helped you through this struggle?	How have your relationships changed since you have stopped using?
What self-talk did you engage in to help you through this rough patch?	How have you tweaked your diet to help you keep on the road to recovery?	How have you created more positive emotions during your recovery?	How have you tried to secure more meaning in your life during this substance free period	What positive aspects of your personal relationships have helped you navigate recovery?

Wellness-based questions help clients zone in on and notice wellness factors that help with recovery. For example, a client may come to realize that when he exercises and follows a solid sleep schedule, cravings for drug use significantly lessen (both exercise and proper sleep have been shown to be promising adjuncts to SUD treatment; Linke & Ussher, 2015). Borrowing from SFT, the client is then encouraged to do more of what is working. Additional factors of wellness can be explored and encouraged, helping the client realize that caring for one's wellness ultimately runs counter to addiction.

The Power of Eliciting Strengths and Reducing Shame

Eliciting client strengths can be a powerful way to build a recovery. The power of this technique comes in its ability to counter feelings of shame. Shame is a negative emotion that encompasses the whole person. Self-talk, such as "I am no good", "I am a failure", and "I am bad", indicates global negative feelings toward oneself and usually suggests shame. Note that shame is a global negative assessment of one's self, irrespective of behavior (i.e., instead of saying "I did something bad", the person says, "I am bad"). Indeed, a struggle with addictions treatment is addressing the underlying shame that may be driving the addiction in the first place. When clients are asked to focus on strengths, they naturally shift away from shame to a more positive mindset. Eliciting strengths can be as simple as asking, "what do you consider your strengths?" or more elaborate exercises such as keeping a detailed journal of strengths.

We realize that most clients struggling with addiction are not eager to offer strengths, especially with mounting consequences of their drug use. When strengths are not forthcoming, WBAC clinicians s *elicit* them from clients. That is, clinicians call forth, promote, and explore client strengths and how they may be used in their recovery. If the client initially cannot provide any, stick with it! In WBAC, we believe that most clients, when given space and time, can reflect on and acknowledge personal assets. If facilitation is needed, clinicians can ask clients about strengths when they were a child (i.e., strengths before addiction set in and are possibly hidden), strengths others have observed or noticed, or simply offer their own clinical assessment of strengths via affirmative or encouraging statements.

Once strengths are acknowledged, the clinician should explore with clients how they can be incorporated more into their lives. For example, if a client states that one of her strengths is perseverance, how can she use this determination to push through difficult times in recovery? Helping clients make the connection between strengths and successful recovery is an important process. This exercise can be enhanced by visualization, having clients write down strengths on 3 × 5 cards for later reference or identifying and addressing barriers to incorporating strengths.

Identifying Positive Emotions

A consistent struggle for individuals with SUDs is the concomitant negative emotions that arise because of their addiction. Clients often find themselves in a reciprocal feedback loop where negative emotions and addictions feed off each other leading to personal misery. Research suggests that upsetting emotions, such as feelings of depression or anxiety, increase the risk of substance misuse (Brenner et al., 2019); it stands to reason, then, that those with a propensity toward positive emotions, such as joy, excitement, happiness, and contentment are associated with less problematic substance use. Our clinical experiences confirm this finding: clients who have a preponderance of positive emotions have fared much better with clinical goals compared to clients struggling with negative feelings. This is not to say that clients must only have positive emotions (which is impossible anyway). Indeed, negative feelings cannot and should not be ignored; however, clients who dwell in these negative emotions are usually in significant pain, which results in acting out behavior (i.e., substance use), which sadly contributes to more pain, and then more using, etc. (Nakken, 1996). This addictive cycle can continue for years without intervention (Nakken, 1996).

The positive psychology framework for eliciting positive emotions (see positive psychology techniques above) helps addicted clients to break this cycle. Shifting clients to focus on positive experiences and emotions, while still acknowledging problems in their lives, lays the groundwork for intentionally experiencing more of these feelings. Positive emotions are like a snowball going down a mountain, gaining speed, momentum, and size over time. In WBAC, building positive emotions, wellness, and strengths are at the heart of successful recovery.

CONCLUSION

Using the principles of strength-based counseling, positive psychology, and SFT, we convey to clients the following message: I will affirm your *positive characteristics*, help you *identify wellness factors* that are creating your successes, and *encourage you to do more of these*. I will encourage you to *identify, use, and build your strengths* so that you can bolster your recovery. I will *help you identify positive emotions* so that you can feel better and live in a more preferred manner. Finally, I will help you *make the connection between how changes in wellness coincide with substance use changes and vice-versa*. Ideally, clients take this overall message and channel it toward lifestyle modifications that may have been neglected.

CLIENT EXAMPLE

We conclude this chapter with an example from the case of Eric to see what strength-based interventions integrated within WBAC might look like clinically. In the excerpt below, assume Eric has been in recovery from an alcohol use disorder for approximately six months; however, he has experienced intense cravings that have caused him to question her commitment to recovery.

CLINICIAN: Hello Eric. It is nice to see you again. Tell me how things have been going.

ERIC: Well, I hit the six months mark being alcohol-free, so that's a plus. But the cravings have been intense. I almost relapsed the other day.

CLINICIAN: You still find yourself struggling a bit with cravings. At the same time, you have shown a lot of perseverance in your recovery (Reflective listening followed by affirmation).

ERIC: It has not been easy, but the threat of losing my family was too much to consider. I had to make a choice – alcohol or my family.

CLINICIAN: Eric, I really want to stress what success getting to six months is. What do you believe have been some of your strengths that you have used to get to this point? (Eliciting strengths).

ERIC: You mentioned perseverance – when I put my mind to something, I go all the way. I also think of my dedication to my family, wanting what is best for them.

CLINICIAN: Perseverance and dedication to family. Two key strengths that you have relied on to get this far. What positive emotions come up for you when you think about not using it for this long? (identifying positive emotions).

ERIC: It does feel different to reach this point, in a positive way. I would say I feel more hopeful, more joyful. They do not last long but I notice a shift.

CLINICIAN: You are noticing a shift in how you are feeling, from more negative to more positive, in general. You also identified two strengths you have relied on to help you get to this point. I am wondering how you might use these strengths to tackle the cravings issue so that you might feel even more of these positive emotions. (Variation of the using your strengths in new ways technique).

ERIC: I just need to remember my family. When cravings hit, through perseverance I know that it will pass and that my family takes precedence. I also have been dedicated to my recovery plan since we first met, and that has not lessened at all. But it is simply hard. The cravings can be overwhelming.

CLINICIAN: Remembering that cravings will pass and how important your family is would be a new way to use your perseverance, and your dedication seems rock solid (Reflecting on how strengths can be used to help with cravings).

In this brief example, the WBAC clinician used many strength-based principles and techniques outlined in this chapter that reflect WBAC. These techniques can be incorporated at any time and need not be difficult to implement. Shifting the focus to wellness, strengths, goals, and successes represent a subtle yet profound way to move clients ahead in recovery.

NOTE

1   Note that there are other strength-based approaches, such as narrative, motivational interviewing, and harm reduction. Apart from narrative, we cover motivational interviewing strategies and harm reduction principles throughout the text.

REFERENCES

Allyn & Bacon Professional (Producer). (2001). Solution-focused therapy for the addictions with Insoo Kim Berg [video tape]. Available from www.abacon.com/professional.

Ackerman, C. E. (2020). What is positive psychology and why is it important? Positivepsychology.com

Berg, I. K., & Miller, S. D. (1992). *Working with the problem drinker: A solution-focused approach.* Norton.

Brenner, P., Brandt, L., Li, G., DiBernardo, A., Boden, R., & Reutfors, J. (2019). Treatment-resistant depression as risk factor for substance use disorders – a nation-wide register-based cohort study. *Addiction, 114,* 1274–1282.

Field, B. (2021). How gratitude makes you happier. *Verywellmind.* Retrieved from https://tinyurl.com/yx8ex36k

Hanson, R. (2011). *Buddha's brain: The practical neuroscience of happiness, love, and wisdom.* PESI Seminars: Online webcast.

Hardy, D. (2012). *The compound effect.* Hachette Books.

Lewis, T. F. (2018). Solution-focused approaches in the treatment of substance addiction. In M. Scholl (Ed.), *Postmodern perspectives on contemporary counseling issues* (Chapter 3, pp. 62–93). Oxford.

Lewis, T. F. (2023). Applying solution-focused therapy in the treatment of substance abuse and addiction. In Lewis, T. F. (Ed.), *Substance abuse and addiction treatment: Practical application of counseling theory* (2nd ed., Chapter 11, pp. 286–310). Cognella.

Linke, S. E., & Ussher, M. (2015). *Exercise-based treatments for substance use disorders: Evidence, theory, and practicality, 41,* 7–15.

Linton, J. (2005). Mental health counselors and substance abuse treatment: Advantages, difficulties, and practical issues to solution-focused interventions. *Journal of Mental Health Counseling, 27,* 297–310.

McCollum, E. E., Trepper, T. S., & Smock, S. (2003). Solution-focused group therapy for substance abuse: Extending competency-based models. *Journal of Family Psychotherapy, 14,* 27–42.

Miller, W. R., & Munoz, R. E. (2005). *Controlling your drinking: Tools to make moderation work for you.* Guilford.

Miller, W. R., & Rollnick, S. (2013). *Motivational interviewing: Preparing people for change.* Guilford.

Nakken, C. (1996). *The addictive personality: Understanding the addictive process and compulsive behavior* (2nd ed.). Hazelden.

Pawelski, J. O. (2020). The elements model: Toward a new generation of positive psychology interventions. *The Journal of Positive Psychology, 15,* 675–679.

Peterson, C. (2008). What is positive psychology, and what is it not? Psychology Today. Retrieved from https://www.psychologytoday.com/us/blog/the-good-life/200805/what-is-positive-psychology-and-what-is-it-not

Prochaska, J. O., & DiClemente, C. C. (1992). Stages of change in the modification of problem behaviors. *Progress in Behavior Modification, 28,* 183–218.

Rosengren, D. B. (2019). *Building motivational interviewing skills* (2nd ed.). Guilford.

Seligman, M. (2012). *Flourish: A visionary new understanding of happiness and well-being.* Atria Books.

Seligman, M. E. P., Steen, T. A., Park, N., & Peterson, C. (2005). Positive psychology progress: Empirical validation of interventions. *American Psychologist, 60,* 410–421.

Smock, S. A., Trepper, T. S., Wetchler, J. L., McCollum, E. E., Ray, R., & Pierce, K. (2008). Solution-focused group therapy for level 1 substance abusers. *Journal of Marital and Family Therapy, 34,* 107–120.

van Wormer, K., & Davis, D. R. (2003). *Addiction treatment: A strengths perspective.* Brooks/Cole.

Wang, C. Y., Zhang, K., & Zhang, M. (2017). Dysfunctional attitudes, learned helplessness, and coping styles among men with substance use disorders. *Social Behavior and Personality: An International Journal, 45,* 269–280.

CHAPTER 6

DEVELOPMENT, CULTURE, AND CONTEXT: THE CROSS-CUTTING FORCES IN WELLNESS

INTRODUCTION

Wellness is often viewed as solely the five dimensions. When we reflect on what wellness is, it can be easy to forget about the person's environment, cultural influences, and developmental considerations. We have intentionally placed this chapter before the five dimensions because these forces must be considered when examining a client's wellness across the five dimensions. This chapter underscores that each client's wellness challenges, goals, and successes will be completely unique because their wellness can be affected positively and negatively by a multitude of variables.

To start, we'd like to introduce recovery as a developmental process in and of itself. As you know, you encounter your clients at different stages of recovery, whether just leaving withdrawal management, or leaving a halfway house after six months of sobriety. Further, the developmental tasks (e.g., identity versus role confusion) that one has navigated in their life or currently struggles with affect one's substance use and vice versa. In this upcoming section, we'll discuss the relationship between one's developmental needs, wellness, and recovery. We propose that developmental wellness encompasses an individual's perception of growing from life tasks and challenges faced across the different stages of one's life (childhood through older adulthood) (Myers & Sweeney, 2005; Walsh, 1996, 2002). Lower developmental wellness is reflected in clients feeling stuck and negatively affects their overall life experiences. Developmental wellness is also related to having one's basic needs met (food, water, and housing) in order to reach additional goals. We elaborate more on the function of needs in wellness in the next section.

MASLOW'S HIERARCHY OF NEEDS

Each wellness dimension that a client addresses should be integrated with the client's basic needs. Taormina and Gao (2013) highlighted Seward and Seward's (1937) conceptualization of the relationship between "drives" and "needs" stating the following:

> ...a drive reflects a "need" that arises from the lack of some particular thing, such that a "need" can be characterized by, and defined as, a lack of something that is essential to an organism's (a person's) existence or well-being.
>
> (p. 156)

Maslow (1943) regarded needs as goals or motivational factors. Here, we'll describe each level of Maslow's hierarchy.

- **Physiological needs** (level 1) entail "air, food, water, shelter, and rest" (Hale, Ricotta, Freed, Smith, & Huang, 2019).
- **Safety** (level 2) involves risk to our physical or emotional well-being such as physical or emotional discomfort.

DOI: 10.4324/9781003147954-6

- **Love and belonging** (level 3) refers to having warm relationships and perceiving that one fits in.
- **Esteem** (level 4) involves holding a positive view of oneself grounded in one's accomplishments (Maslow, 1943).
- **Self-actualization** (level 5) entails maximizing one's abilities and possibilities to obtain power, superiority, and intrinsic satisfaction (Groves, Kahalas, & Erickson, 1975).
- **Self-transcendence** has been defined as pursuing "peak experiences" ("…mystical experiences and certain experiences with nature, esthetic experiences, sexual experiences, and/or other transpersonal experiences, in which the person experiences a sense of identity that transcends or extends beyond the personal self"; Koltko-Rivera, 2006, p. 303).

Theoretically and empirically, effective attending to a prior level (e.g., level 1) makes meeting needs at the ensuing level (e.g., level 2) more attainable (Taormina & Gao, 2013). Individuals may not notice higher level needs until previous levels are moderately addressed (Maslow, 1943). Furthermore, needs at higher levels can masquerade as physiological needs. For example, one may feel tired, but the need may be for meaningful pursuits rather than rest if the weariness was due to boredom that was making one feel worthless (level 4) (Maslow, 1943). Maslow's scholarship from 80 years ago has direct application to current brain disease theories of addiction such as the hijacked brain theory (Goldstein & Volkow, 2011), which purports that changes in the brain from substance use confuse the individual into believing that substance use is a literal life or death need like the requirement of food and water to survive. In WBAC, we incorporate these concepts into relapse prevention by asking clients to self-monitor their needs and goals that are underlying their cravings (see Chapter 5 for more information).

Because minimal additional wellness goals can be pursued unless the client's Maslow's levels 1 and 2 needs are met, these needs are among the first to be assessed and addressed. The WBAC clinician can use assessments such as the Addiction Severity Index (ASI) (McLellan et al., 1992) that inquire about housing, food, finances, and beyond. If the client discloses about suicidal and/or homicidal ideation, domestic violence, or other facets that could affect the safety of the client or others, the clinician's top priority is to assess, safety plan, and refer for assessment for hospitalization or other resources. After this, the next level of urgency pertains to any other level 1 needs or other preferences of the client. We must beware not to jump into wellness goals that are different than the client's due to our own biases (Jack Register, personal communication, May 26, 2022). When the wellness plan is broached with the client during the treatment planning process, the clinician emphasizes that physiological needs and physical and emotional safety needs are primary regarding one's wellness. This allows the clinician to invite the client to share if they have any goals in these realms they would like to pursue as part of their wellness plan. In this way, WBAC is similar to Integrated Dual Disorders Treatment (Mueser, Noordsy, Drake, & Fox, 2003) and Assertive Community Treatment (Stein & Test, 1980) where the client prioritizes their goals which may be related more to basic needs than substance use or other wellness changes.

A constructive rapport with the clinician is invaluable (Jack Register, personal communication, May 26, 2022). Small or large instances of progress in Maslow's level 1 and 2 goals may enhance the client's confidence and interest in substance use and other wellness goals. The clinician enhances motivation by examining how progress in these areas impacts other dimensions of wellness, thereby facilitating additional motivation (Mueser et al., 2003).

ERIKSON'S PSYCHOSOCIAL STAGES

Erik Erikson's psychosocial stages of development hold significant utility in providing WBAC. An evidence-based connection exists between Erikson's stages and well-being. In a sample of 4,487 adults, higher scores on growth for each developmental stage correlated with life satisfaction and positive affect and were inversely related to lower negative affect scores (Dunkel, 2013). Clients present for counseling related to substance use concerns at many ages and stages of life from adolescence through older adulthood. These stages of development must be considered to facilitate effective counseling sessions. Moreover, clients may be wrestling with developmental tasks that are different than their age would suggest if they faced barriers to addressing previous developmental milestones. Trauma, mental health symptoms, and life challenges can disrupt one's movement through these tasks. Substance use also has the potential to keep the client stuck in earlier stages of development. Let's first explore Erikson's Psychosocial Stages of Development and then apply them to WBAC.

In the first stage, *trust versus mistrust*, the caregiver-infant relationship is initiated, in large part based on the child communicating a need via crying and learning that they will be attended to/responded to and consoled (Brooks & McHenry, 2015). If a dependable need-response pattern is not established, the infant will not trust in the support of the parent. Stable nurturing from the caregiver over time empowers the infant to trust that they can self-regulate (calm and console themselves) (Brooks & McHenry, 2015).

In stage 2, *autonomy versus shame and doubt*, caregivers allowing and encouraging the child to delve into their surroundings fosters autonomy (Dunkel & Harbke, 2017) or "self-sufficiency" (Domino & Affonso, 1990). These involvements, which can include potty training and interacting with others outside of the immediate family, aid the child in practicing "free choice as well as self-restraint" (Erikson, 1964). My (Phil) nearly two-year-old daughter at the time of writing this book has uttered one of Hamachek's (1988) indicators of positive autonomy – "I think I can do it" (p. 356). Except my daughter leaves out the "I think". Conversely, Hamachek (1988) stated that children experiencing shame and doubt may "prefer being told what to do rather than make their own decisions" (p. 356). This can result when caregivers constrain the child's chances to learn about their environment or the child perceives failures when exerting autonomy (Karcher & Benne, 2008).

In stage 3, *initiative versus guilt*, initiative is cultivated through the child attaining goals, with support from their caregiver. The child may encounter guilt and purposelessness if they cannot recurrently meet their goals. Erikson wrote that play is fertile ground for the child to practice their purpose, working toward goals, refining their skills, and learning from setbacks (1964). If stage 4, *industry versus inferiority*, is effectively navigated by the child, they will attain "competence...the free exercise of dexterity and intelligence in the completion of tasks, unimpaired by infantile inferiority" (Erikson, 1964, p. 124). Karcher and Benne (2008) stated, based on Erikson (1968), that inferiority is a consequence of setbacks in endeavors that are unavoidable and necessary to feel competent. Erikson (1968) also underscored the developmental benefits of celebrating the child's work when successes occur (Karcher & Benne, 2008).

Identity versus role confusion (stage 4) is the individual's process of self-discovery. Kroger and Marcia (2011) stated that "Faced with the imminence of adult tasks...the late adolescent must relinquish the childhood position of being 'given to' and prepare to be the 'giver'" (p. 32). The individual in this stage seeks to learn delayed gratification (Jack Register, personal communication, May 26, 2022), self-awareness and knowledge, and to create an identity that is within the scope of social norms (Kroger & Marcia, 2011).

Intimacy versus isolation (stage 5) involves the cultivation of relational skills; initiating and maintaining connections with friends and romantic partners. Brooks and McHenry (2015) added that a person's family of origin experiences can have a strong influence on how the person engages with others.

Generativity versus stagnation is a stage of life in which one gives back and provides nurturing and support for others via caregiving and in one's working life in a manner that yields meaning (Slater, 2003). Slater enumerated "conflicts" that can emerge including "pride versus embarrassment", "responsibility versus ambivalence", "career productivity versus inadequacy", "parenthood versus self-absorption", and "being needed versus alienation" (Slater, 2003). van der Kaap-Deeder et al. (2022) described the *integrity versus despair* stage that arises during older adulthood stating, "During this crisis, elderly reflect on their life in an attempt to unify past events into a meaningful 'life puzzle' and they come to terms with past negative events" (p. 118). Feelings of integrity are augmented as the person embraces the aging process and makes sense of their own future death and the death of close others (Slater, 2003; van der Kaap-Deeder et al., 2020). The "courage" to sit with despair and utilize it to inform one's progression toward integrity is imperative (Slater, 2003, p. 64; van der Kaap-Deeder et al., 2020).

Importantly, balance is a feature of the wellness model presented in this book and it pertains not only to attending to the five wellness dimensions but also to Erikson's theory of psychosocial development. Several authors discussing Erikson's theory (e.g., Karcher & Benne, 2008; Knight, 2017) highlighted his hypothesis that discerning when trust is merited versus when mistrust is warranted is more reflective of positive development than exclusively trusting or mistrusting. One may then wonder how experiencing feelings of inferiority (stage 4) or role confusion (stage 5) would be beneficial in counterbalancing industry and identity. Insights, awareness, and skills garnered from laboring to know oneself may enable and facilitate the individual's self-discovery (Karcher & Benne, 2008).

There are a few important directions and options for intervention and exploration with the client using Erikson's theory. The first is that Erikson's theory provides insights that the clinician and client can use for client conceptualization. An understanding of the client's developmental strengths and challenges can be helpful from the moment you greet your client. First, you can identify the client's current developmental tasks via their chronological age. An adolescent client, in theory, would be working through identity versus role confusion. Does a discrepancy exist between the client's age and stage of development? What may have factored into this discrepancy?

Another option is to present information on Erikson's stages to the client and discuss what developmental tasks they believe they have met and other tasks that feel incomplete. Depending on the client's preference and level of stabilization, the client can identify life experiences at various stages that helped them manage tasks or posed problems in task attainment. The clinician also facilitates dialog about how these developmental strengths and struggles have affected their wellness and vice versa. Part of this conversation is devoted to the impact of their substance use on developmental tasks. The clinician inquires about how substance use helped them navigate developmental tasks and how it may have disrupted their growth. The clinician can incorporate a formal assessment as well to concretize the client's examination of their development. The Psychosocial Inventory of Ego Strengths assessment is one formal evaluation tool based on Erikson's theory, which provides insights into the client's developmental strengths and struggles (Markstrom, Sabino, Turner, & Berman, 1997).

From these journeys in counseling, clinician and client may now have a better understanding of stuck points and inner resources to mobilize. The following guidelines can help you actualize developmental principles into WBAC:

1. Identify the stuck point(s) or developmental stages in which the client experienced challenges.

2. Discuss the impact on the client's wellness. Help the client understand the connection between developmental challenges and current wellness and substance use challenges, with an eye toward facilitating self-compassion.

3. Identify the skills and strengths the client possesses in that developmental stage(s) and ones the client has cultivated in order to manage the developmental challenge(s) (Walsh, 1996, 2002).

4. Identify a wellness intervention(s) based on the client's strengths and goals to facilitate development and wellness-enhancement.

In the case of Eric, which will be used throughout the book, both of his parents were highly busy working long hours. Furthermore, his mother suffered from depression and was inconsistently attentive. This may have resulted in a sense of insufficiency during those early years of developing resourcefulness and self-efficacy. Upon exploring impact, Eric noted that he consumes alcohol due to fear of failure in every job and uses drinking as an excuse for failure should he perform poorly at his job. Extended dialog revealed the persistent fear is related to his emotional wellness and that the drinking reduces the worry in the short term and increases it in the long term. Discussing strengths, Eric became aware that he does possess self-efficacy and one factor that helps is for him to take time to recognize progress. Client and clinician arrive upon a wellness intervention that involves identifying someone at work that he can discuss progress with once per month (emotional wellness).

CULTURE, WELLNESS, AND RECOVERY

The client's culture must be valued at every turn throughout WBAC. This is one of the reasons that we aim to elicit the client's own definitions and visions of wellness, and personal models of addiction and recovery. What is the role of culture in wellness? That depends on the client. Regardless, in this section, we will discuss several concepts and approaches involving culture and WBAC that can strengthen the counseling process. We will describe several concepts that facilitate cultural responsiveness and how they are actualized during WBAC sessions. Cultural wellness is present when one's well-being is enhanced by developing their cultural identity, positive feelings about their own culture, and receiving support for their cultural identity both from those with whom they interact and their environment.

Lee (2019) stated that "Culture refers to any group of people who identify or associate with one another on the basis of some common purpose, need, or similarity of background" (p. 31). Thomas and Schwarzbaum (2017) indicated that identity is synonymous with cultural identity. One's self-understanding is grounded in one's culture (Lee, 2019). Ibrahim and Heuer (2016) called attention to the DSM-5's Cultural Formulation Interview (CFI) whose delineation of cultural identity includes one's community, where one was born and raised, language(s), race and ethnicity, gender, sexual orientation, and religion or spirituality (American Psychiatric Association [APA], 2013). Pamela Hays' (2008) ADDRESSING model incorporates other facets of cultural identity not noted in the CFI such as "age and

generational influences, developmental disabilities and disabilities acquired later in life...
socioeconomic status...Indigenous heritage, [and] national origin" (Hays, 2009, p. 355).
Ibrahim (2015) noted additional cultural identity aspects such as birth order and family
structure (e.g., number of parents or caregivers, adopted family members, and stepfamily
members).

Intersectionality reminds us of the holistic nature of cultural identity – that in understanding the whole person, one must learn about the amalgamation of all aspects of their
cultural identity (Lee & Ali, 2019). For instance, clinicians should not reduce a client's cultural identity to age and gender only. Moreover, awareness of the interrelation among the
elements of the client's cultural identity is more important than considering them separately. Take, for example, a clinician utilizing Hays' (2008) ADDRESSING model. An inter-
sectional perspective centers the clinician in exploring the client's experience of being a
16-year-old, able-bodied individual, of Christian faith, identifying as Latinx, upper-middle-
class socioeconomic status, etc.

Another cultural and identity factor is worldview – how we engage with and experience
contextual or environmental forces in our lives (Ibrahim, 1991; Sue, 1978). These include
one's outlook on collectivism and individualism, time orientation, and activity orientation.
Clients with a collectivist worldview assign more worth and effort to the aims of the group
than their own endeavors (McCarthy, 2005). They may prioritize relationships comprising
their personal identity, fitting in, seeking feedback, "harmony" of the group over autonomy,
and compliance and veneration of those with influence (Oyserman et al., 2002). Clients with
an individualistic worldview prize personal achievement, autonomy, assertiveness, and individuality (Oysterman et al., 2002). Regarding time orientation, some clients would appreciate incorporating rituals of historical value into counseling, some clients prefer counseling
to be directed toward the present moment, and others favor goal setting and predicting the
outcomes of our behavior (Carter, 1991).

Cultural identity development is a process. Hence, your clients will be in different stages
of cultural identity development. The stage they are in will have an impact on their wellness. The authors of the Racial Cultural Identity Development model (Atkinson, Morten,
& Sue, 1979; Sue & Sue, 1999) noted five identity statuses: conformity, dissonance, resistance and immersion, introspection, and integration and awareness. The model can be
utilized with clients of any race as well as marginalized clients. Individuals in the *conformity
stage* hold negative perceptions of the worldview and norms of their cultural background
and align with the worldview and norms of the majority (White American) culture. In
this phase, the person espouses biased views of their own culture and other non-majority
cultures (Atkinson et al., 1979; Sue & Sue, 1999; Sue, Sue, Neville, & Smith, 2019). The *dissonance phase* is where the client may begin to experience more negative impact on wellness
related to culture. The individual experiences tension as they notice that negative assumptions about their culture are in error. Sue et al. (2019) remarked that dissonance can develop
over time or abruptly if a traumatic event occurs such as the murder of George Floyd by
a police officer. During the identity crisis, the client commences de-constructing biases and
mindfulness increases regarding worrisome aspects of the majority culture and affirmative
aspects of their culture.

According to Sue et al. (2019), the client in the *resistance and immersion phase* experiences
pride in their cultural identity and guilt, shame, and anger. The individual invests whole-
heartedly in learning about their culture and perceives that the majority culture created
inequities that need to be dismantled. Guilt and shame are caused by the belief that they

abandoned their culture and oppressed individuals from their own culture and anger at the marginalization of their culture. Wariness and negative views of the majority culture are pervasive during this period.

The *introspection phase* entails navigating toward a middle path of prizing one's culture and not evaluating the majority culture as exclusively negative (Atkinson et al., 1998; Sue & Sue, 1999; Sue et al., 2019). The person arrives at this point because strong emotions (guilt, shame, and anger) over time preclude identity development and cultural learning. This person's outlook broadens from treasuring their own culture to treasuring other cultures as well. Stress is experienced in the process of re-establishing trust with the majority culture and its members and worry about over-aligning with the majority culture (Atkinson et al., 1998; Sue & Sue, 1999; Sue et al., 2019). Integrative awareness is the middle path when the person can fully celebrate their cultural identity, other cultures, and majority culture after gleaning insight from journeying through these phases (Atkinson et al., 1998; Sue & Sue, 1999; Sue et al., 2019). Clinicians work with clients who are at different stages of identity development. WBAC clinicians take care to invite the client to reflect on aspects of their culture that strengthen their wellness and recovery and those that do not.

Individuals who are not part of the dominant culture may experience stressors that affect their substance use. These stressors can include discrimination, microaggressions, and macroaggressions. "Discrimination is the unfair or prejudicial treatment of people and groups based on characteristics such as race, gender, age or sexual orientation" (APA, 2019). For example, in a study of 417,754 college students, the past month or past year incidence of the use of 18 substances was higher for those who had faced discrimination (Qeadan et al., 2022). Microaggressions are interpersonal or contextual communications that range from being unfavorable about a culture (microinsults) to antagonistic (microassaults) (Sue et al., 2007). Microaggressions can be beyond the awareness of the communicator and hence, not disclosed to upset the other person, while others can be malicious and premeditated. A third type of microaggression called microinvalidations entails the communicator disregarding the impact of the person's culture on their daily life and worldview (Sue et al., 2007).

SELF-AWARENESS

Multicultural competence consists of knowledge, awareness, and skills (Sue, Arredondo, & McDavis, 1992). Recognition of one's biases and personal culture as it relates to wellness and substance use is essential. It can be easy to unknowingly compel clients to define wellness as one sees it individually, as the clinician. The following prompts may facilitate your self-exploration prior to or concurrent with offering WBAC (Gamby, Burns, & Forristal, 2021; Ratts & Pedersen, 2014).

- How do I personally define wellness? How would I personally define each of its dimensions?
- What people, experiences, etc. have affected my definitions and thoughts/feelings on wellness?
- How do the components of my cultural identity inform my beliefs about wellness?
- How could my thoughts/feelings about wellness bias or negatively affect my work with clients?

Gamby et al. (2021) developed several powerful inquiries for the clinician:

- "Does my own conception of wellness focus heavily on individualism versus collectivism?"
- "When I speak to my clients/supervisees/students about wellness, do I consider context (both historical and current)?"
- "How do my beliefs on wellness address social change?"
- "…When I speak about wellness, do I recognize and identify my own privileges?" (p. 239)

During this self-exploration, reflect on your knowledge of other cultures and their wellness practices and culturally sensitive counseling skills that you possess or need to enrich (Gamby et al., 2021; Ratts & Pedersen, 2014).

CULTURALLY INFORMED APPROACHES

A definition of culture should be discussed between client and clinician. Consider sharing the ADDRESSING Model and Pedersen's (1991) definition that culture encompasses "… demographic variables (e.g. age, sex, place of residence), status variables (e.g. social, educational, economic), and affiliations (formal and informal), as well as ethnographic variables such as nationality, ethnicity, language, and religion …" (p. 7). Furthermore, "…cultural groups…are also organized around shared values, beliefs, customs, and traditions …" (Substance Abuse and Mental Health Services Administration [SAMHSA], 2014, p. 161). You'll notice in Chapter 3 that culture is critical to wellness assessment and treatment planning. For instance, the clinician elicits the client's definition of wellness and each dimension of wellness. The client is invited to add or remove dimensions of wellness from the five-dimension wellness model or other wellness models being used.

The CFI (APA, 2013) has inspired several routes of exploration with the client within WBAC. The CFI can be implemented by adhering to the protocol outlined in the DSM (2022) or its handbook (Lewis-Fernández, Aggarwal, Hinton, Hinton, & Kirmayer, 2016). The CFI contains the following item: "For you, what are the most important aspects of your background or identity?" (APA, 2013, p. 753). This question is an excellent point of departure for ensuring the client's culture is honored throughout counseling. The client's meaning of wellness can be further introduced into WBAC by asking if there are certain wellness dimensions that they value more than others. The clinician can ask about wellness-enriching customs, traditions, "…doctors, helpers, and healers …" and which dimensions of wellness they impact (APA, 2013, p. 754).

The CFI (APA, 2013) directs the clinician to inquire about the effect of the client's culture and the experience of discrimination on the issue that precipitated pursuing counseling (the relationship between the presenting concern and their culture). The clinician may want to note that alcohol and drug use culture and recovery culture can also be components of culture. Alcohol and drug cultures can inform "language", "rituals", "rules", "status", and "values" (SAMHSA, 2014, p. 163). Conversely, there are questions about cultural strengths and resources. In essence, the clinician invites the client to consider how strengths from their cultural identity can be drawn upon to attend to the presenting concerns.

Cultural responsiveness also entails striving to include the client's helping preferences in counseling as much as possible. The Cooper-Norcross Inventory of Preferences (C-NIP)

(Cooper & Norcross, 2016) enables identification of the client's thoughts and feelings on how they would like their counseling to proceed. The 18 items ascertain the client's input on the level of directiveness, processing of emotions, examination of past and present, and challenge and support. The inventory also has 11 qualitative items for clients to elaborate on their preferences and clarify others such as type of counseling approach, duration of sessions and counseling process, and cultural background of the clinician (Cooper & Norcross, 2016). This also permits the clinician to use broaching skills if, for instance, the clinician is of a cultural background that differs from the client's preference and a referral to meet the client's wishes is not feasible.

Contextual Wellness

Forces exist within (intrapersonal and contextual) and outside of the client that interact with the client's wellness and addictive behavior (Merçon-Vargas et al., 2020). These forces can substantially impact your client's well-being. For example, as I (PC) write this chapter, a war is being fought between Russia and Ukraine, the COVID-19 pandemic is transforming into an endemic, a new infectious illness has emerged (monkeypox), multiple school shootings have occurred, and the economy and job market is recovering and shifting in response to the pandemic.

If you have worked in counseling and addictions counseling for any length of time, you are likely quite familiar with clients (as all people) having multiple layers of challenges and strengths. It can be overwhelming for the clinician to decide which client concern to address first. The problem is that we sometimes forget about these contextual forces, neglect to integrate them into our counseling approaches, or parse them out separately from the whole of the individual. The addictions field made this mistake years ago in utilizing separate treatment for clients with co-occurring disorders in which one treatment center provided the addictions counseling and then later or concurrently referred the client for mental health counseling (Mueser et al., 2003).

Contextual wellness pertains to one's environment and its stressors or wellness-enriching factors in the home, workplace, other locations the individual frequents, and their community, nation, and world (Bronfenbrenner, 1977). For individuals with addiction, clinicians also examine intrapersonal contextual wellness factors such as co-occurring mental health, trauma, and medical issues that are part of the client's internal context and affect their inner experience. In this portion of the chapter, we'll start with the topics of co-occurring disorders and trauma; intrapersonal contextual factors that affect the majority of your clients with SUDs.

CO-OCCURRING DISORDERS

Multiple challenges can accompany having a co-occurring disorder. Individuals with co-occurring disorders must attend to both their mental health and substance use issues; dealing with the risk of a relapse into mental health symptoms upending one's substance use recovery and vice versa. Co-occurring disorders can also include variables of physical health problems and diagnoses as well as more than one mental health diagnosis (Miller, Forcehimes, & Zweben, 2019). Research findings suggest that individuals with co-occurring disorders may have more physical health problems than persons with mental health disorders alone (Onyeka, Collier Høegh, Nåheim Eien, Nwaru, & Melle, 2019). They may also be managing trauma symptoms as a study revealed that 77% of individuals with co-occurring disorders who were receiving addictions treatment compared to 40% of the general population had been victims of crime in the past year (de Waal, Dekker & Goudriaan, 2017). These differences were even more pronounced at the crime-specific level in which 38% of those with co-occurring disorders were victims of physical assault in the past year in contrast to 3% for the general population. Additionally, issues of housing insecurity may exist for some individuals with co-occurring disorders (Vallesi, Tuson, Davies, & Wood, 2021). Although there is a high prevalence of persons with co-occurring disorders among individuals with SUDs, there are fewer mutual help groups and media discussions on co-occurring disorders.

Individuals with co-occurring disorders benefit significantly from addiction and integrated treatment (when one treatment team concurrently attends to the mental health disorder and SUD using approaches that pertain to each disorder [Mehta, Hoadley, Ray, Kiluk, Carroll, & Magill, 2021]). In a study with 234 addiction treatment participants, two-thirds of who were evaluated as having a high likelihood of having a co-occurring mental health disorder, the possible co-occurring disorder group's substance use declined to approximately the same amount as the SUD-only group by three months after treatment completion (Cridland, Deane, Hsu, & Kelly, 2012). The same occurred for the degree of the participants' depression, anxiety, and stress symptoms.

COUNSELING INDIVIDUALS WITH CO-OCCURRING DISORDERS

In order to help individuals with SUDs and co-occurring disorders, one must understand their reasons for using substances. For those with co-occurring disorders, the "why" behind the substance use can entail lessening the symptoms from their MHD, decreasing the anxiety of interpersonal interactions (given the anxiety that can manifest in social situations from MHD symptoms), and fitting in (social credibility can be ascribed to the person for their use or provision of substances) (Hendrickson, Schmal, & Ekleberry, 2004). If their co-occurring disorder has resulted in career, relational, educational, or lifestyle instability (which can diminish one's daily activities), the client may pass the time by using a substance. The person may also use substances in lieu of self-harm if they are experiencing suicidal ideation related to their co-occurring disorder. Furthermore, substance use can be the person's outlet for self-harm if they feel hopeless or ambivalent about life but do not want to attempt suicide. Hendrickson et al. (2004) also noted that some individuals would rather attention be directed at their substance use instead of their MHD, which they believe is more stigmatizing. Lastly, substances are used to prevent withdrawal symptoms (Hendrickson et al., 2004).

The WBAC approach aligns effectively and builds upon existing co-occurring disorders counseling approaches. Motivation-Based Treatment has been recommended by Mueser et al., (2003) and others. It includes an Engagement Stage in which the clinician develops the helping relationship and centers treatment on the client's goals, which may not involve substance use. During the Persuasion Stage, the client explores the implications of their use and embarks on their harm reduction or abstinence plan. The Active Treatment Stage falls one month or more into the client's change plan and the clinician supports the client in persisting with any gains that have occurred. Clients in Relapse Prevention cultivate these skills as well as pursue goals that are not directly substance related (Mueser et al., 2003).

WBAC clinicians advance the client's motivation for change by examining their goals across wellness dimensions. Once the client has received an assessment and is aware and prepared to process their co-occurring disorders diagnosis, psychoeducation should be provided including inquiring about the client's MHD symptoms, substance use, and how they impact each other and the client's wellness across dimensions. Lower areas of wellness that have affected the client's co-occurring disorder symptoms should also be discussed. Miller, Forcehimes, and Zweben (2011) suggest "Because of possible cognitive difficulties, give smaller bits of information and use some repetition, particularly by presenting the same thing in different ways or by giving specific examples" (p. 294). WBAC risks being convoluted if not presented clearly. Make sure that the client's definitions of wellness are prized in the process and ensure the client firmly comprehends the topics at hand.

Psychotropic medication should be strongly considered as a component of the wellness plan by clients with co-occurring disorders (Miller et al., 2019). Similar to examining one's myths about emotions (see Chapter 10), the clinician can invite the client to share their perspectives and experiences with psychotropic medications. Potential myths and misinformation can be addressed by the clinicians and apprehensions reviewed further (Miller et al., 2011). Clients may benefit from completing a decisional balance related to medication. If the client currently takes medication or begins medication, the role of the medication in the wellness plan should be frequently evaluated. For instance, inquire about ways in which the medication increases or negatively affects different wellness dimensions. Miller et al. (2011) noted that problem-solving, enlisting the client's support system, and client and clinician partnership with the client's healthcare providers assists in maintenance of the medication regimen. Mutual help groups add to the client's support system, helping clients attain their substance use and mental health goals (McGovern, 2009). Clients can attend the support group of their preference and derive benefit from 12-step programming. Support groups for persons with co-occurring disorders exist but may be more difficult to find. However, the promising news is that 12-step or other addiction mutual help groups will likely be beneficial (Bogenschutz, 2007; Bogenschutz et al., 2014). Assessing for additional crises for clients with co-occurring disorders is critical. This includes domestic violence, suicidal and homicidal ideation and intent, and trauma (SAMHSA, 2020).

TRAUMA

Clinicians and organizations across the United States appear to be taking action in implementing trauma considerations into the clinical work they provide. In the 2020 National Survey of Substance Abuse Treatment Services (NSSATS), researchers found that 83% of 16,066 addictions treatment centers incorporated "trauma-related counseling" and 45% had trauma-specific programming (SAMHSA, 2021, p. 28). This data suggests a recognition of the prevalence of trauma and relevance of supporting clients through trauma as part of their recovery. Ford and Courtois (2020) define traumatic stressors as "…Events, experiences, and exposures – that greatly exceed the individual's capacity to control, cope with, or withstand, and that compromise the individual's psychophysiological equilibrium or stasis" (p. 4).

The above definition underscores the WBAC conceptualization that trauma is another contributor to the client's wellness becoming out of balance, thereby resulting in a need or desire to use substances. Trauma can result in posttraumatic stress disorder (PTSD) or its symptoms which include flashbacks, disturbing and unpredictable surfacing of traumatic memories, dissociation, mood change/low mood, hyperarousal, substantial self-blame for the trauma, shift to an unfavorable perspective about self and one's context, unpleasant mental and physical response to reminders of the trauma, and mental and physical evasion of reminders of the trauma (APA, 2022). Rates of PTSD may be higher among individuals with SUDs than those who do not have a SUD (Gielen, Havermans, Tekelenburg, & Jansen, 2012).

Several hypotheses have surfaced to make sense of the PTSD-SUD association (Mario-Rios & Morrow, 2020): (a) substance misuse precipitates more exposure to violence, (b) substances are used to cope with trauma, (c) genes cause increased likelihood of PTSD and SUD, (d) behavioral traits such as "cue reactivity" incite PTSD and SUD symptoms, (e) developmental stressors affect the brain's capacity to manage stress, and (f) comparable origins of each disorder amplify the other.

Complex PTSD entails continual abuse or neglect perpetrated by people or organizations that hinder efforts to evade the trauma (Ford & Courtois, 2020). Complex trauma affects one's outlook, self-esteem, self-efficacy, and trust. Individuals living with complex PTSD can experience fight, flight, or freeze symptoms (Ford & Courtois, 2020). Furthermore, emotion regulation problems, harmful behaviors (e.g., substance use), interpersonal problems, and shame can ensue (van der Kolk, 2002). SAMHSA (2020) has provided multiple helpful recommendations for effectively counseling clients with co-occurring trauma and SUDs. In addition to listing screening and assessments for trauma and PTSD, the authors of SAMHSA's *Treatment Improvement Protocol* on the topic of co-occurring disorders (2020) supported the use of an integrated care approach to co-occurring trauma and SUD. Although clinicians using WBAC should screen and assess for trauma, you should neither review specific facets of what occurred nor reprocess the trauma with the client.

Clinicians can engage in stabilization phase work as part of WBAC. Phased treatment for trauma begins with a stabilization phase in which physical and psychological safety is solidified prior to embarking on reopening the client's traumatic experiences (Ford & Courtois, 2020; SAMHSA, 2020). Grounding skills that re-center clients when trauma symptoms manifest (see Chapter 10) are presented and practiced during sessions. A safety plan specific to the client should be a part of the wellness plan. Safety plans can aid in the prevention of revictimization (Ford & Courtois, 2020; SAMHSA, 2014, 2020). Safety plans are also customized for different crises (e.g., suicidal ideation and intimate partner violence). During safety planning, assist clients in writing down "behaviors that promote safety and behaviors that feel unsafe for them today" (SAMHSA, 2014, p. 113). The client can use the wellness model as a guide, identifying safety-promoting skills and needs and risky behaviors or factors across the wellness dimensions (e.g., safe/supportive versus unsafe/less supportive others – connection wellness).

WBAC clients will not be relating specifics about their trauma or reprocessing it. Even sharing that a trauma occurred without describing it can increase symptoms (SAMHSA, 2014, 2020). Hence, if and when trauma symptoms and triggers are discussed, attend to evidence of client dissociation or other trauma symptoms. Confirm with clients that they hold the final decision on the topic, breadth, and depth of sharing (SAMHSA, 2014, 2020). WBAC clinicians offer information on trauma, assist the client in outlining their symptoms and triggers and selecting and practicing corresponding coping skills. One of the hallmarks of WBAC, examining relationships among substance use and wellness, is also a helpful approach with trauma as clients can investigate the reciprocal relationships among their substance use, trauma, and wellness (SAMHSA, 2014, 2020).

Because WBAC is not a trauma counseling approach in which trauma reprocessing is conducted, referral to trauma counseling programming and clinicians trained in trauma work may be needed, unless the WBAC clinician holds this background and the client is ready for advanced phases of trauma work. WBAC is not intended to be a substitute for co-occurring disorders or trauma programming. It is intended to be the central structure and content for general addictions programming, outpatient aftercare, or an adjunct to addictions treatment. Most activities throughout this book encourage and make room for the clinician to inquire about the impacts of stressors, mental health disorders, and trauma on wellness and vice versa. However, the clinician must use their professional discretion to decide when and how much to involve trauma into these discussions. With other co-occurring mental health disorders, if the client is aware of the diagnosis or symptoms, is open to talking about them and can benefit from these conversations, and displays minimal signs of decompensation from these conversations, the clinician may proceed (barring other concerns).

CAREER

Career is central to the identity of many Americans. As has been said before, in the United States, people often ask first about what we do before they inquire about who we are. Work supplies both self-esteem and income. The role of career in substance use and wellness concerns typically arises in three forms: lack of employment, dissatisfaction with employment, or income that precipitates stress by (a) possessing funds that facilitate substance use or (b) financial stress from lack of income factoring into substance use and decreased wellness (Tran et al., 2023). Outcomes of one study revealed that unemployment was higher in a sample of individuals with a past but not current substance use issue than those with no substance use issues in their lifetime (Eddie et al., 2020). Unemployment rates were higher among Black participants than those from other racial/ethnic backgrounds. Individuals who had been arrested more than once had a higher rate of unemployment than those who were not. Happiness, quality of life, and self-esteem were higher among employed participants (Eddie et al., 2020). Laudet (2012) recruited a sample of participants who had been diagnosed with a drug use disorder at some point in their lives but had not used it in over a month. Unemployment was considerably higher for individuals with a co-occurring MHD or a long-term medical problem. Specifically, Laudet (2012) stated that "…male gender and Caucasian race enhanced the odds of employment whereas having a comorbid chronic physical and/or mental health condition halved the odds" (p. 1).

Multiple obstacles may be encountered as individuals in recovery seek/pursue satisfying careers that meet their financial needs and goals. These obstacles can include low self-efficacy regarding being successful in a job or career due to substance use limiting prior training, education, employment, and expertise garnered from past employment (Robertson, Sagvaag, Selseng, & Nesvaag, 2021). Robertson et al. (2021) termed this narrative, "starting all over". Similar to relapse, discouragement can ensue if employment experiences in recovery go poorly. Others may have had satisfying employment, were dismissed related to their SUD, and then have optimism about rejoining the job market. Some may attain job training, further education, and/or entry-level employment to boost/increase their self-efficacy and proficiencies (Robertson et al., 2022).

Currently, we are in a period of economic uncertainty and transition to increased opportunities for remote work as the pandemic shifts to endemic. I have yet to identify much research on the topic to this point, but I fear potential downsides of remote work for persons with SUDs. For example, there is a heightened routine in arriving at an office at a certain time, performing tasks while "on the job" and the wellness-enhancing aspects of interactions with colleagues. Remote work could pose increased triggers that can exist in the home, decreased accountability and routine. However, there are multiple wellness and recovery benefits as well and time and research will inform us further.

ADDRESSING CAREER IN WBAC

Earlier we discussed the importance of flow, and at different points in the book, we have discussed the importance of meaning and purpose in life. Without these, it is too easy for your client to turn to the substance for meaning and flow. Hence, we listen carefully for career, flow, and meaning in life concerns and strengths from the start of counseling. When conversing about meaning and flow, inquire about the role of career. Does it boost their sense of meaning or factor into lower satisfaction? How important is employment to their wellness and in what way? The meaning of employment for some may be the finances it provides to support oneself, one's loved ones, and one's lifestyle and wellness (Busacca & Rehfuss, 2017). Conversely, employment can be synonymous with one's identity and be a principal way of deriving meaning. Ensure that you explore what career means to your client. The clinician would also do well to share Fullen's (2019) definition of vocational wellness that "Vocation is related to the pursuit of life calling, regardless of whether the calling is associated with paid work" (p. 69). For clients not seeking paid employment, they can nonetheless benefit from examining options including volunteering and taking classes if these interest them.

Explore the client's career goals, barriers, resources, and actions that will facilitate the attainment of these aims (Center for Substance Abuse Treatment (CSAT), 2000b). For some clients, career may not be of concern or a goal. Scaling questions can facilitate goal setting related to career. For example, "On a 1 to 10 scale, how satisfied are you in your current career/job? On a 1 to 10 scale, how important would it be for us to discuss your career/employment during counseling?" For some clients, the issue is not gainful employment. Rather, working long hours in a job in which one has lower interest or belief that one's pay is below what is deserved can reduce satisfaction (Busacca & Rehfuss, 2017). Employment in a field in which the client's interests, skills, and/or abilities do not align with the nature of the work can result in lower satisfaction. Conversely, work addiction can co-occur with substance addiction and exacerbate the client's substance use. As the client abstains or reduces their substance use, their substance addiction may transfer to engaging addictively with work. Work addiction can entail a loss of control in setting time boundaries with work and managing cognitions about work (similar to craving), resulting in mental health, physical health, and overall wellness consequences (Schaufeli, Bakker, van der Heijden, & Prins, 2009; Schaufeli, Taris, & Van Rhenen, 2008).

First, the clinician needs to listen for the presence of work addiction. The Bergen Work Addiction Scale (Andreassen, Griffiths, Hetland, & Pallesen, 2012) offers potential questions for discussion. For instance, the scale includes a valuable item that states, "Worked in order to reduce feelings of guilt, anxiety, helplessness and depression?" (Andreassen et al., 2012, p. 269). Applying the first three questions from the CAGE questionnaire (Ewing, 1984) and substituting the word "work" for drinking may also be helpful in screening for work addiction. Clinicians using WBAC are well positioned to address work addiction because they can explore the impact of work on the person's cross-dimensional wellness (positive and negative). Clients seeking change can use the wellness plan and relapse prevention skills to help the client select other dimensions of wellness to increase and ways to set constructive boundaries at work.

You and the client will benefit from ascertaining how the client's substance use may have affected previous and current employment. The Lifestyle Health Questionnaire (Martin et al., 2015) has questions that pertain to the impact of substance use on job performance, job search, and employment in unsatisfying jobs to fund one's substance use. Clinicians may discover that clients sold drugs as well. De-constructing the influence of these experiences with your clients can raise the client's awareness about their positive and negative effects. Issues with low career self-efficacy may manifest that the clinician should assess and address. Farr and Stevens (2008) noted several "negative attitudes" to assess for and challenge with destructive thoughts such as "I've made too many mistakes in life" and "I won't find a job that pays enough". Constructive implications can also be derived. For example, it is possible that the client who sold drugs developed certain skills or this involvement helps them recognize certain skills they possess (CSAT, 2000a). If career is a wellness goal for the client, CSAT (2000b) adapted several recommended "prevocational counseling activities" from the Rehabilitation Research and Training Center on Drugs and Disability (1996). These include "career exploration activities" (examine the client's career history which also involves education and training, "visit community resources", survey job search, and career information resources) and "structured activities" (career assessments, "take continuing education courses to determine and validate interests", and "write a resume") (p. 30).

Several online resources can be used by the client or alongside the clinician to locate career information and assess career interests, skills, and abilities. The Occupational Outlook Handbook offered through the Bureau of Labor Statistics (https://www.bls.gov/ooh/) allows one to read information about their career of interest. One can also search for jobs based on how much they pay, how much education is required, and current and future demand for different jobs. The O*NET Online website (https://www.onetonline.org/) allows individuals to search jobs based on their interests, skills, abilities, values, "knowledge", "work styles", and other factors. The website also contains an interest assessment. Career One Stop (https://www.careeronestop.org/) is also comprehensive in including links to training opportunities, interests, skills and work values assessments, and information for military service members and veterans, middle age and older adult job seekers, individuals with disabilities, and criminal justice-involved persons. In personal communication with M. B. Scholl (March 28, 2022) who recommended the above websites, he noted

> When using one of these search engines, I advise clients to enter "fair chance employer" as one of their search terms. For those employers who are not "fair chance employers" also known as "second chance employers" they may automatically disqualify applicants who indicate they have a criminal conviction.

CONTEXT MAPPING

In Chapter 2, we mentioned the Contextual factors of Myers and Sweeney's (2005) Indivisible Self Model of Wellness (IS-Wel) model that includes local (family, neighborhood, and community), institutional (education, religion, government, and business), global (politics, culture, global events, environment, and media), and chronometrical (perpetual, positive, and purposeful) dimensions (p. 35). These considerations (along with additional facets) apply to SUD treatment. The family context will be discussed further in Chapter 12. Bronfenbrenner's ecological system's theory (1979) grounds the Contextual factors of the IS-Wel model. This theory also grounds client conceptualization and interventions in WBAC. The theory reminds the clinician of the external factors in our clients' lives and the interfacing between the client and their environment.

Microsystems involve "a pattern of activities, roles, and interpersonal relations experienced by the developing person in a given setting with particular physical and material characteristics" (Bronfenbrenner, 1979, p. 22). Family, friendships, school relationships, work relationships, and community relationships are examples of microsystems (Myers & Sweeney, 2004; Rogers, Gilbride, & Dew, 2018). Mesosystems entail the interfacing among microsystem settings, for instance, an adult who most often uses substances at home with their romantic partner (Bronfenbrenner, 1977, 1979). The person starts a new job and meets others who use substances, introduces their partner to their colleagues, and friendships develop that involve substance use. The client is not a part of the setting of their exosystem, yet as an *institution* ranging from *media* to *government* to *transportation*, it factors into their well-being because it may collide with a setting of someone in their microsystem (Bronfenbrenner, 1977). Myers and Sweeney (2004) also list the exosystems of *education* and *religion* as contextual wellness variables. Macrosystems are national and international happenings (e.g., COVID-19 pandemic) and beliefs (e.g., politics) that materialize in the other systems (Bronfenbrenner, 1977; Myers & Sweeney, 2005; Rogers et al., 2018). The chronosystem is the client's intrapersonal development and contextual developments during their life course (Bronfenbrenner, 1994; Rogers et al., 2018). Specific to wellness counseling, Myers and Sweeney (2005) purported that attending to wellness in previous phases of life can benefit us during the subsequent phase as current inattention can worsen wellness concerns in later phases.

Rogers et al. (2018) developed a mapping activity based on the work of Williams, McMahon, and Goodman (2015). Mapping may effectively concretize contextual wellness which can appear more abstract to the client. We have modified their approach and propose an additional version of mapping, specifically for exploring contextual wellness. The activity is divided into two parts. The first part involves mapping one's activities, roles, and interactions. The second entails the individual pinpointing/distinguishing/ascertaining (a) intrapersonal contextual wellness factors, (b) environments (e.g., neighborhood, volunteer site, church, and school), and (c) local, national, and international events affecting them. The client's roles should be identified first. One person may be in the roles of mother, work supervisor, volunteer, sister, friend, romantic partner, student, and more. Activities often flow from the roles that we inhabit (Bronfenbrenner, 1979). The client should list every activity that they are currently or were recently involved in on a weekly to monthly basis. Caregiving responsibilities, date nights, volunteering, work, school, hobbies, cooking, household chores, medical, and/or mental health appointments are examples. The client should be specific so that if multiple caregiving duties exist, they should each be noted. If the client is still actively using substances, that should also be noted. The client then enumerates the people they meaningfully interact with on a daily and weekly basis. Meaningful interactions can be positive or negative. Instruct the client to mark the roles, activities, and interactions that have the greatest positive impact on their wellness recovery and the one or two roles, activities, and interactions that have the greatest negative impact on their wellness/recovery. The client should also denote the one or two to which they devote the most time (Marlatt, 1985). The same process can be followed when mapping intrapersonal, environmental, and local/national/international events. Figures 6.1–6.4 are Eric's contextual maps.

Processing the activity is of the utmost importance. It can be helpful to start by examining what resonated with the client from the activity. The clinician can accomplish this by asking what it was like for the client to map aspects of their contextual wellness and see it on the page. Below is a list of processing questions that can accompany the activity:

Eric Context Mapping – Roles

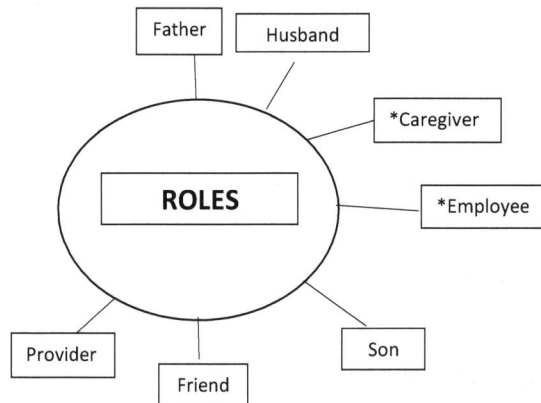

Figure 6.1 Eric Context Mapping – Roles.

Eric Context Mapping – Activities

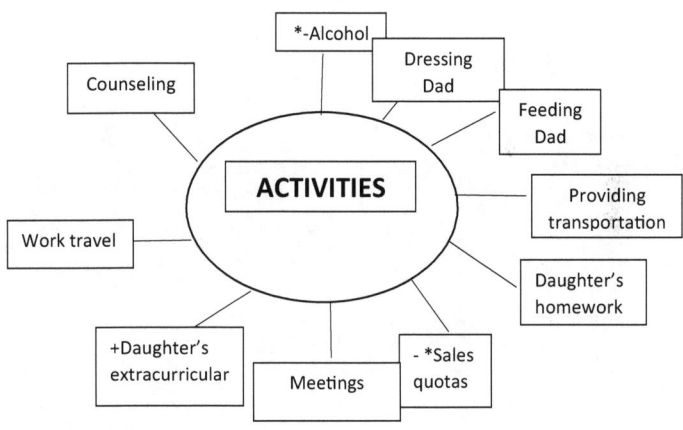

Figure 6.2 Eric Context Mapping – Activities.

- What was something new you learned about yourself and something about your-self that was reinforced that you already knew?
- What existing contextual wellness factors would you like to make a greater part of your life? How could you nurture those positive aspects further? What would that look like?

Eric Context Mapping – Interactions

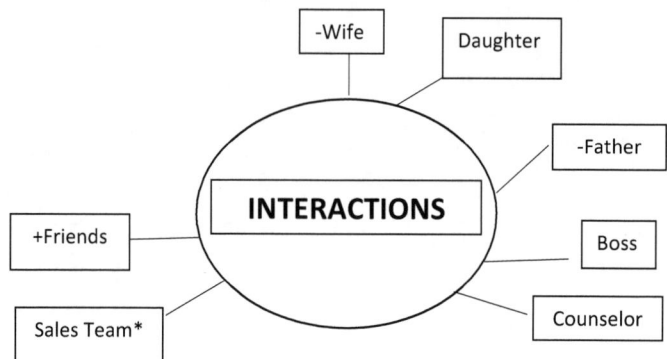

Figure 6.3 Eric Context Mapping – Interactions.

Eric Context Mapping – Intrapersonal, Environmental, and Systemic

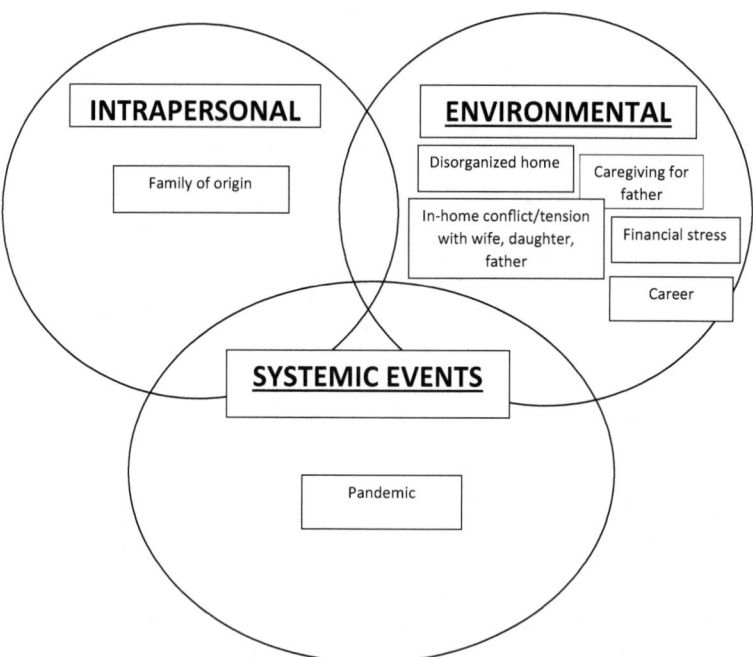

Figure 6.4 Eric Context Mapping – Intrapersonal, Environmental, and Systemic.

- What contextual wellness factors would you like to decrease, change, or eliminate from your life? What impact on your wellness and recovery might occur from these changes?
- How (if at all) does your substance use affect your contextual wellness and vice versa?
- If a negative aspect of your contextual wellness is unchangeable, in what ways might you enhance your coping with them?
- What indirect or hidden wellness benefits may exist to some of the contextual wellness factors you marked as negative?

CONTEXT MAPPING WITH ERIC

During an individual counseling session, Eric and the clinician completed mapping his contextual wellness. This section details some of his responses during the debriefing. Eric's initial response was of how much more helpful it was to map out the contextual wellness rather than discuss it alone. He noted at first, he did not believe contextual wellness really applied much to him when thinking about his wellness plan, but he quickly realized that these factors play a major role in his life, alcohol use, and overall wellness. Below are portions of Eric's responses to the mapping processing questions.

- What was something new you learned about yourself and something about yourself that was reinforced that you already knew? *A couple things. When you said alcohol should be listed as an activity, I was kinda surprised. Even though once I thought about it I was embarrassed, because of course, drinking is an activity and one I've been doing too much of probably. Then I thought about how I do actually spend quite a bit of time drinking and that got me feeling worse. I also noticed that there weren't many fun activities in my map – no trips with Kelly, not many social outings – not without drinking, at least. A lot of stress, I guess.*
- What existing contextual wellness factors would you like to make a greater part of your life? How could you nurture those positive aspects further? What would that look like? *I feel like Kelly and I have grown really distant from each other. Through this process, I realized that we haven't gone on a date in forever. Part of that is the pandemic, but most of that is on us. This reminds me that I really also need to focus on my relationship with Kelly as part of my counseling. I don't really take care of my friendships. My friend who encouraged me to get treatment, along with Kelly, was a friend who lives right here in town but I hadn't spent much time with over the past couple of years. He's a great, motivating person to be around. And he's a straight shooter.*
- What contextual wellness factors would you like to decrease, change, or eliminate from your life? What impact on your wellness and recovery might occur from these changes? *This ties back to your question on what I was surprised about. But you noticed that two of the three factors that are most negative to my wellness are relationships – my wife and father. And I can admit that things aren't perfect with Lia either. I've talked about things with Kelly a bit and not as much my dad. I think the combination of caregiving for my dad and stress from work are too much for me at times. He was rarely there for me when I was a kid and now I feel like I'm taking time away from my wife and daughter to care for him. But I've been completely surprised to see that he actually seems to appreciate it. I really don't have time to make sense of all this because I have to keep my job. Kelly and I both need to be employed to afford bills between raising Lia and dad living with us. Honestly, if these things were less overwhelming, I feel like changing my drinking would be easier and I would be happier.*

- How (if at all) does your substance use affect your contextual wellness and vice versa? *Alcohol makes my life more disorganized. On the days I drink more, especially, I'm just hanging on by a thread to my responsibilities for that day. I'm not as capable of planning ahead or even fully staying on schedule. So my context becomes chaotic. Like, even literally, the house is dirtier and more in chaos and that just makes me feel more stressed out.*

- If a negative aspect of your contextual wellness is unchangeable, in what ways might you enhance your coping with them? *I can't change that I'm a caregiver for my dad and I can't change my work requirements and hours. But I do believe that the plan related to my drinking will be helpful. The drinking makes the situation from these things even worse because then I feel guilty like "how could I put another job at risk by still drinking?" It just adds another thing to worry or feel bad about. Also, we've talked about the importance of thinking and approach to things and a lot of times I put a huge mental pressure on myself to do well or more often, not to mess up. I guess that's a self-talk thing I can work on. And I need to be better about scheduling who is doing what with taking care of my dad and the house. Because half the time, it's unclear who is going to be home with him, or help with bathing, or whatever. Or who is supposed to clean what around the house. And we both end up angry feeling like we're doing more than the other person. And the house, bills, all that stuff, gets jumbled.*

- What indirect or hidden wellness benefits may exist to some of the contextual wellness factors you marked as negative? *I guess in a weird way, there are some opportunities here. Like, maybe dad living with me is a chance to learn more about him and have time with him. And despite all the things I feel like I've messed up, I do have a job and I haven't completely screwed that up yet. And I like the job so far and getting promoted is a possibility. Maybe finding ways to pause every once in a while and realize that I have salvaged some things. And who knows what my life can be if I keep making positive changes?*

CONCLUSION

In this chapter, we have defined development, contextual, and cultural wellness and how these facets intersect with SUDs. We have suggested several WBAC interventions that address these areas of wellness. It should be noted that an entire book could be devoted to any of these three factors as they relate to SUDs. Hence, the information shared is not exhaustive. For instance, other developmental theories can be used in WBAC with your client other than Erickson's Psychosocial Theory. There are multiple theories of cultural development that are critical to review in understanding clients from different cultural backgrounds. More contextual wellness factors exist than those discussed. However, this chapter is a foundation and structure for how these dimensions can effectively be addressed in WBAC.

REFERENCES

American Psychiatric Association (APA) (2013). *Diagnostic and statistical manual of mental disorders* (5th ed.). American Psychiatric Association.
American Psychological Association (APA) (2019). *Discrimination: What it is and how to cope.* American Psychiatric Association. Retrieved March 22, 2023, from https://www.apa.org/topics/racism-bias discrimination/types-stress
American Psychiatric Association (APA) (2022). *Diagnostic and statistical manual of mental disorders* (5th ed., text rev.). American Psychiatric Association.

Andreassen, C. S., Griffiths, M. D., Hetland, J., & Pallesen, S. (2012). Development of a work addiction scale. *Scandinavian Journal of Psychology, 53*(3), 265–272. https://doi.org/10.1111/j.1467-9450.2012.00947.x

Atkinson, D. R., Morten, G., & Sue, D. W. (1979). *Counseling American minorities: A cross cultural perspective.* Brown.

Atkinson, D. R., Morten, G., & Sue, D. W. (1998). *Counseling American minorities* (5th ed.). McGraw Hill.

Bogenschutz, M. P. (2007). 12-step approaches for the dually diagnosed: Mechanisms of change. *Alcoholism: Clinical and Experimental Research, 31,* 64s–66s. https://doi.org/10.1111/j.1530-0277.2007.00496.x

Bogenschutz, M. P., Rice, S. L., Tonigan, J. S., Vogel, H. S., Nowinski, J., Hume, D., & Arenella, P. B. (2014). 12-step facilitation for the dually diagnosed: a randomized clinical trial. *Journal of Substance Abuse Treatment, 46*(4), 403–411. https://doi.org/10.1016/j.jsat.2013.12.009

Bronfenbrenner, U. (1977). Toward an experimental ecology of human development. *American Psychologist, 32*(7), 513. https://doi.org/10.1037/0003-066X.32.7.513

Bronfenbrenner, U. (1979). *The ecology of human development: Experiments by nature and design.* Harvard University Press.

Bronfenbrenner, U. (1994). Ecological models of human development. In T. Husen & T. N. Postlethwaite (Eds.), *International encyclopedia of education, Vol. 3* (2nd ed.). Elsevier. Reprinted in M. Gauvain & M. Cole (Eds)., *Readings on the development of children* (2nd ed.) (1993, pp. 37–43). Freeman.

Brooks, F., & McHenry, B. (2015). *A contemporary approach to substance use disorders and addiction counseling* (2nd ed.). John Wiley & Sons.

Busacca, L. A., & Rehfuss, M. C. (2017). Postmodern career counseling: A new perspective for the 21st century. In L. A. Busacca & M. C. Rehfuss (Eds.), *Postmodern career counseling: A handbook of culture, context, and cases* (pp. 28–47). American Counseling Association.

Carter, R. T. (1991). Cultural values: A review of empirical research and implications for counseling. *Journal of Counseling and Development, 70*(1), 164–173. https://doi.org/10.1002/j.1556-6676.1991.tb01579.x

Center for Substance Abuse Treatment (CSAT) (2000a). *Integrating substance abuse treatment and vocational services.* Treatment improvement protocol (TIP) series, no. 38. HHS publication no. (SMA) 12-4216. Substance Abuse and Mental Health Services Administration.

Center for Substance Abuse Treatment (CSAT) (2000b). *Comprehensive case management for substance abuse treatment.* Treatment improvement protocol (TIP) series, no. 27. HHS publication no. (SMA) 15-4215. Center for Substance Abuse Treatment.

Cooper, M., & Norcross, J. C. (2016). A brief, multidimensional measure of clients' therapy preferences: The Cooper-Norcross Inventory of Preferences (C-NIP). *International Journal of Clinical and Health Psychology, 16*(1), 87–98. https://doi.org/10.1016/j.ijchp.2015.08.003

Cridland, E. K., Deane, F. P., Hsu, C. I., & Kelly, P. J. (2012). A comparison of treatment outcomes for individuals with substance use disorder alone and individuals with probable dual diagnosis. *International Journal of Mental Health and Addiction, 10,* 670–683.

de Waal, M. M., Dekker, J. J. M., & Goudriaan, A. E. (2017). Prevalence of victimization in patients with dual diagnosis. *Journal of Dual Diagnosis, 13*(2), 119–123. https://doi.org/10.10 80/15504263.2016.1274067

Domino, G., & Affonso, D. (1990). The IPB: A personality measure of Erikson's life cycle stages. *Journal of Personality Assessment, 54,* 576–588.

Dunkel, C. S. (2013). Relative and longitudinal evidence for the importance of the general factor of psychosocial development in predicting well-being. *Personality and Individual Differences, 54*(1), 118–122. https://doi.org/10.1016/j.paid.2012.08.022

Dunkel, C. S., & Harbke, C. (2017). A review of measures of Erikson's stages of psychosocial development: Evidence for a general factor. *Journal of Adult Development, 24,* 58–76.

Eddie, D., Vilsaint, C. L., Hoffman, L. A., Bergman, B. G., Kelly, J. F., & Hoeppner, B. B. (2020). From working on recovery to working in recovery: employment status among a nationally representative US sample of individuals who have resolved a significant alcohol or other drug problem. *Journal of Substance Abuse Treatment, 113*, 108000. https://doi.org/10.1016/j.jsat.2020.108000

Erikson, E. H. (1964). *Insight and responsibility.* W. W. Norton and Company.

Erikson, E. (1968/1994). *Identity, youth and crisis.* W. W. Norton & Company.

Ewing, J. A. (1984). Detecting alcoholism: The CAGE questionnaire. *JAMA, 252*(14), 1905–1907. https://doi.org/10.1001/jama.1984.03350140051025

Ford, J. D., & Courtois, C. A. (2020). *Treating complex traumatic stress disorders in adults: Scientific foundations and therapeutic models* (2nd ed.). Guilford Press.

Lewis-Fernández, R., Aggarwal, N. K., Hinton, L., Hinton, D. E., & Kirmayer, L. J. (Eds.). (2016). *DSM-5® handbook on the cultural formulation interview.* American Psychiatric Publishing, Inc.

Farr, M., & Stevens, M. (2008). *Quick job search for ex-offenders: Seven steps to finding a job fast.* JIST Publishing.

Fullen, M. C. (2019). Defining wellness in older adulthood: Toward a comprehensive framework. *Journal of Counseling & Development, 97*(1), 62–74. https://doi.org/10.1002/jcad.12236

Gamby, K., Burns, D., & Forristal, K. (2021). Wellness decolonized: The history of wellness and recommendations for the counseling field. *Journal of Mental Health Counseling, 43*(3), 228–245. https://doi.org/10.17744/mehc.43.3.05

Gielen, N., Havermans, R., Tekelenburg, M., & Jansen, A. (2012). Prevalence of post-traumatic stress disorder among patients with substance use disorder: It is higher than clinicians think it is. *European Journal of Psychotraumatology, 3*(1), 17734. https://doi.org/10.3402/ejpt.v3i0.17734

Goldstein, R. Z., & Volkow, N. D. (2011). Dysfunction of the prefrontal cortex in addiction: Neuroimaging findings and clinical implications. *Nature Reviews Neuroscience, 12*(11), 652–669. https://doi.org/10.1038/nrn3119

Groves, D. L., Kahalas, H., & Erickson, D. L. (1975). A suggested modification to Maslow's need hierarchy. *Social Behavior and Personality: An International Journal, 3*(1), 65–69. https://doi.org/10.2224/sbp.1975.3.1.65

Hale, A. J., Ricotta, D. N., Freed, J., Smith, C. C., & Huang, G. C. (2019). Adapting Maslow's hierarchy of needs as a framework for resident wellness. *Teaching and Learning in Medicine, 31*(1), 109–118. https://doi.org/10.1080/10401334.2018.1456928

Hamachek, D. E. (1988). Evaluating self-concept and ego development within Erikson's psychosocial framework: A formulation. *Journal of Counseling & Development, 66*(8), 354–360. https://doi.org/10.1002/j.1556-6676.1988.tb00886.x

Hays, P. A. (2008). Addressing cultural complexities in practice: Assessment, diagnosis, and therapy (2nd ed.). American Psychological Association.

Hays, P. A. (2009). Integrating evidence-based practice, cognitive–behavior therapy, and multicultural therapy: Ten steps for culturally competent practice. *Professional Psychology: Research and Practice, 40*(4), 354. https://doi.org/10.1037/a0016250

Hendrickson, E. L., Schmal, M. S., & Ekleberry, S. C. (2004). *Treating co-occurring disorders: A handbook for mental health and substance abuse professionals.* Haworth Press.

Ibrahim, F. A. (1991). Contribution of cultural worldview to generic counseling and development. *Journal of Counseling & Development, 70*(1), 13–19. https://doi.org/10.1002/j.1556-6676.1991.tb01556.x

Ibrahim, F. A., & Heuer, J. R. (2016). *Cultural and social justice counseling: Client-specific interventions.* Springer.

Karcher, M. J., & Benne, K. (2008). Erik and Joan Eriksons' approach to human development in counseling. In K. L. Kraus (Ed.), *Lenses: Applying lifespan development theories in counseling* (pp. 199–228). Lahaska Press.

Knight, Z. G. (2017). A proposed model of psychodynamic psychotherapy linked to Erik Erikson's eight stages of psychosocial development. *Clinical Psychology & Psychotherapy, 24*(5), 1047–1058. https://doi.org/10.1002/cpp.2066

Koltko-Rivera, M. E. (2006). Rediscovering the later version of Maslow's hierarchy of needs: Self-transcendence and opportunities for theory, research, and unification. *Review of General Psychology, 10*(4), 302–317. https://doi.org/10.1037/1089-2680.10.4.302

Kroger, J., & Marcia, J. E. (2011). The identity statuses: Origins, meanings, and interpretations. In S. J. Schwartz, K. Luyckx, & V. L. Vignoles (Eds.), *Handbook of identity theory and research* (pp. 31–53). Springer.

Laudet, A. B. (2012). Rate and predictors of employment among formerly polysubstance dependent urban individuals in recovery. *Journal of Addictive Diseases*, *31*(3), 288–302. https://doi.org/10.1080/10550887.2012.694604

Lee, C. C. (2019). Multicultural competency: A conceptual framework for counseling across cultures. In C. C. Lee (Ed.), *Multicultural issues in counseling: New approaches to diversity* (5th ed., pp. 31–41). American Counseling Association.

Lee, C. C., & Ali, S. (2019). Intersectionality: Understanding the complexity of identity in counseling across cultures. In C. C. Lee (Ed.), *Multicultural issues in counseling: New approaches to diversity* (5th ed., pp. 51–60). American Counseling Association.

María-Ríos, C. E., & Morrow, J. D. (2020). Mechanisms of shared vulnerability to post traumatic stress disorder and substance use disorders. *Frontiers in Behavioral Neuroscience*, *14*, 6.

Marlatt, G. A. (1985). Lifestyle modification. In G. A. Marlatt & J. R. Gordon (Eds.), *Relapse prevention: Maintenance strategies in the treatment of addictive behaviors* (pp. 280–348). Guilford Press.

Markstrom, C. A., Sabino, V. M., Turner, B. J., & Berman, R. C. (1997). The psychosocial inventory of ego strengths: Development and validation of a new Eriksonian measure. *Journal of Youth and Adolescence*, *26*(6), 705–732.

Martin, L. M., Triscari, R., Boisvert, R., Hipp, K., Gersten, J., West, R. C., Kisling, E., Donham, A., Kollar, N., & Escobar, P. (2015). Development and evaluation of the lifestyle history questionnaire (LHQ) for people entering treatment for substance addictions. *The American Journal of Occupational Therapy*, *69*(3), 6903250010p1–6903250010p9. https://doi.org/10.5014/ajot.2015.014050

McCarthy, J. (2005). Individualism and collectivism: What do they have to do with counseling? *Journal of Multicultural Counseling and Development*, *33*(2), 108–117. https://doi.org/10.1002/j.2161-1912.2005.tb00009.x

McGovern, (2009). *Living with co-occurring addiction and mental health disorders: A handbook for recovery*. Hazelden Foundation.

McLellan, A. T., Kushner, H., Metzger, D., Peters, R., Smith, I., Grissom, G., Pettinati, H., & Argeriou, M. (1992). The fifth edition of the addiction severity index. *Journal of Substance Abuse Treatment*, *9*(3), 199–213. https://doi.org/10.1016/0740-5472(92)90062-S

Mehta, K., Hoadley, A., Ray, L. A., Kiluk, B. D., Carroll, K. M., & Magill, M. (2021). Cognitive-behavioral interventions targeting alcohol or other drug use and co-occurring mental health disorders: A meta-analysis. *Alcohol and Alcoholism*, *56*(5), 535–544. https://doi.org/10.1093/alcalc/agab016

Merçon-Vargas, E. A., Lima, R. F. F., Rosa, E. M., & Tudge, J. (2020). Processing proximal processes: What Bronfenbrenner meant, what he didn't mean, and what he should have meant. *Journal of Family Theory & Review*, *12*(3), 321–334.

Miller, W. R., Forcehimes, A. A., & Zweben, A. (2011). *Treating addiction: A guide for professionals*. Guilford Press.

Miller, W. R., Forcehimes, A. A., & Zweben, A. (2019). *Treating addiction: A guide for professionals* (2nd ed.). Guilford Press.

Mueser, K. T., Noordsy, D. L., Drake, R. E., & Fox, L. (2003). *Integrated treatment for dual disorders: A guide to effective practice*. Guilford Press.

Myers, J. E., & Sweeney, T. J. (2004). The indivisible self: An evidence-based model of wellness. *Journal of Individual Psychology*, *60*, 234–244.

Myers, J. E., & Sweeney, T. J. (2005). The indivisible self: An evidence-based model of wellness. In J. E. Myers & T. J. Sweeney (Eds.), *Counseling for wellness: Theory, research, and practice* (pp. 29–38). American Counseling Association.

Onyeka, I. N., Collier Høegh, M., Nåheim Eien, E. M., Nwaru, B. I., & Melle, I. (2019). Comorbidity of physical disorders among patients with severe mental illness with and without substance use disorders: A systematic review and meta-analysis. *Journal of Dual Diagnosis*, *15*(3), 192–206. https://doi.org/10.1080/15504263.2019.1619007

Oyserman, D., Coon, H. M., & Kemmelmeier, M. (2002). Rethinking individualism and collec-
   tivism: Evaluation of theoretical assumptions and meta-analyses. *Psychological Bulletin, 128*(1),
   3–72. https://doi.org/10.1037/0033-2909.128.1.3
Pedersen, P. B. (1991). Multiculturalism as a generic approach to counseling. *Journal of Counseling &
   Development, 70*(1), 6–12. https://doi.org/10.1002/j.1556 6676.1991.tb01555.x
Qeadan, F., Azagba, S., Barbeau, W. A., Gu, L. Y., Mensah, N. A., Komaromy, M., English, K., &
   Madden, E. F. (2022). Associations between discrimination and substance use among college
   students in the United States from 2015 to 2019. *Addictive Behaviors, 125*, 107164. https://doi.
   org/10.1016/j.addbeh.2021.107164
Ratts, M. J., & Pedersen, P. B. (2014). *Counseling for multiculturalism and social justice: Integration, theory,
   and application.* John Wiley & Sons.
Rehabilitation Research and Training Center on Drugs and Disability (1996). *Substance abuse, dis-
   ability and vocational rehabilitation.* Rehabilitation Research and Training Center on Drugs and
   Disability.
Robertson, I. E., Sagvaag, H., Selseng, L. B., & Nesvaag, S. (2021). The hunt for a job: Narrating
   the process of gaining employment for people in recovery from lives dominated by drug use.
   Drugs: Education, Prevention and Policy, 29(6), 675–684. https://doi.org/10.1080/09687637.20
   21.1973962
Rogers, J. L., Gilbride, D. D., & Dew, B. J. (2018). Utilizing an ecological framework to enhance
   counselors' understanding of the US opioid epidemic. *Professional Counselor, 8*(3), 226–239.
Schaufeli, W. B., Bakker, A. B., van der Heijden, F. M., & Prins, J. T. (2009). Workaholism among
   medical residents: It is the combination of working excessively and compulsively that counts.
   International Journal of Stress Management, 16(4), 249–272. https://doi.org/10.1037/a0017537
Schaufeli, W. B., Taris, T. W., & Van Rhenen, W. (2008). Workaholism, burnout, and work
   engagement: Three of a kind or three different kinds of employee well-being? *Applied Psychol-
   ogy, 57*(2), 173–203. https://doi.org/10.1111/j.1464-0597.2007.00285.x
Stein, L. I., & Test, M. A. (1980). An alternative to mental hospital treatment. I: Conceptual
   model, treatment program, and clinical evaluation. *Archives of General Psychiatry, 37*, 392–397.
Substance Abuse and Mental Health Services Administration (SAMHSA) (2014). *Improving cultural
   competence. Treatment improvement protocol (TIP) series no. 59.* HHS publication no. (SMA) 14-4849.
Substance Abuse and Mental Health Services Administration (SAMHSA) (2020). *Substance use
   disorder treatment for people with co-occurring disorders. Treatment improvement protocol (TIP) series, No.
   42. SAMHSA publication no. PEP20-02-01-004.* Substance Abuse and Mental Health Services
   Administration.
Substance Abuse and Mental Health Services Administration (SAMHSA) (2021). *National survey
   of substance abuse treatment services (N-SSATS): 2020. Data on substance abuse treatment facilities.* Substance Abuse and Mental Health Services Administration.
Seward, G. H., & Seward, J. P. (1937). Internal and external determinants of drives. *Psychological
   Review, 44*(4), 349. https://doi.org/10.1037/h0059631
Slater, C. L. (2003). Generativity versus stagnation: An elaboration of Erikson's adult
   stage of human development. *Journal of Adult Development, 10*(1), 53–65. https://doi.
   org/10.1023/A:1020790820868
Sue, D. W. (1978). World views and counseling. *The Personnel and Guidance Journal, 56*(8), 458–462.
   https://doi.org/10.1002/j.2164-4918.1978.tb05287.x
Sue, D. W., & Sue, D. (1999). *Counseling the culturally different: Theory and practice.* John Wiley & Sons
   Inc.
Sue, D. W., Arredondo, P., & McDavis, R. J. (1992). Multicultural counseling competencies
   and standards: A call to the profession. *Journal of Counseling & Development, 70*(4), 477–486.
   https://doi.org/10.1002/j.1556-6676.1992.tb01642.x
Sue, D. W., Capodilupo, C. M., Torino, G. C., Bucceri, J. M., Holder, A. M. B., Nadal, K. L., &
   Esquilin, M. (2007). Racial microaggressions in everyday life: Implications for clinical prac-
   tice. *American Psychologist, 62*(4), 271–286. https://doi.org/10.1037/0003 066X.62.4.271
Sue, D. W., Sue, D., Neville, H. A., & Smith, L. (2019). *Counseling the culturally diverse: Theory and
   practice* (8th ed.). Wiley.

Taormina, R. J., & Gao, J. H. (2013). Maslow and the motivation hierarchy: Measuring satisfaction of the needs. *The American Journal of Psychology, 126*(2), 155–177. https://doi.org/10.5406/amerjpsyc.126.2.0155

Thomas, A. J., & Schwarzbaum, S. E. (2017). *Culture and identity: Life stories for counselors and therapists* (3rd ed.). SAGE Publications.

Tran, D. D., Fitzke, R. E., Wang, J., Davis, J. P., & Pedersen, E. R. (2023). Substance use, financial stress, employment disruptions, and anxiety among veterans during the COVID-19 pandemic. *Psychological Reports, 126*(4), 1684–1700. https://doi.org/10.1177/00332941221080413

Vallesi, S., Tuson, M., Davies, A., & Wood, L. (2021). Multimorbidity among people experiencing homelessness—Insights from primary care data. *International Journal of Environmental Research and Public Health, 18*(12), 6498. https://doi.org/10.3390/ijerph18126498

Van der Kaap-Deeder, J., Soenens, B., Van Petegem, S., Neyrinck, B., De Pauw, S., Raemdonck, E., & Vansteenkiste, M. (2020). Live well and die with inner peace: The importance of retrospective need-based experiences, ego integrity and despair for late adults' death attitudes. *Archives of Gerontology and Geriatrics, 91*, 104184. https://doi.org/10.1016/j.archger.2020.104184

van der Kaap-Deeder, J., Vermote, B., Waterschoot, J., Soenens, B., Morbée, S., & Vansteenkiste, M. (2022). The role of ego integrity and despair in older adults' well-being during the COVID-19 crisis: The mediating role of need-based experiences. *European Journal of Ageing, 19*(1), 117–129. https://doi.org/10.1007/s10433-021-00610-0.

van der Kolk, B. A. (2002). Assessment and treatment of complex PTSD. In R. Yehuda (Ed.), *Treating trauma survivors with PTSD* (pp. 127–156). American Psychiatric Publishing.

Walsh, F. (1996). The concept of family resilience: Crisis and challenge. *Family Process, 35*(3), 261–281. https://doi.org/10.1111/j.1545-5300.1996.00261.x

Walsh, F. (2002). A family resilience framework: Innovative practice applications. *Family Relations, 51*(2), 130–137. https://doi.org/10.1111/j.1741-3729.2002.00130.x

Williams, J. M., McMahon, H. G., & Goodman, R. D. (2015). Eco-webbing: A teaching strategy to facilitate critical consciousness and agency. *Counselor Education and Supervision, 54*(2), 82–97. https://doi.org/10.1002/ceas.12006

CHAPTER 7

PUT YOUR MIND TO IT: MENTAL WELLNESS AS A CATALYST FOR HOLISTIC RECOVERY

INTRODUCTION

When I (Todd) was counseling a client struggling with alcohol addiction, I recall being surprised at how much his thinking was getting in the way of his own way of recovery. Within Alcoholics Anonymous (AA) circles, this type of mental behavior is called "stinkin' thinkin'" and is characterized by negative thought patterns, pessimism, and a bevy of "cognitive distortions". His core beliefs about himself seemed to stem from early negative messages from his family. These cognitive mechanisms served as major triggers for relapse. In my estimation, this client needed to strengthen his mental wellness – not only to help reduce his substance use behavior but also to increase his well-being. Mental wellness, including brain health, neurogenesis, and healthy thinking and functioning is the topic of this chapter. As you will see, many elements of mind wellness serve as an important foundation for holistic recovery.

In this chapter, we will define mental wellness and its relation to addiction, and then turn to a basic review of the brain and nervous system. Insights from neuroscience will guide our discussion of the impact of addiction on the brain. From this analysis, we will explore numerous cognitive-behavioral and neuroscientific (aka brain-based) strategies you can employ to improve your clients' overall wellness and reduce or eliminate substance use behavior. Several brain and cognitive concepts and approaches will help your clients meet their wellness and substance use recovery goals. Other dimensions of wellness will be involved in mental wellness approaches; however, the brain and its processes will be the central feature.

MENTAL WELLNESS AND ADDICTION

Mental wellness pertains to the well-being of our brain and thought processes. It is the "positive interaction among genes, neurobiology, experiences, thoughts, and emotions to strengthen the neural circuitry that supports wellness" (Ohrt, Clarke, & Conley, 2019, p. 48). Many existing counseling approaches take a cognitive focus so mental wellness is fertile ground as an intervention point in WBAC. Additionally, neurocounseling scholars and practitioners have noticed that providing information about addiction, recovery, and the brain is engaging and empowering for clients and students (Russell-Chapin, 2016). Mental wellness directly connects to addictive behaviors and use of substances. Cognitive functioning can be largely affected during consumption of the substance and over time when paired with ongoing ingestion of the substance. Adverse childhood and life experiences can affect the brain, rendering one at increased risk for substance use behaviors and/or mental health concerns. Many of the evidence-based relapse prevention approaches rely on helping clients make changes to or be mindful of their cognitions. Even the DSM-5-TR, for instance, portrays cravings as a cognitive process (American Psychiatric Association, 2022). Let's now turn to some basic brain physiology and how that connects to mental wellness and addiction.

DOI: 10.4324/9781003147954-7

Brain Basics and Mental Wellness

Despite the tremendous advances in neuroscience and related research, there is still a lot we do not know about the brain (Jones, 2017). However, researchers are beginning to discover that even relatively simple behaviors require an intricate interplay of neurochemicals and structures that manifest in our everyday experiences. The human brain is a delicate, yet complex structure that weighs about three pounds and has a tofu-like consistency (Hanson, 2011). Three overarching areas make up the structure of the brain: (a) the lower brain, which includes the cerebellum, hypothalamus, and thalamus, (b) the midbrain (limbic region), which contains the hippocampus and amygdala, and the (c) upper brain, which contains the cerebral cortex (Miller & Beeson, 2021).

The lower brain is generally responsible for automatic processes below the threshold of consciousness, such as heart rate, blood pressure, and breathing (Miller & Beeson, 2021). The midbrain plays a key role in memory, emotion, and reward. Later, we will discuss the major influence that drugs and alcohol have on this region of the brain. As noted, the upper brain is composed of the cerebral cortex, which is the folded mass that we most think about when picturing a brain (Jones, 2017). Part of the cerebral cortex is the prefrontal cortex, which covers the frontal lobe, and is a part of the brain in which addictive substances have a direct impact. The prefrontal cortex is responsible for executive functions (Miller & Beeson, 2021), including planning, attention, flexibility, and self-control (Scully, 2022). Within these three overarching components of the brain, there are numerous additional structures and substructures that interconnect and communicate with each other.

The health of the brain is intimately connected to all other dimensions of wellness. Damage to one part or structure of the brain can have profound impacts on personality, behavior, thoughts, emotions, and quality of life. This fact is reflected in the story of Phineas Gage, a railroad worker in the 1800s who had an iron rod shoot through his skull (Ohrt et al., 2019). As a result of his injury, Gage's behavior changed substantially, pointing to the relationship between brain functioning and personality. But it doesn't have to be a serious injury that disrupts brain functioning: stress, lack of exercise, poor sleep, poor diet, and substance misuse also negatively impact the brain. Because the brain is a biological organ that is connected to so many aspects of our lives, clients are encouraged to engage in healthy brain-based behaviors as a beginning point in counseling; taking care of one's brain means taking care of one's life.

You might be wondering how knowledge of brain structures and wellness relates to WBAC. Well, it turns out that substances, depending on type, dosage, etc. have a major influence on one or more of these brain regions. For example, central nervous system depressants (e.g., barbiturates, alcohol) are well known to impact the lower regions of the brain, such that an overdose can produce labored and ineffective breathing, slow pulse, and even organ failure. The reward center of the brain (housed in the midbrain area) has been the focus of intense research on substance addiction, where it is believed that drugs "hijack" this region (more on this later) leading to intense cravings for the rewarding effects of drugs. Finally, drugs and alcohol have significant negative effects on the prefrontal cortex, with scientific evidence suggesting that these regions of the brain atrophy with prolonged use. A weakened prefrontal cortex means poorer ability to sustain attention, use self-control, and make healthy choices.

Brain health and mental wellness, then, is a major component of the WBAC approach and is intimately impacted by substance use. Helping clients to understand the connections between substance use, brain health, and mental functioning can provide insights that make sense of their experiences. These connections can also pave the way for brain-based counseling interventions to limit or even reverse brain damage from substance use disorder. Let's now look at how communication happens within the brain.

Neurons and Neurotransmitters

Neurons are brain cells that communicate with each other to influence our experiences; the primary way a releasing neuron communicates with a receiving neuron is through neurotransmission. That is, the releasing neuron dispenses neurotransmitters, or chemical messengers, that fit into the receiving neuron like how a key fits into a lock. This communication process impacts all mental events and experiences, including thoughts, sensations, perceptions, and movements. The various substances primarily exert their substantial influence within this neurotransmission process.

The structure of the neuron begins with the cell body, which includes the cell nucleus and dendrites, responsible for connecting to other neurons in the brain. Extending from the cell body is the axon, a long, narrow structure surrounded by layers of myelin sheath, which serve to protect the axon and speed up the communication process. At the end of the axon are the terminal buttons, which release neurotransmitters when stimulated within the neuron. Interestingly, neurons within the brain do not directly touch each other, as a tiny gap exists between the dendrites of one cell and the terminal buttons of another. This tiny space is called the synapse and is where neurotransmitters are released and absorbed in the transmission process.

There are several neurotransmitters that are implicated in addiction, but the most common include serotonin (sleep and mood), dopamine (pleasures, motivation, and craving), glutamate (learning and memory), and gamma-aminobutyric acid (GABA; relaxation). As an example, some drugs block a process called reuptake. When a neuron releases a neurotransmitter, not all the neurotransmitter is used by the receiving neuron. Some of the excess neurotransmitter is reabsorbed back into the releasing cell – that is reuptake. Cocaine, a central nervous stimulant, blocks the reuptake process of dopamine, leaving an overabundance of dopamine within the synapse. The net result is excess dopamine in the system, which promotes the effects of cocaine (Plotnik, 1996). Other drugs may block receptor sites, such as lysergic acid (LSD), precluding the neurotransmission process (Plotnik). There are probably thousands of different, specific actions that drugs have on the brain and body, and not everyone responds in the same manner to a particular drug, dose, or drug-taking ritual (Kuhn, Swartzwelder, & Wilson, 2019).

Neuroplasticity

It was once believed that the developing brain had two primary episodes of significant growth – early childhood and adolescence – and that growth in brain structures ceased around early adulthood. Research has now discovered that the human brain can continue to grow, altering its structure and function well into the adult years. This process is called neuroplasticity, and it occurs in response to internal and external environmental changes (Field, Jones, & Russell-Chapin, 2017). That is, the neurons of the brain can rewire, form new connections, and prune old, unused connections based on environmental experiences including relationship quality, levels of stress, and, of course, continuation or cessation of substances.

Neuroplasticity is a concept that can provide hope for those struggling with addiction. We know that drugs and alcohol can confer damage to various structures and functions of the brain. For example, the atrophy of the prefrontal cortex from continued drug use is likely due to the reduced gray matter in this region. Goldstein and Volkow (2011) highlighted how neuroimaging studies have shown how a dysfunctional prefrontal cortex leads to less cognitive flexibility and poorer decision-making. Parvaz et al. (2016) found that reduced gray matter volume in the prefrontal cortex is a consequence of cocaine use; however, the researchers also found that individuals can recover this volume with significant reductions in or abstinence from drug use at six months' follow-up. In other words, through neuroplasticity, clients with substance use disorders can promote and encourage positive influences on their brains that strengthen the recovery process.

Cutting-edge research in neuroscience has demonstrated that the environment can have a significant influence on shaping the neuronal structures and functions within the brain (i.e., promoting neuroplasticity; Galvan, 2010; Miller & Beeson, 2021). In conjunction with limiting or stopping substance use, this means that, through a WBAC recovery plan, clients can establish healthier behavioral habits to promote physical, emotional, spiritual, and mental wellness. These positive influences can heal and support a healthier brain.

Cramer et al. (2011) listed "cognitive training" through cognitive-behavioral therapy (CBT) as one of several avenues for promoting neuroplasticity. However, most likely any therapeutic endeavor that can help clients shift viewpoints, adopt new wellness patterns, promote a strong recovery mindset, and feel better emotionally would likely have an impact on neuroplasticity (Lewis, 2023). Cramer et al. also listed exercise as a positive habit to promote neuroplasticity. Exercise fits squarely within physical wellness (Chapter 8) and is something that WBAC clinicians can encourage for their clients in recovery. All of this is good news for clinicians and the work we do to help clients in recovery. WBAC clinicians, in particular, are well suited to promote health across all wellness dimensions, which can have a significant impact on a person's recovery as they return to and restore brain health.

Hijacking of the Reward Center

Most, if not all, addictive substances target the brain's "reward center" (Brown-Rice & Moro, 2018), also called the mesolimbic dopamine pathway (MDP; Thombs & Osborn, 2019). The MDP is made of several structures and neurons that primarily respond to the neurotransmitter dopamine (Thombs & Osborn, 2019). When one consumes drugs, a flood of dopamine is released, leading to euphoric impacts (Brown-Rice & Moro, 2018), and overwhelms structures in the MDP. Through the memory structures in our brains (e.g., the amygdala), pleasurable experiences are easily encoded and remembered. The net effect is the cycle of addiction: positive reinforcement from drug use motivates individuals to chase the high (Brown-Rice & Moro, 2018).

The reward from drug use is significantly more intense than natural rewards, such as watching a nice sunset or reading a good book (Brown-Rice & Moro, 2019). Because the release of dopamine from drugs is far beyond any natural release, the body will compensate by producing less dopamine itself and/or shutting down dopamine receptors. With less dopamine, individuals will have a blunted response to any natural experiences of pleasure. Sadly, the only way they can regain pleasurable feelings (albeit in an attenuated form) is to continue using (Brown-Rice & Moro, 2018; Polk, 2015). This is one mechanism by which drug use "hijacks" the reward center of the brain.

Having a basic understanding of how the brain works and implications for how addiction compromises brain health and mental wellness is important for both clinicians and clients to know. With this understanding, clients can create new narratives that better explain what is happening in their brains and what they can do to help themselves heal. Let's now turn to some treatment strategies that can help clients strengthen their mental wellness. These strategies focus primarily on thoughts, behaviors, emotions, and brain health to not only promote mind wellness but also overall wellness.

TREATMENT STRATEGIES USING COGNITIVE AND NEUROSCIENCE METHODS

Cognitive Behavioral Approaches

Cognitive-behavioral (CBT) approaches have been utilized with individuals with a range of mental health, substance use, and co-occurring disorders concerns (Beck, 2011). These approaches that engage mental wellness require the client to reflect on their mental experience as it relates to other dimensions that comprise the gestalt of their life (mind, body, spirit, emotions, and connection). A foundation of cognitive concepts and skills enables the client to identify what is going through their mind, the beliefs they hold, and how these cognitive constructs are linked to their substance use and wellness.

ABC Model and Corresponding Interventions

Empowering clients by first informing them about cognitive concepts prior to or concurrent with implementing these interventions is an important starting point. We recommend that clinicians present the ABC model, which depicts the associations among thoughts, feelings, and behaviors (referred to as antecedents, beliefs and thoughts, and consequences). The ABC model represents a series of triggers leading with antecedents: events that occur within the person or outside of the person that evoke thoughts, images, and/or beliefs that spark "emotions, behaviors, and physiological responses" or consequences (Liese & Beck, 2022, p. 22). Liese and Beck cited that the relapse precipitants ("high risk situations") from Marlatt's (1985) relapse taxonomy are examples of within-person antecedents such as a negative or positive emotional state. Peer pressure is an example of an external antecedent.

Distinguishing between thoughts, beliefs, and core beliefs is important for clinicians and clients. A thought is "an idea or image that may manifest as an impression, prediction, judgment, memory, plan, and so forth" (Liese & Beck, 2022, p. 15). Automatic thoughts (ATs) arise quickly and occur involuntarily. Meditation serves as a window into understanding this concept as many authors have noted that when one must focus on one thing such as the breath, one notices the mind vaulting to different thoughts (e.g., Bowen, Chawla, Grow, & Marlatt, 2021). ATs can advance through the mind and dissipate. Authors have used the metaphor of a ticker tape that runs across the screen of the mind. Some ATs are thus benign while others can precipitate further disconcerting thoughts, feelings, and behaviors. Beliefs are thoughts that have taken longer to form than ATs due to being contemplated for longer than an AT. Core beliefs are the foundation of who we are as they represent our perspectives on ourselves, the world, our future, others, and relationships (Liese & Beck, 2022). The following statement speaks to the relationship among thoughts, substance use, and mental health for individuals with co-occurring disorders:

For those who have a severe mental health problem and misuse drugs or alcohol, the beliefs they hold about the substances they use are sometimes linked to their experience of severe mental health problems. These beliefs may help the person to feel he/she can self-manage or regulate both the symptoms and the experience of having a severe mental health problem....

(Graham, 2004, p. 25)

THOUGHT DIARY AND GUIDED DISCOVERY

Life experiences (across mind, body, spirit, emotion, and connection), substance use, mental health and wellness experiences, and thoughts and beliefs are all interrelated (Graham, 2004). These experiences can become embedded into one's thoughts and beliefs. Hence, any given individual will have an assortment of positive and negative thoughts or beliefs about themselves, the world, others, the future, and relationships (Liese & Beck, 2022). Similarly, any given individual will have thoughts or beliefs about their SUD or co-occurring disorder that can be helpful or not helpful to their recovery.

To begin sorting through these thoughts and beliefs with the client, the clinician can use a "Thought Diary". Clients must be attentive to the internal or external events (antecedent). Advise the client that experiencing stress, craving, low wellness, and/or mental health symptoms are a signal that an antecedent has occurred. The diary prompts the client to note the thoughts and beliefs arising about the antecedents. Clients then document the consequences to their mental, emotional, physical, spiritual, and/or connection wellness. Next, the client identifies a more helpful thought or belief with which to challenge the less helpful thought or belief. The final column signifies how the "effect" of the consequence changes (in one or more of the wellness dimensions) concurrent with a change in thinking (Beck, 1976; Ellis, 1991). Table 7.1 is an example of a "thought diary" with one entry completed.

De-constructing beliefs that manifest during sessions or via the thought diary can be accomplished using Guided Discovery questions. This line of inquiry makes it possible for the client to apply a critical lens to the beliefs that come into their awareness. A few questions from Mitcheson et al. (2010, p. 116) to help the client identify indicators substantiating their beliefs include: "What are your reasons for thinking that will happen?" Regarding the latter question, the clinician can use follow-up prompts or questions such as "What experiences may have influenced you forming this belief?" or "What messages have you received from others in your life that have factored into this belief?" When seeking information that runs contrary to the belief, the clinician can inquire, "What has happened to you that doesn't fit with this?" (Mitcheson et al., 2010, p. 118) The last step is like the "thought diary" in which

Table 7.1 Wellness-Based Thought Disputation Example

Antecedents	Beliefs	Wellness Consequences	Disputation	Effect (Current or Possible)
Did not exercise as I had planned	I'm a failure.	**Mental:** Ended up having a bunch of other negative thoughts **Physical:** I didn't exercise for the rest of the week **Emotion**: Irritable Spiritual: N/A Connection: N/A	I am not a failure because of one missed exercise session. I have been exercising a lot more over the past weeks.	**Mental:** Fewer negative thoughts **Physical:** Calm in my body **Emotion:** Hope, proud Spiritual: N/A Connection: N/A

the client creates a more helpful thought or belief with which to challenge the belief being examined.

Another option when a client is wed to a belief that has yielded unfavorable consequences is to assess the benefits and costs of holding that belief. The clinician can make two columns on a page: one for the benefits of adhering to the belief (living one's life in accordance with the belief) and another for the costs of adhering to the belief. Thus, even if a client espouses that belief, they may recognize that it is unhelpful and potentially damaging, thereby incentivizing them to develop a new belief (Burns, 1999; Liese & Beck, 2022).

The clinician using WBAC also wants to unearth and crystallize the thoughts and beliefs that have or could enhance the client's wellness and recovery. The clinician can thus ask the client about beliefs they hold about self, the world, others, their future, and relationships that have or could benefit their wellness and substance use goals (Liese & Beck, 2022). Kuyken, Padesky, and Dudley (2009, p. 108) have operationalized this approach into the following questions:

- "What rules or beliefs can help you be resilient in this situation?"
- "Ideally, what qualities would you like to show in the face of these obstacles?"
- "What beliefs [about you/others/the world] help you show these qualities?"
- "If you coped in the best way you can imagine, what would you be thinking [about yourself/others/the world]?"

Substantial therapeutic value using cognitive and behavioral techniques derives from the client being able to identify their thoughts. As J. S. Beck (2011) noted, the essential question in cognitive therapy is "what was going through your mind?" (p. 142) Informing clients about cognitive distortions that are prevalent and often precipitate distress prepares clients to access and understand the thoughts that affect them. The following are examples of cognitive distortions:

The Escape: Thoughts that one cannot manage a stressor, issue, and emotion, and have no choice but to escape using a behavior or addictive behavior (Najavits, 1993 as cited in Najavits, Gotthardt, Weiss, & Epstein, 2004).

Beating Yourself Up: Unhelpful and inaccurate blaming of oneself (Najavits, 1993 as cited in Najavits et al., 2004).

Time Warp: Thinking that an uncomfortable emotion and/or craving will persist with no endpoint (Najavits, 1993 as cited in Najavits et al., 2004).

Disqualifying or Discounting the Positive: Thinking that when good things or accomplishments occur, or favorable attributes are brought to one's attention, they are not important (Beck, 2021).

Catastrophizing: Assuming that what has occurred or what one is thinking or feeling will have consequences that cannot be managed (Beck, 2021).

Emotional Reasoning: One's feelings represent reality (e.g. "My feeling is that my relationship is broken which means that it is broken") (Beck, 2021).

Blaming Others: A denial thought in which one defers blame and disregards their accountability for what has occurred (Barriga, Gibbs, Potter, & Liau, 2001).

Negative Expectations: Assuming the outcome of an endeavor or occurrence will be negative (Hollon & Kendall, 1980).

Comparison: "The tendency to compare oneself whereby by the outcome typically results in the conclusion that one is inferior or worse off than others" (Freeman & DeWolf, 1992; Freeman & Oster, 1999; Yurica & DiTomasso, 2005, p. 119).

Perfectionism: "A constant striving to live up to some internal or external representation of perfection without examining the evidence for the reasonableness of these perfect standards…" (Freeman & DeWolf, 1992; Freeman & Oster, 1999; Yurica & DiTomasso, 2005, p. 119).

Multiple avenues can be explored utilizing the cognitive distortions. The clinician can request that the client highlight the two or three cognitive distortions that they perceive they experience most often and/or that have the most negative impact on their wellness or substance use. Encourage the client to provide specific examples of the antecedent, the thought or belief, the consequence, helpful thoughts with which to dispute the distortion, and any effect (change in wellness following the disputation). The cognitive distortions can be integrated into the "thought diary", giving the client the opportunity to practice labeling and challenging the thought distortions and noticing the outcomes of this process (Beck, 2011). We have included an additional activity on positive affirmations. See below in Handout 7.3.

Handout 7.3   Validation Exercise by M.K. Curry

It is important to note that when looking to incorporate any of the mindfulness techniques and approaches outlined here (or from other sources) into a session with a client, the practitioner is also aware of best practices from a trauma-informed perspective. Many persons with substance use issues have also experienced high levels of trauma. While most clinicians may be aware of some trauma from client disclosure, there always remains the possibility that a client has not disclosed a traumatic event or events, whether that be a conscious or unconscious decision on the part of the client. It serves the client best for an engaged practitioner to integrate trauma-informed care out of respect for any trauma the client may have experienced.

Some aspects of trauma-informed praxis include principles of safety, choice, collaboration, trustworthiness, and empowerment. For example, before implementing an intervention in a session, make sure to provide the client with some background on the intervention, including but not limited to why this technique might be of service; an explanation or walkthrough of how the technique unfolds and what to expect structurally; and, perhaps most critically, making sure the client knows they can stop the intervention or technique at any time during the session. By including the client in the decision-making process for the integration of the technique, aspects of safety, collaboration, choice, trustworthiness, and empowerment are all demonstrated to be of value to you and in this therapeutic alliance. Checking in with the client afterward and providing space for processing feelings of safety is also crucial in maintaining a trauma-informed approach.

Many mindfulness-based guided body scans and progressive muscle relaxation scripts begin by asking a client to close their eyes. For a person with an activated nervous system, or who is living with high levels of unprocessed trauma, doing these exercises in an unfamiliar room or among unfamiliar people might rouse a response very counter to the relaxation or mindfulness that the practitioner is attempting to offer the client, and could end up unintentionally harming the client or re-activating trauma responses. This is a space in which including a trauma-informed approach and offering choices such as keeping eyes open or closed, or making sure the client knows they can choose a different seat in the room, afford the client some empowerment and might even illuminate something about their own responses of which they had not been previously aware.

The following is a validation script with options for both neutral acceptance and positive affirmations designed around a strength-based approach. Neutral acceptance does not require positivity to honor and respect the self or body that one has; rather, it is about noticing any feelings around oneself non-judgmentally. At the end is a sample outline for processing the activity in a trauma-informed way that connects the activity to wellness-based addiction counseling.

Script for: Validation Exercise Rationale: This exercise can be used for clients who have difficulty articulating positive things about themselves, who engage in negative self-talk, or who are learning how to accept things about themselves or their wellness journey without judgment. This exercise can be used with a client in session; can be adapted or co-developed with a client to more personalize the statements; or can be given to a client to use as part of a daily practice. Clients can choose one or two that resonate and be invited to explore integrating those statements into space around them (written at the top of journal entries; used as a mantra while walking; notes on a mirror, etc.)

There are options for both positive affirmations and neutral acceptance. Positive affirmations are strength-based statements that validate; neutral acceptances are statements that remind clients to suspend judgments and criticisms and to use rational statements to challenge negativity.

Positive Affirmation Validation:
I am worth the time it takes to become well.

I am strong for choosing to take my wellness seriously.

I am resilient in choosing to return to difficult spaces.

I am able to accept love, love myself, and love others.

I am capable of growing toward the person I know I can become.

I deserve recovery.

I deserve a fulfilling life.

Neutral Acceptance Script:
Today is a hard day and I am doing my best.

Everyone must ask for help sometimes.

With time, I can do this.

With support, I can do this.

I will try again today.

One bad experience does not make the whole day worthless.

I am not feeling strong today, and I know that I do not have to be strong every day.

I am still working on becoming who I want to be, even if the progress feels small today.

Script for: Processing Mindfulness Activities
We have just engaged in a vulnerable activity. With your permission, I would like to take time to process some of what you experienced, and make sure that you know you have space to explore some of the space you went to and to voice any concerns or discomforts you may have had with the activity.

Did you notice any places in your body that felt particularly tense? ...If so, please tell me more about this.

Did you find it difficult to stay present with the activity? ...If so, where did your mind wander to?

Did you push through any moments of discomfort? ...If so, did you have an interior narration for this?

What has this activity taught you or shown you about yourself?

Note. This handout was authored by M.K. Curry.

MINDFULNESS

Mindfulness of one's experiences facilitates clients' recognition of the mind-body-spirit-emotion-connection relationships. Urge surfing is a technique in which the client learns to identify cravings and apply mindfulness and/or cognitive-behavioral approaches to navigate them. Some research support exists for the use of urge surfing. For example, a randomized control trial with adolescents demonstrated that urge surfing corresponded with decreases in alcohol consumption (Harris, Stewart, & Stanton, 2017). Urge surfing begins by providing information to the client (Lloyd, 2003) (a) suggesting that urges are comparable to waves, starting lower, reaching a point of highest craving (e.g., the peak of a wave), and then declining and fading away (Carroll, 1996; Ito, McNair, Donovan, & Marlatt, 1984), (b) "Urges typically last only a few minutes, and rarely more than 10 minutes" (p. 453), (c) indulging in the urge via addictive behavior exacerbates future urges and not responding to the urge with addictive behavior can lessen its strength over time. Clinicians also normalize for clients that consistent and strong cravings may arise during recovery, sometimes years later, and that managing urges can be a taxing endeavor (Lloyd, 2003). Furthermore, clinicians can reframe that the client's awareness of these cravings is a positive sign as it suggests they are able to observe their experience and are therefore empowered to select their response.

The clinician should then help the client unpack their experience of an urge via self-monitoring or in conversation with you. The self-monitoring handout from Chapter 4 can serve this purpose. Clients should rehearse urge surfing with smaller cravings to increase their preparedness for larger ones and implement urge surfing once they have removed themselves from any external triggers, if possible (Carroll, 1996; Ito et al., 1984). Lloyd (2003) advised that

> While experiencing an urge the client should sit in a comfortable position with feet flat on the floor, take some deep breaths, turn his or her attention inward, and focus on where in the body the urge is being experienced.
>
> (p. 454)

The client then observes the craving and describes it comprehensively, exhausting all the qualities they can identify.

The process of observing and describing continues, incorporating updates on where the urge resides and how it feels, until the urge ends. Instead of getting swept away in the wave of the urge, the client remains grounded due to mindfulness of their bodily experience rather than attachment to pleasurable qualities of or cognitive distortions about the addictive behavior (Lloyd, 2003). Carroll (1996) integrated self-monitoring into her urge surfing using a 5-column handout in which the client writes down the date of the urge or craving, the triggering event, thoughts, and feelings, the intensity of the urge on a 1–100 scale, the duration of the urge, and coping behaviors (and coping thoughts).

This is an excellent time to pause and remind yourself that the techniques presented in this chapter should be used toward your clients' overall wellness goals and not just substance use or addictive behaviors. In fact, clients and clinicians should constantly look for instances in which a technique can be used to target substance use or addictive behavior *and* other wellness goals. For example, the client may discover a belief or cognitive distortion that not only has resulted in relapse regarding their substance use but also relates to their mood disorder or connection wellness. Therefore, it is advisable, when appropriate, for the clinician to ask

- In what other dimensions of your life does _____ issue show up?
- How can your insights from this activity/discussion be applied to other areas of your life?
- Now that you are noticing progress from using this activity/approach, what other dimensions of wellness have benefited from using this approach to address _____?

Further, several of these activities can be used to address addictive behaviors as well as other mental health and wellness concerns. Urge surfing, for instance, may be able to generalize to other urges a client may experience such as a client working on a dimension of wellness and seeking to manage desires to engage in behavior incongruent with their behavior goals.

Cognitive Stimulation

Intellectual or cognitive stimulation is another important facet of mental wellness. Participating in activities that captivate the mind and provide meaning affects one's level of wellness. Marlatt and others have noted this in their work, and there are areas of study dedicated to research exploring the benefits of stimulating activity ranging from leisure science scholarship to positive psychology literature. Evidence for the role of meaningful stimulation for individuals with SUDs is no different. For example, multiple researchers have reported correlations between boredom and increased substance use (e.g., Berg et al., 2019). Additionally, employment is a significant factor in reducing substance use (e.g., Henkel, 2011), and working can be a flow activity (Csikszentmihalyi, 2014).

Flow

Flow can be defined as "a subjective state people report when they are completely involved in something to the point of forgetting time, fatigue, and everything else but the activity itself" (Csikszentmihalyi, 2009, p. 394). We have included Flow in the Mind chapter because of the association between Flow and cognition. Pursuits that induce flow states capture attention, which is needed for goal attainment. Flow is possible when (a) the purpose of the activity is evident, (b) the activity is attainable, and (c) feedback is built into the activity (Csikszentmihalyi, 2014).

Researchers are beginning to uncover a link between flow and behavioral addiction. For example, a study on gaming addiction revealed that one of the aspects of flow, "distortion of time perception when playing the game", was a predictor of the intensity of addictive engagement with a game played prior to survey participation (Hull, Williams, & Griffiths,

2013, p. 148). It is thus possible that flow can be constructive or destructive. It is also plausible that deficits in constructive flow can precipitate seeking flow from potentially destructive behaviors or substances. This notion has some empirical support given research showing boredom as a risk factor for addictive engagement with the internet (Wang, 2019).

The WBAC clinician would thus do well to assist their clients in identifying healthy opportunities for flow. Ragheb (1980) divided leisure activities into mass media, sports, social, cultural, outdoor, and hobbies (Perkins & Nakamura, 2013). The clinician can present these areas to the client who can note the activities they are already involved in that fit in each leisure type and rate the level of satisfaction derived from each activity. Client and clinician can brainstorm activities from among the leisure types that the client would like to try. The clinician then helps the client select one or two activities, make plans regarding the frequency and duration of weekly involvement, and rate their wellness prior to and after the activity.

We recommend that the clinician and client evaluate the client's current leisure activities and note the ratio of time engaged in passive leisure (e.g., watching television) to active leisure activities (e.g., participating in one's hobby of restoring classic cars). Csikszentmihalyi (1997) contends that passive leisure can be helpful in moderation and harmful if used to the exclusion of active leisure. This should be considered as the client develops their weekly leisure plans. The clinician can inform the client that, at times, it may not feel worth it to muster the increased effort for active leisure as opposed to passive; however, if the client can follow through with the activity, they stand to gain more meaning and pleasure (Csikszentmihalyi, 1997). To concretize this concept, the clinician can have the client rate their mood, stress level, or well-being before and after activities, comparing personal passive versus active leisure outcomes.

Additionally, the flow concept allows for meaningful discussion about the role of substance use in the client's life. For example, the client can process ways in which their addictive behavior was similar or dissimilar to the definition of flow experiences. The clinician can inquire, "In what ways did your addictive behavior temporarily grab your attention to the point of taking away your feelings of stress and boredom?" and "In what ways was your addictive behavior like passive leisure, for instance, making you feel relaxed?" The clinician then normalizes that the similarities between addictive behaviors and flow are part of what makes these activities so addictive. The conversation can now shift to ways in which addictive behavior is actually false flow. The clinician does this by eliciting examples of how over time, the addictive behavior becomes less compelling, causes negative thoughts and feelings, impedes their ability to pursue other leisure, flow, and meaningful experiences, and does not compel them to apply their skills. These developments are in stark contrast to the outcomes from health flow experiences.

Some clients may benefit from processing the difficulty of abstaining or pursuing harm reduction because the addictive behavior appeared to enhance their ability to experience genuine flow. For instance, individuals with co-occurring concerns who experience anxiety may have found that the substance use erased some of their anxiety so that they could become engrossed in the activity at hand. Learning that this perceived enhancement of flow delivered this added benefit can normalize why it can be extremely difficult to change one's behavior. The clinician can then point to this as another example of false flow by asking about the adverse consequences that ensued over time for the client and about positive flow experiences when the person is not under the influence of an addictive behavior. Clients may report that it is more gratifying to long-term wellness when they can achieve flow without the use of a mind-altering substance.

Employment

As noted earlier, employment can be a key component of recovery. It serves multiple pur-poses of potentially alleviating boredom, reducing exposure to triggers, providing mental stimulation and flow experiences, meaning, self-esteem, and the finances to support improv-ing wellness across other dimensions. Csikszentmihalyi's recommendations for enhancing flow at work include being mindful of all actions that accompany one's duties and reflecting on the following:

- Is this step necessary?
- Who needs it?
- If it is really necessary, can it be done better, faster, and more efficiently?
- What additional steps could make my contribution more valuable? (1997, p. 104)

For these reasons and more, employment is a significant aspect of recovery capital and men-tal wellness.

Brain-Based Approaches in Working with Addictions

There are several atheoretical strategies for working with clients in recovery from a brain-based, or neuroscience, perspective. Like the mental wellness strategies discussed earlier, these can offer clients an alternative narrative related to their addiction and recovery, pro-mote neuroplasticity, and encourage positive habit formation that can substitute for con-suming drugs. They also can be combined with any theoretical counseling approach. The WBAC clinician has a bevy of options in their application of approaches to promote brain and mental wellness.

1. Neuroeducation (Miller & Beeson, 2021). Neuroeducation simply means educating clients about neuroscientific concepts related to addiction. For example, clients can be taught how the reward center of the brain becomes compromised with addiction, leading to ever-increasing intensity of craving. They also can be taught the principles of neuroplasticity, to encourage changes in behavioral habits to promote healing. Neuroeducation does not need to be intricate and complicated. Basic, easily understandable concepts can be shared with clients without overly technical language or discussions about complex research. In my (Todd) experience, I had to overcome the fear that discussions of neuroscience would be seen as uninteresting or not applicable; however, the more I discussed brain-based issues with students and clients, the more interested they became. Several great resources online can help you articulate neurosci-entific concepts to your clients, starting with the online publication, *Drugs, Brains, and Behavior: The Science of Addiction* (National Institute on Drug Abuse [NIDA], 2020).

2. Stress Management and Coping. Stress plays a key role in substance addiction and relapse (Worden, 2015). This is primarily because stress releases a brain chemical called corticotropin-releasing factor (CRF; Worden). CRF, in turn, releases dopamine, which is implicated in seeking reward. As such, a person who is under stress may seek the reward of drugs to lower levels of stress (Koob & LeMoal, 2005, as cited in Worden). This process makes sense, because for those addicted to drugs, the craving from the dopamine release will lead to an automatic desire for substances (Worden). The takeaway from this process is that stress needs to be managed for those to have a successful recovery. Of course, that is easier said than done, given that stress not only can contribute to substance use but result from it as well.

Stress and craving can also negatively impact the prefrontal cortex and frontal lobe functioning (Worden, 2015). This region of the brain is responsible for our human characteristics: reasoning, judgment, making rational choices, and emotional regulation (Worden). This condition leads to *hypofrontality*, which is characterized by deficits in judgment and making long-term, sustainable decisions. In other words, a person under stress feels compelled to seek short-term, more reckless goals, instead of longer term, life objectives (Worden). This explains why many individuals struggling with addiction make rash, impulsive decisions to misuse substances seemingly without any forethought.

Stress also has an impact on our central and peripheral nervous systems. The central nervous system comprises the brain and spinal cord. However, our focus here is on a subdivision of the peripheral nervous system: the autonomic nervous system (ANS). The ANS is further subdivided into the sympathetic and parasympathetic divisions. The sympathetic division houses the body's fight-or-flight response to stress. That is, when one experiences real or imagined stress, the sympathetic nervous system kicks in by directing the release of stress hormones (e.g., cortisol) and increasing heart and breathing rates. This is all a very natural and important process for our survival. Problems develop, however, when our bodies are in a constant state of stress, which can take a toll on all the systems of the body, including the brain and mind, leading to compromises in functioning and wellness.

The amount of stress one experiences with a substance use disorder can be mind-boggling. For example, substance use itself is a significant stressor, and on top of this is the stress from dysfunctional relationships, poor job performance, anxiety, financial concerns, health challenges, and ever-increasing isolation. The constant release of cortisol can damage body systems and organs over time. In other words, individuals struggling with addiction live with too much "sympathetic tone", which means their sympathetic nervous system is on overdrive, leading to a vicious cycle of pain, addiction, more pain, etc. (Nakken, 1996). This impacts all dimensions of wellness, including mental wellness.

Stress management techniques can help clients cope with daily stressors and emotional dysregulation, quiet their sympathetic nervous systems, and promote more parasympathetic functioning. Such activities are often called *bottom-up neuromodulation* because they are designed to calm the deeper limbic structures of the brain (Gintner, 2021). Strategies such as deep, diaphragmatic breathing, meditation, yoga, and listening to relaxing music are examples of activities to accomplish these goals (Canbeyli, 2013, as cited in Ginter). Bottom-up neuromodulation are also excellent strategies to start treatment with as they "set the stage" for more top-down activities, such as cognitive restructuring and CBT (Gintner). With a more relaxed nervous system, clients are in a better position to make healthier choices in accordance with their recovery plans. Stress no longer becomes such an intense trigger for relapse; in a more relaxed state, a person can calmly evaluate situations and turn to healthier coping skills.

3. Associate Dopamine with Natural Rewarding Activities. As noted above, the reward center of the brain becomes hijacked due to continued substance use. This is due to the unnatural flood of dopamine, ultimately leading to a combination of a numbed pleasure response with heightened experiences of craving. Natural, everyday rewards no longer produce feelings of joy and pleasure. A key task of addiction treatment, then, is to help clients reset their reward/motivational system (Worden, 2015).

The first step to accomplish this is for clients to remain abstinent from substances (or adherent to an ideal use plan of reduced and non-addictive substance use) and engage fully in the recovery process. The client and counselor can then explore alternative activities the client enjoys (or used to enjoy). Focus should be placed on creating a rewarding life without substances and enhancing life satisfaction (Worden, 2015). Some themes to consider include helping the client to feel safe, increasing leisure, finding ways to be productive, and working on building resilience. Resilience encompasses six dimensions, including (a) vision (sense of meaning, goals); (b) composure (staying calm, focused); (c) reasoning (creativity, planning for difficulties); (d) tenacity (persistence); (e) collaboration (social connections and skills); and (f) health (bodily wellness; Rossouw, 2021). According to Rossouw, building resilience strengthens the prefrontal cortex so that it does not become overwhelmed by signals from the deeper, more primitive regions of the brain (i.e., limbic brain). A stronger prefrontal cortex means more rational choices rather than operating completely on emotional processes.

Due to neuroplasticity, over time new neural pathways and connections are made, old connections are pruned, new habits are formed, and the client begins to reclaim the natural joys of living a well-lived life.

4. Pivot Towards Your Values (Hayes, 2019). Acceptance and Commitment Therapy (ACT) has had a significant impact on the counseling and psychotherapy world. ACT is considered a "third wave" intervention strategy (Ohrt et al., 2019) that builds on previous psychoanalytic, cognitive, and behavioral approaches (although in many ways ACT is an improvement on what Hayes views as inadequacies within the traditional CBT approach). A review of the ACT approach is beyond the scope of this chapter; however, the concept of "cognitive flexibility" is a useful construct for those struggling with addiction. Cognitive flexibility can be established by helping clients accept rather than avoid, as avoidance (of life experiences) is a potent trigger for substance use (Hayes). For example, when clients experience a negative emotion, they are instructed to accept the feeling rather than avoid it. One strategy is to help clients "sit with" an emotion, exploring where it is in the body, and what it looks and feels like. If the client can give it a voice, what would it say? This type of emotional processing encourages clients to complete the gestalt contact cycle with their emotions allowing them to emerge, rise, and then dissipate over time. This process is far different than avoiding or covering up emotions through distractions, such as substance use. Once the distractions are removed, the difficult, intense emotions are still there, prompting the person to return to substance use. Another strategy to achieve cognitive flexibility is acting according to your values. We can't think of a more relevant action for clients struggling with addiction to consider than engaging in behaviors that are consistent with what is important to them. Indeed, Hayes (2019) noted that of all the ACT processes to encourage cognitive flexibility, focusing on one's values should be a consistent practice as clients work on other cognitive and behavioral skills. This is because seeing how substance use is precluding one from living their highest values can be a powerful motivator to endure the occasional painful parts of the recovery process (Hayes).

The previous cognitive and brain-based strategies can be implemented within the WBAC approach. The goals of their use are not only to strengthen mental wellness but also to promote holistic wellness. We would now like to turn to our case study and show how mental wellness strategies can be incorporated into the case of Eric.

CLIENT EXAMPLE

Eric would benefit from interventions to help with the mental wellness dimension, which in turn will help with his alcohol consumption, especially cravings. One of the first issues that sticks out in the case is Eric's level of stress. Bottom-up neuroadaptation strategies, such as deep, diaphragmatic breathing, meditation, and/or yoga could be implemented to help calm Eric's overactive sympathetic nervous system and establish a calmer presence in his life. This enhanced relaxation will help Eric make better choices when it comes to relating to his family, work, and drinking.

Another strategy that would help Eric is turning toward his values. It is clear from the case that Eric values his family and wants to have strong, positive relationships with his wife, daughter, and father. He values hard work and providing for his family. The WBAC clinician could explore with Eric other values that he holds in high regard, perhaps through a values clarification exercise. In this exercise, Eric could be presented with several values, and he could pick out the top five or ten that resonate most with him. Once his top values are established, the clinician can explore how his current drinking and associated consequences fit or do not fit with his current values. From this exercise, Eric may see the disconnect between his behaviors and values and be encouraged to pivot more toward living his life according to his highest ideals. Such an activity contributes to cognitive flexibility, giving Eric the motivation he needs to persevere through the rough patches of recovery.

Eric has made several attempts to stop or cut down on his drinking. However, he also has relapsed several times due to cravings for alcohol, especially when he is stressed. Recently, his drinking has increased because of stressors both at home and at work. A third mental wellness intervention that would be beneficial to Eric would be to establish a mindfulness practice, with an emphasis on urge surfing. Because stress can exacerbate cravings for alcohol, Eric could be taught mindfulness and self-monitoring using the 5-column handout (Carroll, 1996). In this handout, Eric would write down when he experienced a craving, the preceding event that triggered this craving, his thoughts and feelings going on at the time of the craving, the intensity of the craving on a scale of 1–100, how long the craving lasted, and what coping behaviors he implemented. An example of the five-column technique is shown in Table 7.2.

Table 7.2 Example of the 5-Column Technique in the Case of Eric

Date	Column 1 Precipitating Event	Column 2 Thoughts and Feelings	Column 3 Craving Intensity (1–100)	Column 4 Length of Craving	Column 5 Coping Behaviors
6/4/22	Fight with Kelly	I am going to lose her; why can't I get my life figured out; anxiety	85	About 12 minutes	Deep breathing, Urge surfing
7/2/22	Overdraft in bank account	I am failing my family; thoughts of miscarriage were triggered; deep sadness	90	About 10 minutes	Pivoting toward values; challenging automatic negative thoughts

In addition to addressing Eric's stress level, urge surfing, and mindfulness, cognitive-behavioral strategies as outlined above would be useful to build Eric's mental wellness. Consider the vignette below which outlines several of these techniques.

CLINICIAN: You mentioned that you had a close call this past week to drinking. We will definitely explore how you were able to remain abstinent in spite of the strong cravings that you mentioned. But first…. I was struck by the tone of your voice when you shared about the close call. You sound, "down". [Preparing to explore the thoughts associated with his affect].

ERIC: I'm alright. It's just that I feel like I relapsed even though I didn't. And I'm disappointed in myself that I let myself get so close to that line. I just feel like…….

CLINICIAN: What are you saying to yourself at this moment? [eliciting self-talk].

ERIC: That I'm not strong…. It's ridiculous that I'm still craving and almost drank. I'm going to mess up my wellness plan and the progress I've made at home.

CLINICIAN: Let's tease apart this thought. "I'm not strong". How is that thought affecting you or how could it affect you in mind, body, spirit, emotion, connection? [Explore the Consequence portion of the ABC model].

ERIC: Like you said, it must be affecting my mood. It's affecting my feelings, because at this moment, I kinda want to quit on my wellness plan. I was thinking like this yesterday and at the time I didn't want to be around Kelly or Lia and when I was, I was not present and I said some mean things.

CLINICIAN: So holding onto this thought affected your wellness in multiple ways including your emotional wellness and connection wellness [reflection linking the thoughts to their wellness consequences].

ERIC: Yes. Absolutely.

CLINICIAN: Let me challenge you, Eric. Given that these particular thoughts have not been wellness-enhancing for you, can you come up with a more helpful thought with which to challenge the thought of "I'm not strong"?

ERIC: I'm stuck. I'm not really sure what would be a good challenge thought.

CLINICIAN: We recently talked about the effects of substances on the brain and it seemed to hit home for you in a big way. I'm wondering if any ideas from these discussions could help you identify a challenge thought.

ERIC: I remember some of the things you said about addiction and the brain. You said that cravings are out of my control and that they're normal. The brain is trying to heal and it's easy for triggers to happen.

CLINICIAN: OK. Put those ideas into a thought that will hold some real power when the thought of "I'm not strong" pops up.

ERIC: Cravings are a part of recovery. I have done things in my life that show me I can be a strong person

CLINICIAN: Now, I'll sit quietly and I'd like you to say that thought to yourself a few times. [Clinician will then ask the client about any positive effects from the thought disputation and any potential positive effects on their wellness if they utilize this thought outside of session when less helpful thoughts occur].

CONCLUSION

Mental wellness is a vast dimension for exploration and intervention with your clients. Constructs in mental wellness range from mental stimulation to brain health. Discussions with your clients about brain changes that manifest through addiction and recovery can transform into an empowering resource. Cognitive-behavioral techniques that direct clients to take a closer look at their thoughts and to challenge ones that are not helpful have been methodically researched. However, WBAC complements these approaches as clients can now use the dimensions of wellness as cues for the occurrence of negative thoughts and recognize the holistic impact of negative and positive thoughts.

The above examples with Eric demonstrate how the cognitive-behavioral interventions employed in mental wellness work can be the difference between maintaining and abandoning one's wellness goals. Conversely, traditional cognitive-behavioral techniques can be mobilized toward increasing wellness across dimensions. Lastly, the positive psychology concept of flow is critical to mental wellness. When you interface with your clients, ask yourself, "what flow activities does this person engage in? How often do they engage in these activities? In what ways are they seeking flow that result in decreased wellness?"

Handout 7.1   Wellness-Based Thought Disputation

Antecedents	Beliefs	Wellness Consequences	Disputation	Effect (Current or Possible)
		Mental: Physical: Emotional: Spiritual: Connection:		Mental: Physical: Emotional: Spiritual: Connection:
		Mental: Physical: Emotional: Spiritual: Connection:		Mental: Physical: Emotional: Spiritual: Connection:
		Mental: Physical: Emotional: Spiritual: Connection:		Mental: Physical: Emotional: Spiritual: Connection:
		Mental: Physical: Emotional: Spiritual Connection:		Mental: Physical: Emotional: Spiritual: Connection:

Handout 7.2 5-Column Technique

Date	Column 1 Precipitating Event	Column 2 Thoughts and Feelings	Column 3 Craving Intensity (1-100)	Column 4 Length of Craving	Column 5 Coping Behaviors
6/4/22	Fight with Kelly	I am going to lose her; why can't I get my life figured out; anxiety	85	About 12 minutes	Deep breathing, Urge surfing
7/2/22	Overdraft in bank account	I am failing my family; thoughts of miscarriage were triggered; deep sadness	90	About 10 minutes	Pivoting toward values; challenging automatic negative thoughts

REFERENCES

American Psychiatric Association (2022). *Diagnostic and statistical manual of mental disorders* (5th ed., text rev.). American Psychiatric Association.

Barriga, A. Q., Gibbs, J. C., Potter, G. B., & Liau, A. K. (2001). *How I think (HIT) questionnaire manual*. Champaign, IL: Research Press.

Beck, A. T. (1976). *Cognitive therapy and the emotional disorders*. Meridian/Penguin Group.

Beck, J. S. (2011). *Cognitive behavior therapy: Basics and beyond* (2nd ed.). Guilford Press.

Beck, J. S. (2021). *Cognitive behavior therapy: Basics and beyond* (3rd ed.). Guilford Press.

Berg, C. J., Haardörfer, R., Payne, J. B., Getachew, B., Vu, M., Guttentag, A., & Kirchner, T. R. (2019). Ecological momentary assessment of various tobacco product use among young adults. *Addictive Behaviors, 92,* 38–46. https://doi.org/10.1016/j.addbeh.2018.12.014

Bowen, S., Chawla, N., Grow, J., & Marlatt, G. A. (2021). *Mindfulness-based relapse prevention for addictive behaviors: A clinician's guide* (2nd ed). Guilford Press.

Brown-Rice, K., & Moro, R. R. (2018). Biological theory: Genetics and brain chemistry. In P. S. Lassiter & J. R. Culbreth (Eds.), *Theory and Practice of Addiction Counseling* (pp. 47–75). Sage.

Burns, D. D. (1999). *Feeling good: The new mood therapy*. Harper Collins.

Canbeyli, R. (2013). Sensorimotor modulation of mood and depression: In search of an optimal mode of stimulation. *Frontiers in Human Neuroscience, 7,* 428. https://doi.org/10.3389/fnhum.2013.00428

Carroll, K. M. (1996). *Cognitive-behavioral coping skills treatment for cocaine dependence*. Yale University Psychotherapy Development Center Substance Abuse Center.

Cramer, S. C., Sur, M., Dobkin, B. H., O'Brien, C., Sanger, T. D., Trojanowski, J. Q., Rumsey, J. M., Ramona, H., Cameron, J., Chen, D., Chen, W. G., Cohen, L. G., DeCharms, C., Duffy, C. J., Guinevere, E. F., Fetz, E. E., Filart, R., Freund, M., Grant, S. J., Haber, S., Kalivas, P. W., … Vinogradov (2011). Harnessing neuroplasticity for clinical applications. *Brain, 134*, 1591–1609.

Csikszentmihalyi, M. (1997). *Finding flow: The psychology of engagement with everyday life*. Basic Books.

Csikszentmihalyi, M. (2009). Flow. In S. Lopez (Ed.), *The encyclopedia of positive psychology* (pp. 394–400). Blackwell Publishing Ltd.

Csikszentmihalyi, M. (2014). *Flow and the foundations of positive psychology: The collected works of Mihaly Csikszentmihalyi*. Springer.

Ellis, A. (1991). The revised ABC's of rational-emotive therapy (RET). *Journal of Rational Emotive and Cognitive-Behavior Therapy, 9*(3), 139–172.

Field, T. A., Jones, L. K., & Russell-Chapin, L. A. (2017). *Neurocounseling: Brain based clinical approaches*. American Counseling Association.

Freeman, A., & DeWolf, R. (1992). *The 10 dumbest mistakes smart people make and how to avoid them*. HarperCollins.

Freeman, A., & Oster, C. (1999). Cognitive behavior therapy. In M. Hersen & A. S. Bellack (Eds.), *Handbook of comparative interventions for adult disorders* (2nd ed., pp. 108–138). Wiley.

Galvan, A. (2010). Neural plasticity of development and learning. *Human Brain Mapping, 31*, 879–890. https://doi.org/10.1002/hbm.21029

Gintner, G. (2021). Bottom-up neuromodulation: Calming from below. In R. Miller & E. T. Beeson (Eds.), *The neuroeducation toolbox: Practical translations of neuroscience in counseling and psychotherapy* (pp. 243–251). Cognella.

Goldstein, R. Z., & Volkow, N. D. (2011). Dysfunction of the prefrontal cortex in addiction: Neuroimaging findings and clinical implications. *Nature Reviews Neuroscience, 12*, 652–669.

Graham, H. L. (2004). *Cognitive-behavioural integrated treatment (C-BIT): A treatment manual for substance misuse in people with severe mental health problems*. John Wiley & Sons.

Hanson, R. (2011). *Buddha's brain: The practical neuroscience of happiness, love, and wisdom*. PESI Seminars.

Harris, J. S., Stewart, D. G., & Stanton, B. C. (2017). Urge surfing as aftercare in adolescent alcohol use: A randomized control trial. *Mindfulness, 8*, 144–149.

Hayes, S. C. (2019). *A liberated mind: How to pivot toward what matters*. Avery.

Henkel, D. (2011). Unemployment and substance use: A review of the literature (1990 2010). *Current Drug Abuse Reviews, 4*(1), 4–27.

Hollon, S. D. & Kendall, P. C. (1980). Cognitive self-statements in depression: Development of an automatic thoughts questionnaire. *Cognitive Therapy and Research, 4*, 383–395.

Hull, D. C., Williams, G. A., & Griffiths, M. D. (2013). Video game characteristics, happiness and flow as predictors of addiction among video game players: A pilot study. *Journal of Behavioral Addictions, 2*(3), 145–152. https://doi.org/10.1556/jba.2.2013.005

Ito, J. R., McNair, L., Donovan, D. M., & Marlatt, G.A. (1984). *Relapse prevention for alcoholism aftercare: Treatment manual*. Unpublished manuscript, Health Services Research and Development Service, VA Medical Center.

Jones, L. K. (2017). Anatomy and brain development. In T. A. Field, L. K. Jones, & L. A. Russell-Chapin (Eds.), *Neurocounseling: Brain based clinical approaches* (pp. 19–43). American Counseling Association.

Koob, G. F., & Le Moal, M. (2005). Plasticity of reward neurocircuitry and the 'dark side' of drug addiction. *Nature Neuroscience, 8*(11), 1442–1444.

Kuhn, C., Swartzwelder, S., & Wilson, W. (2019). *Buzzed: The straight facts about the most used and abused drugs from alcohol to ecstasy* (5th ed.). W.W. Norton & Company.

Kuyken, W., Padesky, C. A., & Dudley, R. (2009). *Collaborative case conceptualization: Working effectively with clients in cognitive-behavioral therapy*. Guilford Press.

Lewis, T. F. (2023). *Substance abuse and addiction treatment: Practical application of counseling theory* (2nd ed.). Cognella.

Liese, B. S., & Beck, A. T. (2022). *Cognitive-behavioral therapy of addictive disorders*. Guilford Press.

Lloyd, A. (2003). Urge surfing. In W. O'Donohue, J. E. Fisher, & S.C. Hayes (Eds.), *Cognitive behavior therapy: Applying empirically supported techniques in your practice* (pp. 451–455). John Wiley & Sons, Inc.

Marlatt, G. A. (1985). Relapse prevention: Theoretical rationale and overview of the model. In G. A. Marlatt & J. R. Gordon (Eds.), *Relapse prevention: Maintenance strategies in the treatment of addictive behaviors* (pp. 3–70). Guilford Press.

Miller, R., & Beeson, E. T. (2021). *The neuroeducation toolbox: Practical translations of neuroscience in counseling and psychotherapy*. Cognella.

Mitcheson, L., Maslin, J., Meynen, T., Morrison, T., Hill, R., & Wanigaratne, S. (2010). *Applied cognitive and behavioural approaches to the treatment of addiction: A practical treatment guide*. John Wiley & Sons.

Najavits, L. M. (1993). *Cognitive distortions scale*. Unpublished measure. Harvard Medical School/McLean Hospital, Boston, MA.

Najavits, L. M., Gotthardt, S., Weiss, R. D., & Epstein, M. (2004). Cognitive distortions in the dual diagnosis of PTSD and substance use disorder. *Cognitive Therapy and Research, 28*, 159–172.

National Institute on Drug Abuse [NIDA] (2020). *Drugs, brain, and behavior: The science of addiction*. Retrieved from https://nida.nih.gov/publications/drugs-brains-behavior-science-addiction/preface on 2022, June 6.

Ohrt, J. H., Clarke, P. B., Conley, A. H. (2019). *Wellness counseling: A holistic approach to prevention and intervention*. American Counseling Association.

Parvaz, M. A., Moeller, S. J., d'Oleire Uquillas, F., Pflumm, A., Maloney, T., Alia-Klein, N., & Goldstein, R. Z. (2016). Prefrontal gray matter volume recovery in treatment-seeking cocaine-addicted individuals: A longitudinal study. *Addiction Biology, 22*, 1391–1401.

Perkins, K., & Nakamura, J. (2013). Flow and leisure. In T. Freire (Ed.), *Positive leisure science: From subjective experience to social contexts* (pp. 141–157). Springer.

Plotnik, R. (1996). *Introduction to psychology* (4th ed.). Cengage Learning.

Polk, T. A. (2015). *The addictive brain*. The Teaching Company.

Ragheb, M. G. (1980). Interrelationships among leisure participation leisure satisfaction and leisure attitudes. *Journal of Leisure Research, 12*(2), 138–149. https://doi.org/10.1080/0022221 6.1980.11969433

Rossouw, J. (2021). Advancing despite adversity: Building neuro-informed resilience. In R. Miller & E. T. Beeson (Eds.), *The neuroeducation toolbox: Practical translations of neuroscience in counseling and psychotherapy* (pp. 60–69). Cognella.

Russell-Chapin, L. A. (2016). Integrating neurocounseling into the counseling profession: An introduction. *Journal of Mental Health Counseling, 38*(2), 93–102.

Scully, K. (2022). *10 executive functioning skills: The ultimate guide*. Retrieved from https://www.thepathway2success.com/10-executive-functioning-skills-the-ultimate-guide/.

Thombs, D. L., & Osborn, C. J. (2019). *Introduction to addictive behaviors* (5th ed.). Guilford.

Wang, W. C. (2019). Exploring the relationship among free-time management, leisure boredom, and internet addiction in undergraduates in Taiwan. *Psychological Reports, 122*(5), 1651–1665. doi:10.1177/0033294118789034

Worden, T. (2015). *The neurobiology of addiction and brain-based relapse prevention* (PESI Seminar). PESI, Inc.

Yurica, C. L., & DiTomasso, R. A. (2005). Cognitive distortions. In A. F. Freeman, S. H. Felgoise, A. M. Nezu, C. M. Nezu, & M. A. Reinecke (Eds.), *Encyclopedia of cognitive behavior therapy* (pp. 117–122). Springer.

CHAPTER 8

BODY WELLNESS: NURTURING THE INSTRUMENT OF RECOVERY

INTRODUCTION

Of all domains of wellness, the impact of substance addiction on the body is probably the most understood. From the effects on brain integrity and functioning, to problems with multiple physiological systems (e.g., cardiovascular), substance addiction has the potential to cause irreparable damage to the physical body. A body out of balance is a body that is compromised and in pain, and this compromise becomes a central reason for continued use. Substance addiction often results in poor health, which is a strain on the body (Ford, 2014); that is, a significant stressor that has an enormous influence on our physical integrity. Sadly, the body is often neglected within the ravages of addiction and is ignored as a foundation of recovery. In WBAC, we are committed to helping clients reclaim their lives and find inner peace and wellness that are on the other side of incapacitating addiction. Body wellness is an important key to this reclamation. Through proper nutrition, exercise, and quality sleep, there is no limit to the potential for personal growth and meaningful recovery. In this chapter, we dive into the topic of body wellness and its implications for helping clients reduce or abstain from substances and thrive in recovery. We first define body wellness and then explore typical resistances to physical health. The topic then turns to nutrition, physical activity, and sleep as important conduits to body wellness. Finally, we end the chapter with sample protocols and a brief case study.

DEFINING BODY WELLNESS IN RECOVERY

Ohrt, Clarke, and Conley (2019) defined body wellness as, "growth toward intentional behaviors and thought processes related to integrating how you nourish, move, and express gratitude toward your body" (p. 71). As such, the components of body wellness include nutrition, physical activity, and body image. Although body image is considered an internal phenomenon (i.e., how a person feels about his or her body), it can have an enormous impact on one's physical health (Ohrt et al., 2019). Applied to addiction, we can expand the body wellness definition to include behaviors and thoughts specifically designed to recover and heal the body from the misuse of harmful substances.

In WBAC, the body is the first place we look to start the healing and recovery process. Clinicians focus on helping clients cut down or eliminate harmful drugs from their lives, establish important support systems, and encourage healthy activities to assist them in feeling physically better. As the body begins to recover, other factors of wellness start to improve. The interplay of physical, emotional, mental, and spiritual wellness builds on each other to create momentum in recovery. Indeed, body wellness is a logical place to begin in helping clients on the road to recovery. This includes exploring topics such as the physical fall-out of drug use, psychoeducation on the bodily dangers of use, the importance of nutrition, physical activity, and sleep, and the connection between body wellness and the other wellness

DOI: 10.4324/9781003147954-8

The Addictive Cycle

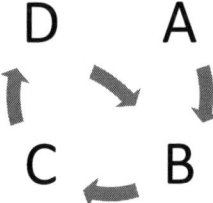

A = pain (physical or mental); B = feel pressure to use; C = use, start to feel relief; D = pain resulting from using (e.g., guilt, fear, more physical pain); B = feel pressure to use; C = use, start to feel relief, etc.

Figure 8.1 The Addictive Cycle.

factors. However, before we can begin to help clients physically heal from the effects of addiction, we need to address some of the typical resistances to body wellness.

RESISTANCE TO BODY WELLNESS

Clients with substance use disorders sacrifice body wellness for the sake of assuaging deep-seated pain, whether physical or emotional (Nakken, 1996). Pain sets off an addictive cycle, which can spiral out of control, leading to more pain (see Figure 8.1; Nakken). The urge to cover up pain becomes so strong that individuals resist efforts to promote body wellness – nutrition suffers, physical activity declines, and body image, integrity, and self-esteem deteriorate. Resistance to body wellness is inherent in the addictive process because the most important issue for those struggling with addiction is avoiding pain, no matter the physical costs and other consequences.

In WBAC, we strive to interrupt the addictive cycle by embracing body wellness as a conduit to overall wellness. Through small successes, clients come to learn how physical well-being provides the undergirding for a life well-lived. From a foundation of body wellness, we can then explore deeper emotional and cognitive issues that also play a role in maintaining an addiction.

The Body as a Road to Recovery

Healing the body from the ravages of substance use begins when the chemical is no longer causing damage in the body's systems. Because the body has adapted to the ingestion of drugs through physical tolerance, cessation of chemical use usually brings about withdrawal symptoms. Withdrawal symptoms, unfortunately, can be so unpleasant that they serve as a primary negative reinforcement for why clients relapse. That is, client's major aim is to avoid the pain of withdrawal, usually by relapsing or continuing to use. Withdrawal is a critical time in the recovery process for clients to receive support (including medical supervision, if necessary).

With nutrition, physical activity, and sleep as the foundation for physical recovery from addiction, alternative and complementary therapies, such as yoga, therapeutic touch, meditation, energy work, and massage, also can assist in helping to strengthen body systems.

In WBAC, we actively explore and consider many different paths to body wellness through psychoeducation, collaboration, and counseling. Indeed, proper recovery and care of the body are considered a foundation to the road to recovery. However, when the body is out of balance, clients can take a detour on that road and move straight on to relapse. Let us now explore the common body-based relapse triggers.

Body-Based Relapse Triggers

A *relapse trigger* is an experience that places a person at risk for relapsing into pre-treatment levels of substance use. In general, there are two types of relapse triggers: intrapersonal-environmental and interpersonal. In this chapter, we will focus on intrapersonal-environmental triggers such as how individuals can cope with negative physical states. Negative physical states place the body out of balance, which leads to symptoms of pain, discomfort, anxiety, agitation, and tension. These experiences also can be exacerbated by negative mental and emotional states. Below, we examine three significant body-based relapse triggers: issues related to blood sugar, physical pain, and physical anxiety, tension, and stress.

Blood Sugar Issues

Blood sugar, or the concentration of glucose found in the blood, is an important indicator of metabolic health and, if disrupted, impacts our physical experiences. According to WebMD (2020), glucose is one of the most important fuel sources for our body when present at normal levels. However, at high levels, it acts as a toxic drain on virtually every bodily system. Particularly hard hit is the pancreas, where the ability to make insulin is compromised. As a result, the pancreas overcompensates by making more insulin (WebMD), but the insulin levels stay too high as the body becomes *insulin resistant* (i.e., insulin loses its ability to shuttle glucose into cells for energy, leaving too much glucose circulating in the blood). Consistently high blood sugar, often manifesting as type 2 diabetes, can create major disruptions in the nervous, circulatory, immune, and other bodily systems. The opposite of high blood sugar, hypoglycemia, is when glucose concentrations in the body are low. Too low blood sugar can lead to feelings of dizziness, anxiety, lack of energy, blurred vision, and body weakness (WebMD). Interestingly, diabetic individuals might experience hypoglycemic symptoms if, in managing their disease, blood sugar drops too low. These issues become more complicated if clients also struggle with a substance addiction: blood sugar levels can lead to physical discomfort, thus triggering relapse and substance use, which can lead to problems with high blood sugar. Managing this bi-directional relationship, although challenging, paves a smoother road to recovery.

Checking in with clients regarding physical issues such as blood sugar levels is an important step in managing this relapse trigger. Clinicians are encouraged to educate clients on the signs and symptoms of high or low blood sugar and explore how these experiences may be a trigger for relapse. For example, if a client experiences signs of hypoglycemia, she may feel irritable and anxious, which may trigger the desire to use a substance to calm her down. The client may erroneously believe that she is simply an "anxious person" when in fact she has chronic low blood sugar in which the body responds with physical anxiety. Encouraging clients to meet with their physicians and working closely with these professionals is consistent with body wellness and the WBAC approach. Managing blood glucose can go a long way in helping individuals better manage their symptoms and reducing the risk of relapse.

Body Pain

Physical pain is another significant trigger for substance use behaviors. Clients who experience substantial body pain seek to escape their experiences by altering how they feel physically. Although body pain can have complex causes, including a combination of physical, emotional, and mental components, many clients with substance use disorders clearly and distinctly feel pain in their bodies. Potter, Prather, and Weiss (2008) found that patients experiencing physical pain within the previous 12 months were more likely to report weekly heroin and narcotics use, as well as increases in depressive symptoms compared to those without physical pain. The researchers concluded that pain assessments may need to be a consistent part of client's substance use disorder (SUD) treatment. In another study, Jakubczyk et al. (2016) found a significant correlation between decreases in perceived levels of physical pain and lower risk of alcohol relapse among a sample of clients from an inpatient alcohol treatment center. These studies highlight that it is not just feeling pain that has implications for substance use; the ability to reduce pain also has a measurable impact on lowering relapse risk.

Inquiring about bodily pain, then, is an important component of assessment, treatment, and recovery. Successful management of pain may help in removing a potential trigger to relapse. Often, however, clients have legitimate medical concerns related to pain and are prescribed pain medication. Unfortunately, most pain medications fall within the opiate class of drugs and are extremely addictive. When I (TFL) worked with clients struggling with pain medication addiction, I was struck by their difficulties in titrating off their medications. The risk of relapse was ever-present. Pain medication was a necessity in their minds, even if their physical pain had significantly lessened. They developed tolerance and found themselves physically dependent on the medications. Helping these clients learn healthy ways to manage pain, manage cravings, and safely withdrawal for prescription pain pills was a major part of our work moving forward.

A full overview of treatment protocols for pain is outside the scope of this book. However, we strongly encourage clinicians to consult with pain specialists if working with clients whose pain symptoms serve as a serious relapse risk. Physicians need to be aware of clients who may be at risk of addiction to monitor prescription pain medication. Although controversial in some circles, opiate agonist medications (e.g., Suboxone and Subutex) have been developed that are much less addictive and ease withdrawal symptoms from opioid substances. Alternative methods for pain reduction, such as acupuncture, relaxation training, and deep breathing, also hold promise for the treatment of pain symptoms. The astute WBAC clinician explores the role of pain in recovery, assesses pain as a relapse trigger, and collaborates with the client and other professionals to establish a pain management and relapse prevention protocol.

Physical Anxiety, Tension, and Stress

Anxiety problems are far more common than once believed (Balch, 2010). In general, anxiety manifests in two ways: as a diffuse, somewhat vague sense of dread (e.g., generalized anxiety disorder), or an intense, strong physical response or experience (e.g., panic disorder or specific phobia). Avoidant behavior is a common adjunct to anxiety, fueled by anticipatory fear of having another anxiety attack or confronting a feared stimulus. Although anxiety is listed as a "mental health disorder", there are concomitant physical symptoms, such as increased heart rate, nervousness, rapid breathing, tightness in chest, and shakiness, that many people describe as uncomfortable. Upwards of 10%–20% of Americans will have a panic attack in their lives, according to Mayo Clinic researchers (Balch). To assuage anxiety, many clients turn to medications or illegal substances, usually in the form of central nervous system depressants (e.g., benzodiazepines, barbiturates).

Anxiety is a significant relapse trigger because it produces uncomfortable sensations that individuals want to avoid or escape. The physical symptoms of panic, for example, can cause some people to fear they are having heart attack, despite having no risk of heart problems. Drugs are a powerful way to lessen the physical symptoms of anxiety, followed by a sense of mental and emotional calm. As with opiate-based medications, however, drugs used to assuage anxiety can be extremely addictive.

In WBAC, we assess for signs of anxiety and its potential to trigger relapse. Clients often use terms such as "stressed", "afraid", "nervous", or "tense" to describe the experience of anxiety. Thankfully, there are numerous alternative, complementary, and effective activities to help clients manage anxiety and associated physical tension. For example, relaxation training, breathwork, meditation, and yoga are some excellent ways to calm the nervous system and mental tension. As the client withdrawals from drug use, anxiety may be an initial symptom to monitor but over time should diminish as physiological balance is restored. There is a strong connection between anxiety and nutritional deficiency (Korn, 2016); a nutrient-dense diet with select supplementation can complement other methods to cope with anxiety. If the client continues to need medication to help manage anxiety, close monitoring and communication with their primary care physician is warranted. If clients in recovery become aware of how anxiety serves as a trigger for relapse, they can be empowered to incorporate wellness-based strategies (as outlined below) to better manage their emotions and recovery.

Watch Out for H.A.L.T.: Reducing Relapse Through Care for the Body

A common refrain within addiction circles is H.A.L.T., meaning that recovering persons should not get too hungry, angry, lonely, and tired. Each of these experiences has a bodily or physical component. For example, although anger is a core emotion, it can manifest physically as tense muscles, stomach discomfort, and tightness in the chest. Of course, all people experience hunger, anger, loneliness, and fatigue from time to time. However, with H.A.L.T., it is the intensity of these experiences that matter. Despite its simplicity, H.A.L.T. can be a useful mnemonic for recovering persons. Clinicians should be aware that any one of these components can create bodily discomfort and place one at heightened risk for relapse.

Taking care of the body's physical needs reduces the intensity of H.A.L.T. For example, eating nutrient-dense meals with select supplementation helps manage the body's nutritional needs, avoiding the "hangry" (i.e., hungry, and angry) experience that may trigger relapse. To effectively deal with H.A.L.T., recovery should include body wellness components with a focus on minimizing or eliminating physical symptoms that place one at risk to reengage with substance use. In the sections below, we consider several body-wellness factors, including nutrition, physical activity, sleep hygiene, and self-care. Approaching these factors, the WBAC counselor operates within an atmosphere of collaboration and compassion. MI philosophy and techniques ground the counselor's approach as body wellness and addiction issues are explored. We now turn to common wellness factors and behaviors that can help clients avoid H.A.L.T., relapse, and associated consequences.

Nutrition

Nutrition has a significant impact on our health and well-being. Indeed, Hippocrates, the father of medicine, memorably stated, "Let food be thy medicine and medicine be thy food". Proper nutrition provides us with the vitamins, minerals, and other nutrients to function optimally. Without these critical nutrients, the body compensates in all sorts of ways, which can eventually lead to breakdown and disease. The Standard American Diet (S.A.D.), filled with too much sugar, saturated fats, and processed foods, has resulted in a nutritional crisis in the United States. This is reflected in the fact that two out of every three Americans are overweight and chronic diseases such as type 2 diabetes continue to rise at alarming rates (Ohrt et al., 2019).

There is an undeniable connection between food and physical and mental health. However, so much information is available through the internet, social media, and other outlets that it can be dizzying to sort through all the (often contradictory) data (Ohrt et al.). WBAC adopts the counseling approach to nutrition and wellness outlined by Ohrt et al., who stated that no matter the dietetic system (e.g., keto, paleo, and raw), the best path forward is for clinicians to gain a foundational knowledge of how food and nutrition contribute to health. Clinicians should avoid focusing on what foods are "taboo" or "bad" with their clients so as not to create more guilt and shame, two emotions that are already high for some individuals with SUDs.

Many clinicianss are reluctant to discuss dietary issues in recovery (Ohrt et al.). In the case of opiate addiction, Chavez and Rigg (2020) noted that addiction providers give little, if any, nutritional information to clients, and this knowledge is seldom incorporated into treatment programs. The reasons for this reluctance often come down to not feeling competent to provide such information or beliefs that providing nutritional information will not work. Whereas it is true that providing dietary advice or developing nutritional treatment programs is outside the practice scope of many mental health professionals, they can make the link between what clients consume and how it impacts their cognitive and emotional well-being (Korn, 2018). Korn noted that nutritional self-care is *psychoeducation*, which fits squarely within clinician skills (see Table 8.1). Clinicians are encouraged to assess their own competency levels and state laws to determine their scope of practice. For example, in some states, the combination of competency, credentials, and state law allows some clinicians s to fully integrate nutritional interventions into their mental health counseling practice (Korn). In others, clinicians may need to promote collaboration by working with and referring to professionals licensed to prescribe and/or administer nutritional programs. Either way, WBAC affirms the vital role clinicians can make in helping clients make important connections between their nutrition, mental health, and substance use behavior.

Unfortunately, negative beliefs about the effectiveness of providing nutritional information to clients in recovery can hinder the process. Specifically, it is not that nutritional assessment and information are unimportant but rather beliefs that clients will not follow through on nutritional recommendations. However, WBAC is well-suited to address issues of low motivation using MI as a foundational technique (and this holds for the remaining body wellness factors discussed below). We advocate inviting clients to consider nutritional aspects into their recovery plan. Making the "food-mood" connection (Korn) is a critical, yet often overlooked, ingredient to helping clients recover from drug use problems.

Table 8.1 Examples of Nutritional Supplements and their Effects on Recovery and Mood[a]

Nutritional Food or Supplement	*Uses*
Bone/broth chicken broth	Alcohol and drug recovery
Lithium orotate	Alcohol recovery and addiction; balancing circadian rhythm; mineral of choice for mood disorders
CDP choline	Cocaine cravings
Myer's cocktail (magnesium, calcium, vitamins B12, B6, C) – intravenous protocol	Overall recovery; helps to jumpstart recovery
Phenibut	Acts on GABA and dopamine receptors; alternative for benzodiazepines; useful for short-term treatment of anxiety
Niacin and niacinamide (Vitamin B3)	Alcohol addiction; depression and anxiety
Ibogaine (from West Africa)	Treatment for opiate addiction
Chromium	Helps with hypoglycemia (low blood sugar) as most individuals with alcohol use disorders are hypoglycemic

Adapted from Korn, L. (2018). Korn, L. (2018). *Certified mental health integrative medicine provider (CMHIMP) training course: Nutritional and integrative medicine for mental health professionals [online course]*. Pesi.com.
[a]Many of the recommended dosages for the supplements in this table vary greatly from client to client. In addition, contraindications with nutritional supplements can occur and may interact with medications or certain medical conditions. Follow all guidelines for recommend dosage levels. For specific recommendations, contraindications, and dosage ranges for your clients, please consult Korn (2016) or a nutritional specialist.

NUTRITION AND ADDICTION

Drug use, and its physical consequences such as metabolic changes, cardiovascular damage, constipation, and weight loss, often leads to nutritional deficiencies and a lifestyle of unhealthy eating devoid of adequate, healthy food (Chavez & Rigg, 2020). These nutritional problems are roadblocks to successful recovery and treatment (Chavez & Rigg). Virtually all addictive substances deplete the body of specific nutrients, although which nutrients are impacted depends on the specific substance (Balch, 2010). For example, barbiturate drugs rob the body of vitamin C, a critical nutrient that detoxifies and reduces drug cravings (Balch). Excessive alcohol drains the body of important nutrients, including the B vitamins, magnesium, and vitamins C, D, E, and K. This may explain why those with severe alcohol addiction struggle with energy production (lack of B vitamins) and weakened immunity (lack of vitamins C, D, E, and K). According to Balch, correcting these nutritional imbalances begins with eating a well-balanced, nutrient-dense diet that emphasizes fresh fruits and vegetables, adding protein to the diet, and avoiding heavily processed food with high levels of sugar and salt. Although processed foods can provide rapid energy, the inevitable blood sugar crash may intensify drug cravings. Guided and smart use of supplements also may help clients regain physical balance in recovery.

Supplementation   As Korn (2018) noted, proper diet is essential but usually not sufficient to meet nutritional needs and optimal functioning. This is especially the case for clients in

Table 8.2 Common Nutritional Supplements and their Recovery Benefits

Supplement	Examples	Health and/or Recovery Benefits[a]
Vitamins	Vitamins A, B complex, C, D, E, and K	*Helps and supports* healthy metabolism; immune system; maintaining cell membrane and structure; production of red blood cells; hair, skin, nails; hormone production; bone development; nervous system
Minerals	Zinc, Selenium, Magnesium, Calcium	*Helps and supports* strong teeth and bones; lowering cholesterol; healthy brain function; the body utilizing various nutrients; regulating blood pressure, heartbeat, and muscle function
Amino Acids	L-tryptophan, L-theanine, L-tyrosine	*Helps and supports* positive mood; muscle growth; strength; skin and hair health; cognitive performance; increased energy
Herbs	Ashwagandha, nettle root, ginseng, ginkgo biloba	*Helps and supports* cognitive function; bowel function; reducing risk of cancer; anti-inflammation; positive mood; cardiovascular health

[a]These are some general health and/or recovery benefits of nutritional supplements in general. Specific benefits are individualized depending on the nutrient (e.g., calcium helps in strengthening bone and teeth) and individual. This list is not exhaustive of all health benefits.

recovery due to potentially severe dietary deficiencies from years of heavy drug use. Nutritional supplements include vitamins, minerals, amino acids, and herbs that can serve to restore, balance, and assist in recovery efforts. As the name suggests, supplements work by *supplementing* existing dietary protocols by filling in any nutritional gaps. They come in many forms, including powders, tinctures, drinks, tablets, and capsules. Supplements can ease withdrawal symptoms, strengthen the body's internal systems, and reduce cravings. In addition, most supplements do not produce the physical dependency that is often the case with medications. Many herbal formulations (e.g., ashwagandha) are *adaptogens*, which work to help the body lower cortisol and adapt to stress. Key supplements and their general health benefits are highlighted in Table 8.2.

Another benefit of supplementation within a recovery wellness plan is it removes the controversy of using medication to treat addiction. For example, Suboxone is a highly effective medication for opiate use disorders, primarily helping clients to reduce cravings. However, Suboxone also has been found to be addictive (American Addiction Centers, 2020); critics argue that the medical community is simply substituting one addiction for another (the same can be said for methadone maintenance programs, where clients consume methadone daily to stave off craving for the more severe drug heroin). Nutritional supplements largely stay out of this argument because the mechanisms of action are natural, slower, and gentler and have a less severe side effect profile.

A complete review of supplementation protocols for addiction, withdrawal, and recovery is outside the scope of this chapter. However, we would like to stress the importance of targeted supplementation as an adjunct in recovery efforts.

A word of caution is warranted at this point. Whereas we are enthusiastic about the potential for nutritional supplements to be a part of any addiction treatment plan in WBAC, we also want to stress that medication for addiction has been shown to be successful at different points in the recovery process. I (TFL) have seen firsthand how effective Suboxone has been with clients struggling with pain pill addiction, despite its mild addictive potential. As such, we are not advocating for the substitution of nutritional supplements in place of medication. Indeed, a valid option for clients in recovery may be a combination of medication and supplementation under the supervision of qualified professionals. However utilized, the synergistic benefit of targeted supplementation and nutrition can be of great value in recovery efforts and promoting wellness.

PROMOTING NUTRITION IN WBAC

We advocate promoting nutritional food and supplementation as an important component of the WBAC recovery plan. As noted earlier, clinicians are within their scope of practice to review, explore, educate, and refer clients for nutritional help if their current credentials and state laws do not allow for primary or autonomous nutritional counseling. Other professional options include certifications, such as the *Certified Mental Health Integrative Medicine Provider* (CMHIMP) credential, that can build upon existing licensures and competencies. Keep in mind that dietary and supplemental protocols are but one portion of a comprehensive wellness plan for recovering clients.

So, what does a nutritional plan (dietary and supplemental) look like for a client in recovery? Based on the work of Korn (2016) and Balch (2010), core nutritional and supplemental protocols form the foundation for general substance use problems. Addiction to specific drugs may need more targeted considerations. As always, unless specifically qualified, mental health professionals are encouraged to consult and work collaboratively with a licensed nutritionist or other integrative professional.

Dietary Recommendations   All clients in recovery are encouraged to follow a nutrient-dense diet emphasizing fresh, whole, and raw foods (plenty of fruits and vegetables; Balch, 2010). A high protein intake is also recommended because protein helps stabilize energy and reduces cravings by naturally increasing dopamine in the body. Processed foods, including all junk foods, are to be avoided. Although these foods provide quick energy, the resulting crash from a sugar rush may increase cravings for drugs (Balch).

Supplemental Recommendations   As noted, a nutritious diet is essential for health but often is not enough; dietary supplements can address many nutritional deficiencies. For optimum mental health during recovery, the following supplements form a core nutritional foundation for a client in recovery from a range of addictive substances. Some of these nutrients may not have a direct effect on addiction but rather promote overall health and well-being as one progresses through recovery. Additional herbs or other supplements can be added as needed and/or depending on the substance (Korn, 2016).[1]

1. *Complex vitamins and minerals with L-methylfolate (Vitamin B9 or folic acid).* Usually, this can be in the form of a multi-vitamin complex. Addresses micronutrient deficiencies. Vitamin B9 has positive effects on mental health, liver health, and cardiovascular function.

2. *Omega 3 fish oil (DHA/EPA).* Promotes heart and brain health. DHA promotes restful sleep.

3. *Gamma linoleic acid (GLA)*. Typically found in seed oils such as borage, evening primrose, and black currant. Positive impacts on blood pressure, depression, fatigue, and back pain.

4. *Free amino acids.* Greatly aids in muscle tissue building, nervous system maintenance, and enzymatic and hormonal balance.

5. *Probiotics*: May reduce negative thoughts that lead to sad mood.

6. *Vitamin D.* The sunshine vitamin, vitamin D has numerous health benefits including building strong bones, muscles, supporting the immune system, and hormonal health. Encourage clients to choose vitamin D3, which is a more potent version of the nutrient.

7. *Chromium – glucose tolerance factor (GTF).* Especially useful for diabetics as chromium has been found to help regulate blood sugar levels (Balch, 2010). Also useful for sugar cravings, appetite suppression, and weight loss, although more research is needed to substantiate these claims.

8. *CDP – Choline.* May help reduce cravings.

NUTRITION IN THE FACE OF FOOD INSECURITY

Many clients struggling with addiction live in poverty, are unemployed, or have such low income that access to healthy, nutritious food is not possible. Economic conditions, such as record high inflation, also can impact access to healthy food, as individuals and families try to live within restricted budgets. Food insecurity, defined as lack of consistent access to food for every family member to be healthy and thrive, effects approximately 34 million people, including 5 million children in the United States (United States Department of Agriculture, 2022). A related concern is the concept of "food deserts", which are living areas, often socioeconomically disadvantaged, that lack reasonable access to affordable healthy fruits, vegetables, whole grains, and other nutritious foods (Beaulac, Kristjansson, & Cummins, 2009). If food is available, it is often processed, high in sugar, fat, and sodium, and low in nutritional quality. Within the United States, Beaulac et al. (2009) found clear-cut evidence for differences in food access stratified by socioeconomic status and race. Clearly, clinicians need to be sensitive to economic, physical, and other barriers to adequate nutrition.

Promoting a healthy diet and appropriate supplementation may seem out of touch among those who struggle daily with food insecurity. In WBAC, we believe in advocating for clients by acknowledging their struggles and helping them to find ways to overcome systematic barriers to nutrition. For example, the clinician could help the client explore community resources, methods of public transportation, and employment opportunities to promote financial gain and access to food. Putting clients in touch with public assistance employees may help them gain access to resources that can ease financial burdens. Clinicians themselves can advocate for clients by contacting local ordinances and political leaders to spotlight troublesome issues. Educating clients on healthy food choices when they are available could also help. Within addiction, stable housing, gainful employment, and healed relationships can go a long way in bolstering the client's life, including access to nutritious and healthy foods.

Physical Activity and Exercise

It goes without saying that physical activity and exercise are important components of overall body wellness (and mental health). Ohrt et al. (2019) defined physical activity as body movement where muscles contract and use energy and exercise as intentional body movement for sustaining and improving health and fitness. For our purposes, we will use these terms interchangeably and suggest that movement of any kind is what is important. The benefits of physical activity are so ubiquitous that it is reasonable to assume there are biological, psychological, and social reasons for direct and indirect benefits to those in recovery (Alessi, Rash, & Pescatello, 2020). That is, as one's health improves through physical activity (and improved nutrition), addictive tendencies begin to dissipate (e.g., through less craving and improved mood). Increasing physical activity can be a great starting point for addiction recovery. As a positive feedback loop, the benefits of exercise build motivation, which leads to continued physical movement. New physical habits can then take the place of old, addictive, and less useful ways of living. For these and other reasons, in WBAC, we encourage clients to engage in physical activity as part of their recovery plan.

Physical activity comes in two forms, aerobic and anaerobic, based on how the body uses oxygen. Aerobic exercise is associated with the typical "cardio" workouts where the heart rate raises to a relatively high percentage of the maximum rate for an extended period. In aerobic exercise, the intent is to improve the efficiency of the cardiovascular system in using oxygen. Anaerobic activity is often associated with weight and power training, muscles are stressed, and the heart rate does not go above a certain threshold for a lengthy period. Both forms of activity are important for overall body wellness. When we think about physical activity, most people have images of intense gym workouts where attendees are sweating it out on a cardio machine (aerobic work) or lifting weights (anaerobic work). However, being in a gym is not required to attain the gains of physical activity. Simply walking for 30 minutes a day, for example, has been found to have numerous health benefits, including improved mood, weight loss, lowered blood pressure, stress relief, improved sleep, and much more.

As part of addiction recovery, it makes sense that physical activity has potential to be a positive adjunct to any treatment protocol. Despite the health benefits, however, epidemiological evidence suggests an inverse relationship between high-risk substance use and physical activity (Linke & Ussher, 2015): on the one hand, clients in the throes of an addiction tend to engage in little, if any, exercise. On the other hand, there is an emerging body of evidence suggesting *increased interest* in physical activity and exercise among those in the recovery community, for both general health and substance-related reasons (Linke & Ussher). Researchers are exploring how to tap into this potential to increase intrinsic motivation to engage in physical activity. Let us take a closer look at how physical activity benefits those struggling with addiction or in recovery.

PHYSICAL ACTIVITY AND ADDICTION

There are three avenues from which physical activity has positive impacts on substance use. First, exercise interventions may impact substance use directly, by promoting reduced craving, easing of withdrawal symptoms, and reduction in stress (Alessi et al., 2020). Second, negative emotional states (e.g., anxiety and depression) are often concomitant problems and precipitators to relapse. Exercise-based interventions have been found to reduce these negative emotional states (Ohrt et al., 2019; Wipfli, Rethorst, & Landers, 2008). Third, physical activity and exercise promote feelings of well-being that tend to counter the addiction mindset. Physical activity leads to increased feelings of accomplishment and self-efficacy, improves self-perception, increases feelings of joy, and improves self-esteem (Ohrt et al.). With time and support, these benefits become self-fulfilling and neutralize the negative self-narratives surrounding substance use behavior.

Empirical evidence is generally supportive of using exercise as an adjunct to SUD treatment. Ellingsen, Johannesen, Martinsen, and Hallgren (2018) found that activities such as football, circuit training, and walking were associated with short-term reductions in drug craving and brief improvements in mood and affect among inpatients with polysubstance dependence. Relatedly, research suggests that exercise may have a reducing effect on craving, especially with alcohol (Ussher, Sampuran, Doshi, West, & Drummond, 2004). In a study that examined the "lived experiences" of substance-using adolescents who engaged in twice-weekly exercise sessions, More et al. (2018) found several important themes, including establishing a healthy routine in recovery, more positive body perceptions, improved sleep and interpersonal relationships, physical release of tension, and a sense of achievement. Related to substance use, structured exercise improved the recovery factors, such as craving and withdrawal, among these youth (More et al.). Similar findings were found by Wang, Wang, Wang, Li, and Zhou (2014).

In a meta-analysis of 22 studies examining whether long-term physical exercise could be an effective treatment for SUDs, Wang et al. (2014) found that physical exercise positively impacts abstinence rate, lessens withdrawal symptoms, and reduces markers of anxiety and depression. Treatment effects were found among three categories of exercise: intensity, type, and follow-up. The researchers concluded that moderate and high-intensity aerobic exercises can be an effective, long-term treatment for clients struggling with SUDs. Clearly, it seems that exercise can have both general wellness and recovery-specific benefits.

The connection between physical activity and reductions in markers of substance use, however, may be more complicated when it comes to long-term improvements. Preliminary evidence suggests that engaging in an aerobic exercise program leads to reduced drinking behavior; however, in one study, gains were not maintained at follow-up and some indices of fitness were no different between exercisers and non-exercisers (Franklin, Whaley, Howley, & Balady, 2000). Another potential issue is compliance; research suggests that whereas exercise holds promise to help reduce substance use as part of an overall treatment plan, sustained engagement in exercise is challenging (Alessi et al., 2020). As with any complex health behavior change, starting and maintaining an exercise program takes time and energy, and adherence to such protocols can be difficult for clients recovering from addiction. As such, clinicians should be mindful of these potential challenges when promoting physical activities for their clients. Ideally, lifestyle changes to enhance wellness are introduced gradually but promoted as long-term commitments.

PROMOTING PHYSICAL ACTIVITY IN WBAC

Physical activity is another staple of the WBAC treatment plan. As noted above, those in recovery have taken a greater interest in exercise as an adjunct to their recovery due to the potential overall health and recovery-specific benefits. Of course, clinicians cannot force clients to exercise; however, they can tap into this level of interest and engage clients in a dialogue about the benefits of physical activity on their recovery. In addition, exercise is an effective substitute for using drugs. With our clients, we often ask the question, "what will you be doing *instead* of using?" The client can consider engaging in an exercise routine or program *instead* of hanging out with old using buddies. The natural endorphins produced by exercise are another benefit that satisfies and reduces urges to return to previous patterns. The concomitant increases in self-esteem and mood from exercise, and improvements in virtually all aspects of well-being, translate into reduced substance use.

Whereas it is important for all individuals to consult with a physician before starting an exercise program, it is especially important for clients in recovery. This is because of the well-known connection between the misuse of drugs and negative impacts on the cardiovascular system, as well as other organ systems in the body. In WBAC, we encourage clients to secure a physical and discuss appropriate exercise activities with a physician before starting. Clients in recovery, for example, may need to begin in moderation before slowly increasing exercise intensity. In addition, clinicians need to be mindful of clients engaging in exercise as a substitute for addiction.

Issues of Compliance and Motivation   A consistent finding in the research literature is difficulties with adherence to an exercise program among those in recovery. To mitigate these issues, we advocate collaborating with clients to find out what form of physical activity best fits their level of fitness, situation, and motivation. We caution clinicians to not force exercise into a treatment plan and assume clients are ready to start from day one. It is important to explore barriers to physical activity, whether they be physical, motivational, psychological, or environmental. For example, a client may not feel safe walking in their neighborhood and cannot afford an expensive gym membership. Such barriers should be respected and explored, while helping clients reconceptualize exercise as *any* movement or physical activity. Some clients may simply loathe exercise. In these cases, it may be worth exploring ambivalence as well as barriers, and collaborating on a physical activity plan from which the client can get on board. We suggest promoting physical activity among those actively using or in recovery by following specific WBAC guidelines

1. *Provide psychoeducation.* With permission, share with client the benefits of exercise, in terms of both general health and recovery. Inquire about their perspective and likelihood to engage in physical activity.

2. *Determine what activity best fits the client's situation, motivation, and goals.* Help the client explore what activities they enjoy, keeping in mind that fancy equipment or a gym membership is not required. We have had many clients surprised at how refreshing a simple 30-minute daily walk can be.

3. *Assess and explore barriers.* What might get in the way of the client pursuing an exercise program? Negative influences and barriers need to be anticipated, explored, and addressed. Help clients navigate difficult situations in which they might be pulled away from their recovery plan into relapse. Reinforce times when they were able to overcome barriers.

4. *Track adherence and reinforce success.* Although we advocate incorporating physical activity into WBAC, how structured the plan is depends on many factors. Some clients may have high motivation, join a gym the next day, and keep to a program of daily physical activity. Others may walk 30 minutes two to three times a week. Regardless of how structured the physical activity is, we support tracking progress or brief "check ins" each session to see how the client fared from the previous session. Tracking progress may include adherence to the plan, perceived benefits, impacts on recovery, perceived barriers, and additional physical activity ideas.

Clients who meet nutritional needs and get adequate amounts of physical activity find mental, emotional, and physical balance, making them better able to handle stress. Lowered stress leads to lower stress hormone (i.e., cortisol) in the body, resulting in a greater sense of inner calm. It is this inner calm that is on the other side of the inner chaos of addiction. As clients progress through recovery, nutrition and exercise become indispensable in reducing cravings, minimizing H.A.L.T., and finding balance. Another important body wellness consideration for those struggling with addiction is adequate and proper sleep, a topic we turn to next.

Sleep Hygiene

Simply put, everything runs smoother with proper sleep (Ohrt et al., 2019). Good sleep helps regulate appetite and hunger, promotes emotional regulation and better relationships, and banishes fatigue (Stevenson, 2016) – in other words, sleep addresses all components of H.A.L.T. Unfortunately, the role of sleep in substance addiction is underappreciated and under-researched (Valentino & Volkow, 2020). However, as with nutrition and physical activity, we consider sleep hygiene an *essential* ingredient in WBAC. Let us dive a bit more into why this is the case.

SLEEP AND ADDICTION

Sleep plays a critical role in overall health and wellness and lack of sleep has implications for a wide swath of adverse health outcomes, including SUDs (Logan et al., 2018). In a review of the neurobiology of brain reward systems and the impact of sleep changes on addiction, Logan et al. found that chronic circadian misalignment (i.e., disrupted sleep cycles) enhances tendencies toward increased impulsivity, exacerbating the susceptibility to SUDs among adolescents. Sleep quality and its impact on substance addiction also is not a one-way phenomenon, as alternation in one behavior has consequences for the other (Valentino & Volkow, 2020). As such, exposure to addictive substances has been found to disrupt sleep latency, duration, and quality (Valentino & Volkow). If chronic drug use patterns continue, a negative cycle is established where substance use leads to more severe sleep disruption, which in turn drives up drug craving and impulse to use. It stands to reason, then, that if a client improves in one area (e.g., sleep hygiene), then we can expect improvements in drug craving, impulsivity, and overall use. Therefore, improving sleep hygiene is an important wellness consideration in WBAC.

Chronic sleep disruption is a risk factor for substance use issues, and the severity of sleep problems is predictive of treatment outcomes (Dolsen & Harvey, 2017). Sleep has important implications for memory consolidation, emotional regulation, and willpower. As sleep quality decreases, susceptibility to drug use becomes more likely, manifesting in increased drive to use, greater sensitivity to pain, inability to effectively handle stress, and being biased toward negative emotion. In a commentary on drugs, sleep, and the brain, Valentino and Volkow (2020) stated, "Recognizing and treating sleep disorders may be an important preventative measure against future drug misuse and SUD" (p. 3).

PROMOTING SLEEP IN WBAC

Assessing and correcting for deficiencies in sleep hygiene or circadian disruption is a part of the WBAC treatment plan. Assessing for sleep difficulties can be as simple as inquiring about sleep patterns, quality, and satisfaction. Clients in active withdrawal and in the beginning phases of recovery may find sleep especially difficult. It is during this time that clinicians should help clients manage sleep problems that arise. Aside from practical considerations (e.g., keeping a consistent sleep schedule and turning off mobile devices an hour before bedtime), clinicians can offer psychoeducation about the importance of sleep, brainstorm a plan to get back on track, or refer the client to a sleep specialist who can provide additional recommendations and/or medical interventions. Clients in early recovery need to be reassured that as drugs leave their bodies and they begin to physically heal, achieving quality sleep will become easier. An important consideration, however, is to help clients avoid overly obsessing and worrying about sleep, which would only make the problem worse; reassure clients that, in time, sleep will naturally improve.

In WBAC, the connection between lack of sleep and increased drug craving is emphasized in a psychoeducational manner. Remember that craving for drugs is a key reason for relapse; craving is so ubiquitous, that the *Diagnostic and Statistical Manual of Mental Disorders* (APA, 2013) defines "full remission" as going at least 12 months without meeting any criteria for a SUD, *except* for craving. This exception points to the fact that craving is a stubborn symptom, even when the client does not meet any other criteria for a substance disorder. Although there are many cognitive-behavioral techniques to help clients manage cravings (see Chapter 5), starting with proper sleep will provide a solid foundation.

Trauma-Informed Considerations

Before we move on to wellness and self-care protocols, a quick word about addiction, trauma, and the body. Based on the work of Bessel Van Der Kolk (2014), trauma can be "held" in the body and manifest as numerous physical, psychological, and behavioral symptoms, including substance use and addiction. Although WBAC is not specifically a trauma-based treatment, it adopts a trauma-*informed* approach to care. Trauma-informed treatment is where clinicians seek to understand that trauma people experience can negatively impact their current lives. A trauma-informed approach emphasizes understanding and sensitivity to issues of trauma and adopting principles that provide effective treatment without re-traumatization.

The National Center for Trauma-Informed Care (2015), as part of SAMHSA, is a national organization funded by the U.S. government that provides free information on the interface among mental health, substance use, and treatment, provides six principles of the trauma-informed approach: (a) safety; (b) trustworthiness and transparency; (c) peer support; (d) collaboration and mutuality; (e) empowerment, voice, and choice; and (f) cultural, historical, and gender awareness. WBAC affirms these principles in working with clients in a trauma-informed manner. The physical experiences of emptiness, violation, and pain from past trauma can manifest as substance use behaviors, as clients try to fill the void they feel in their bodies. The WBAC counselor uses strategic questioning to inquire about the trauma and its possible relation to addictive behaviors. Safety, trust, and collaboration, along with MI spirit, undergird this approach. Questions such as, "in what ways has trauma impacted your body wellness?" can help clients gently explore the connection between their substance use and past trauma, and ways to heal their bodies without using substances.

Body Positivity

Up to this point, we have explored how body wellness stems from activities such as eating a healthy diet, exercising, and ensuring enough sleep. However, body wellness is more than what we do, it also entails how we think about and perceive our physical selves (Ohrt et al., 2019). *Body image* is related to how we look and feel physically but is grounded in the thoughts and emotions we have about our bodies (Ohrt et al.). As such, body wellness is intimately connected with mind and emotional wellness. *Body positivity* refers to having a healthy, positive body image, whereas *body negativity* refers to having a negative body image.

There is some evidence that negative body image correlates with substance use. Nieri, Kulis, Keith, and Hurdle (2005) found that, among more acculturated Mexican American middle school youth, those with poor body image had the greatest risk for substance use. Among a sample of 289 young adult women, Carr and Szymanski (2011) found that everyday body evaluations and sexual objectification experiences positively correlated with substance misuse. The authors found support for how self-objectification, body shame, and depression mediated a direct relationship between sexual objectification and substance misuse. These studies suggest that negative body image may be a trigger for the development or continuation of substance use.

Negative body image can also come as a result of substance use. Signs of physical deterioration can be enough to propel clients to consider treatment or stop using on their own. As we have explored in this chapter, the toll that addiction takes on the physical body is enormous, and clients often find it difficult to stay positive about how they look and feel physically. Thus, body negativity leads to negative self-esteem, shame, and can adversely impact the recovery process.

Whether negative body image occurs before or after substance use, the WBAC clinician should be prepared to address these issues with clients, as part of an overall body wellness plan. Ohrt et al. (2019) suggested strength-based and cognitive behavioral approaches to address poor body image. For example, clinicians can help clients set physical goals for themselves rather than rely on unrealistic and stereotypical ideals presented on social or other forms of media (Ohrt et al., 2019). WBAC clinicians need to stay trauma-informed and understand the link between sexual abuse and its negative message that one's body does not have significance nor deserves respect (Ohrt et al., 2019). Clinicians can help clients honor and respect their physical selves with positive affirmations, exploring what their body does rather than simply how it looks (Ohrt et al., 2019), and journaling and replacing negative cognitions to root out underlying thoughts that lead to negative self-evaluations. Handout 8.1 includes clinician scripts for two physical wellness activities (body scan and progressive muscle relaxation). Please refer to the trauma-informed considerations in Chapter 7, Handout 7.3, before using the body scan and progressive muscle relaxation activities with clients.

Other Co-Morbid Health Conditions

Several co-morbid health conditions can complicate the substance addiction treatment picture. Examples of health conditions may include cardiac problems, diabetes, liver disease, kidney disease, weakened immune system, and communicable diseases (e.g., hepatitis from sharing needles). Although treatment of these problems falls under the realm of medicine, the WBAC clinician should not hesitate to assess for health issues the client may be experiencing. We advocate assessing medical or physical health issues as part of a standard addictions counseling intake. Questions such as, "Tell me about any physical problems you may be having" or "Have you ever been diagnosed with a medical condition?" can be good places to start. Clients may benefit from referrals to appropriate medical care if needed. In WBAC, client goals need not just be about stopping or reducing substance use; in collaboration with a medical specialist, goals also can center on improving or even reversing physical problems.

Considerations in a Wellness and Self-Care Protocol

In this chapter, we have focused on body wellness and suggested steps for intentionally involving physical health components in addiction treatment and in a manner that directly connects to relapse or recovery. Early in recovery, the focus of both client and clinician is usually on how to abstain from substances; however, so much focus on not using may lead to overlooking the importance of body wellness as an adjunct to recovery. The key is to integrate body wellness into a recovery plan that is manageable, motivating, and impactful. This integration may include interventions that assist clients in understanding the connection between body wellness, triggers, relapse, and meaningful recovery. Nutrition, exercise, sleep hygiene, and self-care considerations all play a crucial role in helping clients find their physical integrity, manage cravings, and prevent relapse. MI and the strength-based components of wellness counseling inform all these interventions.

We recognize that the sheer amount of information related to body wellness, including many of the recommended interventions in this chapter, can seem overwhelming. Clients may become resistant to so much data and clinicians may not know where to begin. Our advice is to start slowly by incorporating body wellness principles and realize that *any improvement* in body wellness, however small, is progress. For example, instead of covering the intricacies of nutrition, exercise, and sleep in one session, consider taking one body wellness factor, such as exercise, and exploring what types of physical activity the client would be willing to incorporate. Include other aspects of body wellness in subsequent sessions.

In addition, do not assume that clients already know about body wellness and its connection to recovery. When I (TFL) counseled a client in recovery from severe alcohol addiction, a quick assessment of his diet revealed a lot of highly processed, high-sugar/salt foods that had little to no nutritional value. He seemed completely unaware of how this was tied into his feelings and overall recovery. With permission, I offered him some basic nutritional psychoeducation pointing out the connection between diet, mood, and cravings. He was initially skeptical that diet could play such an important role but agreed to incorporate two to three servings of fruits and vegetables every day until the next session (with a goal of increasing this amount over time). When the client returned the following week, he was surprised that his mood improved, and he experienced fewer cravings. Although he was not sure if more fruits and vegetables led to feeling better, he was intrigued by the idea and wanted to learn more. As this brief example illustrates, recovery status, clinical intuition, and client knowledge, motivation, and readiness may require clinicians to start slowly and incorporate body wellness principles over time.

CLIENT EXAMPLE

We conclude this chapter with a review of the case study of Eric to see what body-based interventions integrated within WBAC might look like clinically. The excerpt below included work with Eric after one year of abstaining from alcohol. Years of alcohol misuse has seriously compromised Eric's physical health, including potential blood sugar and blood pressure issues. Based on initial clinical interviews, Eric did not report past trauma, although he did consistently fear his parents would get a divorce based on his father often staying out after work. In the excerpt below, the WBAC clinician explores the benefits of optimizing his diet to address underlying nutritional deficiencies. Note how this discussion is framed within a wellness perspective.

CLINICIAN: Hello Eric. It is nice to see you again. How has this past week gone for you?

ERIC: Oh, ya know, the typical ups and downs of recovery. I can't believe that it has been one year since I stopped alcohol. It has gone fast. Although it is something to be proud of, I continue to struggle with low energy and other health issues.

CLINICIAN: You have come a long way, Eric, and have shown courage in the face of normal adversities when starting a recovery plan (affirmation focused on the client's courage).

ERIC: I think I'm ready to take next step. Being off alcohol has had a lot of benefits, but I still struggle with things like craving, and I know my diet is not the best.

CLINICIAN: You mentioned that before; how have you made the connection, if any, to your diet, nutrition, and wellness/recovery? (exploring what the client already knows before offering information).

ERIC: Well, I have thought a lot about our wellness discussions, and how wellness in recovery starts in the body. Makes sense. The word that comes up for me includes *healing*. I am not there yet but taking a closer look at diet might help start the healing process.

CLINICIAN: And healing is what recovery is all about, as we have discussed. Is that something you would like to focus on today – how you can improve nutrition as part of a recovery, healing, and wellness plan? (strategic wellness question designed to focus the client on benefits of nutrition in recovery).

ERIC: Sure. Anything is probably better than what I eat now.

CLINICIAN: If it is alright with you, I would like to provide some information on nutrition and its role in recovery? (Asking for permission to provide information; client nods in agreement). First, you are not alone in struggling with diet. For many in recovery, past drug use and poor diet can lead to nutritional problems where the person may currently turn to unhealthy food to satisfy cravings. However, once nutritional deficiencies are met through healthier diet, cravings seem to improve, and the person feels more balanced. What do you make of that? (checking in with client after providing information).

ERIC: Interesting. I had no idea that what I ate played such an important role. Honestly, at first, I was just trying to survive and stay off alcohol. Food, diet, nutrition was off the radar. Now that am a year in recovery, it makes more sense to focus on this now.

CLINICIAN: That is great, it feels right to me as well, although you are the ultimate one who decides when and if you make a change. How about we move forward with some recommendations? (stress client autonomy; asking permission again to offer specific recommendations).

ERIC: That sounds like a plan.

CLINICIAN: Ok, as you know I am not a nutritionist, but I can offer an assessment and provide some education on the connection between diet, wellness, and recovery. The first item we should look at is getting a sense of your diet throughout a typical day and where you can make some changes. We can accomplish this through a Food/Mood Inventory, which is an assessment that looks at a typical day of eating and from that deciding where you might be able to improve.

ERIC: Ok, sounds fine.

CLINICIAN: From there, I would encourage you to meet with your physician and secure some tests to look at important markers of health, such as blood glucose levels, blood pressure, triglycerides, and so forth.

ERIC: Are you saying that I am diabetic?

CLINICIAN: No, not at all. Just encouraging these tests so that we know where you are in terms of body wellness. However, we do know that those who struggle or have struggled with alcohol use disorder often have blood sugar issues – either too high or too low – which can impact your emotions, mood, and energy. Often blood sugar issues can be resolved by healthy diet and, like mentioned before, you will feel more stabilized and balanced. What do you think about all this? (provided information with permission; asking the client how they make sense of it all).

ERIC: It does seem a bit overwhelming. At the same time, I kind of already knew that if I eat better, I'll feel better. This may help light a fire under me!

CLINICIAN: [laughing] There does seem to be something motivating about getting feedback from a doctor. In this case, you would be getting some feedback about physical measures of health, which sets the stage to explore how to correct any potential issues. We also have a nutritionist on staff, who can help provide some dietary guidelines.

In this brief example, the clinician focuses on only one aspect of body wellness – nutrition. Most of the interventions were psychoeducational in nature, with brief mention of possible referrals for the client (physician and nutritionist). The MI style of WBAC also was illustrated. For example, the clinician asked for permission before providing information and then checked in with the client after the information was provided. This case example illustrates the typical WBAC clinician approach to body wellness issues that may lie outside their scope of practice; offer psychoeducation and consult/refer to specialists who can provide specific recommendations and/or prescriptions as needed.

Handout 8.1 Body Scan and Progressive Muscle Relaxation Scripts by M.K. Curry

Please refer to the trauma-informed considerations in Chapter 7, Handout 7.3, before using the body scan and progressive muscle relaxation activities with clients.

Script for: Body Scan

Rationale: Body scans can allow a client to notice, connect, and integrate the dimensions of wellness in their somatic self, and this body scan looks toward identifying strengths as well as growth edges and tender spaces in an individual. This activity is best used in individual sessions because there is a vulnerable component to this kind of exercise, though, with caution, it may be adaptable for use in small groups. Body scans can be used to help a client notice spaces where they are holding tensions or anxieties and can be a helpful addition when talk therapy approaches stagnate.

Read the script below aloud to the client, adapting to your own style and approach. Allow time to pass between prompts and remain present to the non-verbal responses of your client.

If you are comfortable doing so, you may close your eyes for this. There is no requirement that you must, and at any point you can choose to open or close your eyes.

I am going to guide you through a scan of your body, asking you to pay attention to any feeling- positive, neutral, or negative, that arises. If at any point you feel unsafe or uncomfortable in a particular space, know that you can ask to move on from that place, or to stop entirely.

Settle into a position that feels comfortable and safe for you.

Pause to take a deep inhale through your nose, holding the breath for a count of 1...2...3...4...5. Exhale slowly through your mouth, feeling free to do so as loudly or quietly as you wish, for a count of; 1...2...3...4...5.

Repeat the deep inhale through your nose and slow exhalation through your mouth.

Take a moment to think about your feet.

Are you gripping the ground with your feet? Are your feet relaxed in your shoes?

Take a moment or two to wiggle your toes, and gently lift each foot from the ground a few times, releasing any tension or pressure.

Move your thoughts from foot to leg.

Are you aware of the connection between your foot and leg?

Pick your feet up and flex toward and away from your body.

Do you feel tension as you pull up and push away?

Notice what the neutral feels like, in between the flex and the push.

Keep breathing deeply in and out for a count of...1...2...3...4...5

Your legs support your core, the center of your body.

Deeply breathing still, turn your thoughts toward your lungs and heart.

Notice how the deep inhale fills your lungs and expands your chest.

Notice how the exhale empties your lungs.

Now, examine how you are holding your neck.

Is there tension? Are your shoulders shrugged up?

Consciously, exhale and relax your shoulders down from your face,

Keep breathing deeply in and out for a count of...1...2...3...4...5

Move your attention to your face.

Notice if you are holding tension.

If you are clenching your jaws or holding tightly, exhale and relax.

Continue deep inhaling and exhaling until you feel fully ready to stop.

Script for: Progressive Muscle Relaxation

Rationale: This exercise has been developed to notice, control, and relax tension within the body. Throughout this exercise, the client will be asked to tense certain parts of their body, and then relax them, paying attention to the differences between tension and relaxation. This kind of exercise can be particularly helpful for a client who might feel out of control or disempowered, or is experiencing anxieties. With any exercise, the more it is practiced, the more available it is to one in times of stress and anxiety.

If you are comfortable doing so, you may close your eyes for this. There is no requirement that you must, and at any point you can choose to open or close your eyes.

I am going to guide you through a progressive muscle relaxation of your body, asking you to pay attention to any feeling-positive, neutral, or negative, that arises. If at any point you feel unsafe or uncomfortable in a particular space, know that you can ask to move on from that place, or to stop entirely.

We begin with a deep inhalation. Notice the feeling of your lungs as breath in expands them. Hold this breath for a count of 1...2...3.

Release this breath and feel your lungs emptying, stomach coming in toward your spine.

Take another deep breath, longer than the first.

Hold it, for a count of 1...2...3...4.

Slowly release the air.

Take an even longer breath in, expanding your lungs, filling and holding the air, for a count of 1...2...3..4...5

As you release this breath, imagine tension emptying from your body.

Put your focus on your feet – pull your toes in, feeling the arch in your feet as you pull them closer. Hold this tension for as long as you can, and notice what this tension feels like.

Release the tension in your feet – notice your breath as you relax the tension. Feel the relaxation beginning in your feet, spreading upwards through your body.

Move your attention from your feet to your lower legs, slowly squeezing the muscles in each calf. Notice the pulling in of your muscles and tendons from your feet into your lower legs. Hold the tension for a count of 1...2...3...4...5.

Exhale any held breath and release this tension from your lower legs. Again, notice the feeling of relaxation.

Move your attention from your lower legs and shift into your upper legs and pelvis. Squeeze your thighs together, paying attention to the tension you are holding. Hold the tension for a count of 1...2...3...4...5.

Exhale any held breath and release the tension from your muscles.

Move your attention from your pelvis to your stomach and chest. Inhale deeply and pull your stomach to your spine. Hold this tension tighter, tighter, tighter. Hold the tension for a count of 1...2...3...4...5.

Exhale any held breath and release the tension from your muscles.

Allow your body to go limp, holding nothing tightly. Notice the way total relaxation feels in your body.

Move your attention to your upper back, squeezing your shoulder blades in toward each other, imagining them touching. Hold the tension for a count of 1...2...3...4...5.

Exhale any held breath and release the tension from your muscles, dropping your shoulders down away from your ears

Take a moment to notice how your body feels in this relaxation

Move your attention to your arms; from your fingers all the way through your elbow, up to your shoulders.

Pull in each fingers one at a time, and make tight fist with both hands. Feel the tension move up your forearms, into your biceps, up to your shoulders. Hold the tension for a count of 1...2...3...4...5.

Exhale any held breath and release the tension from your muscles, again dropping your shoulders down away from your ears

Take a moment to notice the softness in your hands, fingers, arms.

Now, tense your entire body. Tense your feet, legs, stomach, chest, arms. Squeeze each muscle as hard as your can. Hold the tension for a count of 1...2...3...4...5.

Exhale any held breath and release the tension from your muscles.

Notice this feeling of relaxation, and how different it is from the feeling of full tension.

Begin to wake your body up by slowly moving your muscles, lifting feet up from the ground and placing them back down. Gently wiggle your fingers and rotate your wrists. Roll your shoulders up and down again.

Script for: Processing Mindfulness Activities

We have just engaged in a vulnerable activity. With your permission, I would like to take time to process some of what you experienced, and make sure that you know you have space to explore some of the space you went to and to voice any concerns or discomforts you may have had with the activity.

Did you notice any places in your body that felt particularly tense? ...If so, please tell me more about this.

> **Did you find it difficult to stay present with the activity? ... If so, where did your mind wander to?**
> *Did you push through any moments of discomfort? ...If so, did you have an interior narration for this?*
> **What has this activity taught you or shown you about yourself?**
> *Note.* This handout was authored by M.K. Curry.

NOTE

1   Many of the recommended dosages for the supplements below vary greatly from client to client. For specific recommendations and ranges for your clients, please consult Korn (2016) or a nutritional specialist.

REFERENCES

Alessi, S. M., Rash, C. J., & Pescatello, L. S. (2020). Reinforcing exercise to improve drug abuse treatment outcomes: A randomized controlled study in a substance use disorder outpatient treatment setting. *Psychology of Addictive Behavior, 34,* 52–64.

American Addiction Centers (2020, December 7). *Is Suboxone addictive?* Retrieved from https://americanaddictioncenters.org/suboxone/addicitve

Balch, P. A. (2010). *Prescription for nutritional healing: A practical A-to-Z reference to drug-free remedies using vitamins, minerals, herbs, & food supplements* (5th ed.). Avery.

Beaulac, J., Kirstjansson, E., & Cummins, S. (2009). A systematic review of food deserts, 1966–2007. *Preventing Chronic Disease, 6,* A105.

Carr, E. R., & Szymanski, D. M. (2011). Sexual objectification and substance abuse in young adult women. *The Counseling Psychologist, 39,* 39–66.

Chavez, M. N., & Rigg, K. K. (2020). Nutritional implications of opioid use disorder: A guide for drug treatment providers. *Psychology of Addictive Behaviors, 34,* 699–707.

Dolsen, M. R., & Harvey, A. G. (2017). Life-time history of insomnia and hypersomnia symptoms as correlates of alcohol, cocaine, and heroin use relapse among adults seeking substance use treatment in the United States from 1991 to 1994. *Addiction, 112,* 1104–1111.

Ellington, M. M., Johannesen, S. L., Martinsen, E. W., & Hallgren, M. (2018). Effects of acute exercise on drug craving, self-esteem, mood, and affect in adults with poly-substance dependence: Feasibility and preliminary findings. *Drug and Alcohol Review, 37,* 789–793.

Ford, J. A. (2014). Poor health, strain, and substance use. *Deviant Behavior, 35,* 654–667.

Jakubczyk, A., Ilgen, M. A., Kopera, M., Krasowska, A., Klimkiewicz, A., Bohnert, A., Blow, F. C., Brower, K. J., & Wojnar, M. (2016). Reductions in physical pain predict lower risk of relapse following alcohol treatment. *Drug and Alcohol Dependence, 158,* 167–171.

Korn, L. (2016). *Nutrition essentials for mental health: A complete guide to the food-mood connection.* W.W. Norton.

Korn, L. (2018). *Certified mental health integrative medicine provider (CMHIMP) training course: Nutritional and integrative medicine for mental health professionals* [online course]. Pesi.com.

Linke, S. E., & Ussher, M. (2015). Exercise-based treatments for substance use disorders: Evidence, theory, practicality. *The American Journal of Drug and Alcohol Abuse, 41,* 7–15.

Logan, R. W., Hasler, B. P., Forbes, E. E., Franzen, P. L., Torregrossa, M. M., Huang, Y. H., Buysse, D. J., Clark, D. B., & McClung, C. A. (2018). Impact of sleep and circadian rhythms on addiction vulnerability in adolescents. *Biological Psychiatry, 83,* 987–996.

More, A., Jackson, B., Dimmock, J. A., Thornton, A. L., Colthart, A. & Furzer, B. J. (2018). It's like a counselling session ... but you don't need to say anything': Exercise program outcomes for youth with drug and alcohol treatment service. *Psychology of Sport and Exercise, 39,* 1–9.

Nakken, C. (1996). *The addictive personality: Understanding the addictive process and compulsive behavior.* Hazelden.

National Center for Trauma-Informed Care (2015). *Trauma-informed approach and trauma-specific interventions.* Substance Abuse and Mental Health Services Administration. Retrieved from https://tinyurl.com/54mbyvs5

Nieri, T., Kulis, S., Keith, V. M., & Hurdle, D. (2005). Body image, acculturation, and substance abuse among boys and girls in the Southwest. *The American Journal of Drug and Alcohol Abuse, 31*, 617–639.

Ohrt, J. H., Clarke, P. B., & Conley, A. H. (2019). *Wellness counseling: A holistic approach to prevention and intervention.* American Counseling Association.

Potter, J. S., Prather, K., & Weiss, R. D. (2008). Physical pain and associated clinical characteristics in treatment-seeking patients in four substance use disorder treatment modalities. The *American Journal on Addictions, 17*, 121–125.

Stevenson, S. (2016). *Sleep smarter: 21 essential strategies to sleep your way to a better body, better health, and bigger success.* Rodale.

United States Department of Agriculture (2022, September 12). *Key statistics & graphics.* Retrieved from https://www.ers.usda.gov/topics/food-nutrition-assistance/food-security-in-the-u-s/key-statistics-graphics/#insecure

Ussher, M., Sampuran, A. K., Doshi, R., West, R., & Drummond, D. C. (2004). Acute effect of a brief bout of exercise on alcohol urges. *Addiction, 99*, 542–547.

Valentino, R. J., & Volkow, N. D. (2020). Drugs, sleep, and the addicted brain. *Neuropsychopharmacology, 45*, 3–5.

Van der Kolk, B. A. (2014). *The body keeps score: Brain, mind, and body in the healing of trauma.* Penguin Books.

Wang, D., Wang, Y., Wang, Y., Li, R., & Zhou, C. (2014). Impact of physical exercise on substance use disorders: A meta-analysis. *Journal of PLoS One, 9*, e110728.

WebMD (2020, November 17). *High blood sugar, diabetes, and your body.* Retrieved from https://www.webmd.com/diabetes/how-sugar-affects-diabetes

Wipfli, B. M., Rethorst, C. D., & Landers, D. M. (2008). The anxiolytic effects of exercise: A meta-analysis of randomized trials and dose response analysis. *Journal of Sport & Exercise Psychology, 30*, 392–410. http://doi.org/10.1123/jsep.30.4.39

CHAPTER 9

A SPIRITED RECOVERY: SPIRITUAL WELLNESS IN ADDICTIONS COUNSELING

INTRODUCTION

Spirituality is a critical component of wellness and an important part of recovery from substance use disorders (SUDs). Some scholars believe spirituality is at the center of wellness, serving as the foundational element of all other wellness dimensions (Myers, Sweeney, & Witmer, 2000). Before moving forward with our discussion of spiritual wellness in addiction counseling, it is important to provide a definition of spirituality. Myers and Williard (2003) defined *spirituality* as, "the capacity and tendency present in all human beings to find and construct meaning about life and existence and to move toward personal growth, responsibility, and relationship with others" (p. 49). This definition highlights the universality of spirituality, the role of spirituality in meaning-making, and the importance of personal growth, responsibility, and social connections. As individuals pursue long-term recovery from SUDs, each of these elements becomes imperative; thus, spiritual wellness is a natural component of the recovery process. Additionally, the definition is broad enough to encompass expressing one's spirituality through religion or expressing one's spirituality through secular paradigms (Myers & Williard, 2003). Thus, regardless of whether or not a client identifies with a particular religious tradition, they can pursue spiritual wellness in SUD recovery.

SPIRITUALITY AND RELIGION

Although spirituality is conceptualized as a universal capacity, ways of expressing one's spirituality vary considerably. Some individuals express their spirituality through organized *religion*, which is the case for the majority of individuals in the United States. According to the Pew Research Center (2021), 69% of American adults identify with a religious tradition. Religions represented in the United States are many (e.g., Islam, Judaism, Buddhism, and Hinduism), with Christianity as the most prevalent (63% of Americans identify as Christian; Pew Research Center, 2021). However, only assessing a client's religious affiliation is insufficient for conceptualizing a client's spiritual and religious identity. There are numerous denominations within religious traditions (it is estimated that there are 200 denominations of Christianity in the United States) and diverse religious practices (e.g., prayer, meditation, corporate worship, fasting, recitations, celebrating religious holidays, reading sacred texts, dietary restrictions, pilgrimages, tithing, service, meeting with other members of one's religious community, and chanting). Therefore, when broaching a client's spiritual and/or religious identity, it is important for clinicians to ask questions such as, "What does Judaism mean to you?", "How do you practice your Christian faith?", or "In what ways does Islam affect your life?".

Along with open questions, clinicians may choose to use one of the many spiritual assessments that exist including spiritual histories (semi-structured interview to explore client's spiritual narrative over time), spiritual lifemaps (illustration of client's spiritual journey over time), spiritual genograms (depiction of spirituality in client's family system), spiritual

DOI: 10.4324/9781003147954-9

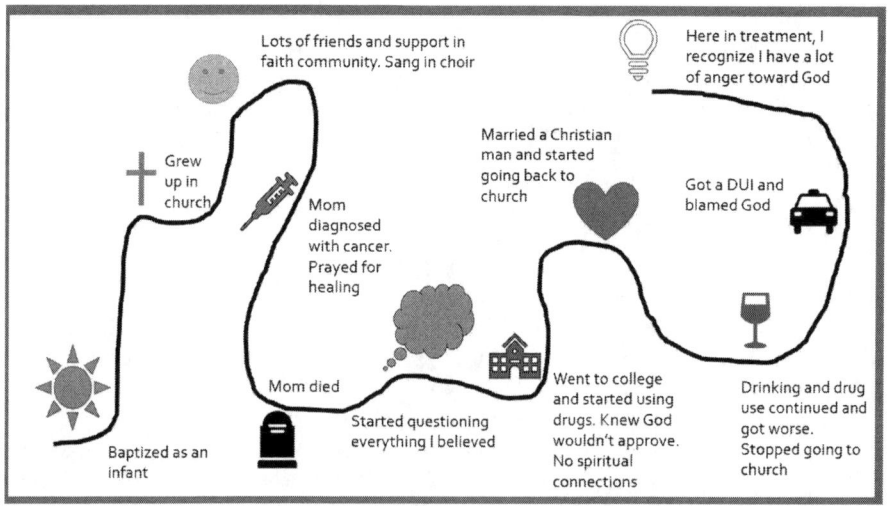

Lots of friends and support in faith community. Sang in choir

Here in treatment, I recognize I have a lot of anger toward God

Grew up in church

Mom diagnosed with cancer. Prayed for healing

Married a Christian man and started going back to church

Got a DUI and blamed God

Mom died

Started questioning everything I believed

Went to college and started using drugs. Knew God wouldn't approve. No spiritual connections

Drinking and drug use continued and got worse. Stopped going to church

Baptized as an infant

Figure 9.1 Spiritual Lifemap.

ecomaps (diagram of client's current relationships with significant spiritual systems), and spiritual ecograms (diagram of spirituality in client's family system and current relationships with significant spiritual systems) (Hodge, 2015). In particular, the spiritual lifemap is described as a "client-constructed pictorial narrative of a spiritual journey" (Hodge, 2005, p. 77). Clients sketch or draw spiritually significant events that they have experienced throughout their lives. This client-directed assessment strategy empowers clients to depict what they consider spiritually significant moments (Hodge, 2005). An example of a spiritual lifemap is shown in Figure 9.1.

These aforementioned spiritual assessments offer clients the opportunity to explore their spiritual identities in ways that have varying degrees of structure. In addition, formal instruments such as the Spirituality Assessment Scale (Howden, 1992), Religious and Spiritual Struggles Scale (Exline, Pargament, Grubbs, & Yali, 2014), and Brief RCOPE (Pargament, Feuille, & Burdzy, 2011) can provide quantitative data regarding multiple dimensions of spirituality, domains of spiritual struggle, and degrees of positive and negative religious coping, respectively.

In contrast to individuals who express their spirituality through religion, some individuals practice their spirituality through secular paradigms. These clients may identify as spiritual but not religious, atheist, agnostic, or may select the answer choice "none" when asked to describe their spiritual affiliation. Currently, 29% of American adults identify as religiously unaffiliated (Pew Research Center, 2021), meaning that about one-third of Americans create purpose and meaning, a sense of values, and a worldview outside of organized religious traditions. There can be great diversity in how each person conceptualizes and practices their spirituality through secular paradigms, thus a curious, humble approach to the subject will be helpful as clinicians seek to understand their client's worldview. Importantly, it would be erroneous to assume that spiritual but not religious clients are not interested in discussing spiritual matters. Per Myers and Williard's (2003) definition, spirituality is a tendency inherent in all human beings. Therefore, non-religiously affiliated clients may desire to examine and develop their beliefs, values, and their connection to something greater than the self without utilizing religious language. Finally, regardless of how a client self-identifies at the initiation of addiction counseling, it is important to note that an individual's spiritual journey can develop and change over time. Clinicians should not assume that clients' spiritual and/ or religious identities are stagnant, but rather dynamic processes that grow and shift across the lifespan.

SPIRITUALITY AND WELLNESS

Clinicians cannot conceptualize wellness without considering spirituality. According to a prominent definition, wellness is a "way of life oriented toward optimal health and well-being in which body, mind, and spirit are integrated" (Myers et al., 2000, p. 252). Oftentimes, we divide up these elements and presume that physicians attend to the body, clinicians attend to the mind, and religious leaders attend to the spirit; yet one of the foundational premises of wellness counseling is that human beings cannot be compartmentalized into distinct segments. Instead, "the wellness counseling approach reminds the clinician to attend to multiple aspects of each client" (Ohrt, Clarke, & Conley, 2019, p. 8). Wellness counseling, therefore, is holistic and addresses the body, mind, and spirit simultaneously. Indeed, given the centrality of spirituality in wellness, the topic correlates with multiple other dimensions in a person's life. Myers and colleagues (2000) stated, "If spirituality is healthy…[it] provides a firm foundation or core for the rest of the components of wellness" (p. 258). Furthermore, in the Wheel of Wellness model, spirituality is one of five interrelated life tasks representing characteristics of wellness, in addition to self-regulation, work, love, and friendship (Witmer & Sweeney, 1992). The life task of spirituality consists of a person's sense of purpose and meaning in life, hope and optimism for the future, values guiding behaviors and decisions, sense of wholeness or oneness, and inner wisdom or spiritual guidance. According to the Wheel of Wellness model, spirituality is a vital component of an individual's wellness across the lifespan (Witmer & Sweeney, 1992).

In addition to theoretical conceptualizations, research has consistently found spirituality to be associated with wellness-related outcomes such as decreased anxiety and depression (Brown, Carney, Parish, & Klem, 2013), increased well-being (Wilt, Grubbs, Exline, & Pargament, 2016), more empathy (Giordano, Prosek, & Lankford, 2014), less substance use (Chitwood, Weiss, & Leukefeld, 2008), and positive affect and better physical health (McIntosh, Paulin, Silver, & Holman, 2011). Moreover, spirituality and religion provide individuals with new ways of coping with life's adversities, which can be an important feature of wellness. Pargament and Abu-Raiya (2007) defined religious coping as "ways of understanding and dealing with life events that are related to the sacred" (p. 743). Positive religious coping encompasses depending upon God's care in the midst of difficulty, seeking support from one's faith community, and drawing closer to the Divine to overcome trouble (Pargament & Abu-Raiya, 2007). Thus, whether by providing new coping strategies, a support system, a sense of community, purpose, meaning, or identity, spirituality is instrumental in an individual's wellness.

SPIRITUALITY AMONG INDIVIDUALS WITH SUDS

Perhaps more than any other mental health concern, spiritual concepts emerge in counseling with individuals with SUDs. This could be due to the influence of 12-Step mutual help programs (discussed below), which are spiritual in nature, or the existential questions that accompany living with the chronic disease of addiction. For example, clients with SUDs may ask questions such as:

- Why is this happening to me?
- How does God feel about me?
- Can I be forgiven for all that I have done?
- Where is God in all of this?
- Why can't I live according to my values?
- What will my religious community think about my addiction?
- What is my purpose?
- Would God even listen to me if I prayed?
- Is there anything after this life?

Along with spiritual inquiries, spirituality also can be an important part of the process of reaching sustained recovery for clients. For instance, among a nationally representative sample of adults who reported being in recovery from an alcohol or other drug (AOD) problem, almost 80% of the sample noted that spirituality helped in their recovery process to some degree (Kelly & Eddie, 2020). Only 22.7% of participants said spirituality did not help them at all to overcome their AOD problem (Kelly & Eddie, 2020). In addition, 76.5% reported experiencing a spiritual awakening while residents of Oxford House Recovery Homes (Bell, Islam, Bobak, Ferrari, & Jason, 2022). Those who had a spiritual awakening had higher scores on coping self-efficacy and hope, both of which are important components of recovery from a SUD (Bell et al., 2022).

Therefore, spiritual wellness can be an important part of reaching and maintaining long-term recovery from a SUD. Spiritual development provides individuals with new, effective coping strategies, new core beliefs about the self, others, and the world, a sense of purpose, and social support. In fact, clients with a history of addiction who reported having a vital spiritual experience noted that the spiritual experience strengthened their commitment to recovery, motivation, and hope (Gutierrez, Mason, Dorais, & Fox, 2021). Thus, spirituality can equip clients with important tools to aid in the recovery process. Yet, how do clinicians ethically and effectively integrate spirituality into addiction counseling?

Utilizing a Multicultural Competence Framework

An individual's spiritual and/or religious identity is a significant aspect of their culture, along with race, ethnicity, sexual orientation, ability status, social class, and other dimensions. Therefore, Giordano (2020) described the importance of considering clients' spirituality through the lens of the Multicultural and Social Justice Counseling Competencies (MSJCC; Ratts, Singh, Nassar-McMillan, Butler, & McCullough, 2016) endorsed by the American Counseling Association (ACA). The MSJCCs comprise four domains necessary for cultural competence: (a) clinician self-awareness, (b) client worldview, (c) counseling relationship, and (d) counseling and advocacy interventions. Each of these domains can help guide clinicians' work with spiritual wellness in addiction counseling.

The first domain, *clinician self-awareness*, charges clinicians with understanding their own cultural identities, including their spiritual identities, values, beliefs, and biases. For example, clinicians should have a clear understanding of their own spirituality to help recognize countertransference issues and the risk of overidentification with clients. Indeed, the spiritual competencies developed by the Association for Spiritual, Ethical, and Religious Values in Counseling (ASERVIC, 2022) note that professional clinicians should actively explore their own values, beliefs, and attitudes pertaining to spirituality and religion. Additionally, the ACA (2014) *Code of Ethics* implores clinicians to engage in self-care to promote their own spiritual well-being. If a clinician's spiritual identity is unexamined, bias, countertransference, or overidentification could affect their clinical work. For example, addiction clinicians could have a bias against 12-Step programs due to their location in a church building or their spiritual foundation. Alternatively, a clinician may overemphasize spiritual themes in counseling due to the importance of spirituality in the clinician's own life, despite lacking importance to the client. Thorough examination of one's own spiritual cultural identity is necessary for effective work with clients' spiritual identities in addiction counseling.

In the second domain of the MSJCC, clinicians are charged with understanding *clients' worldview*. This worldview is influenced by all cultural identities, including spiritual identities. Clinicians are called to understand a client's spiritual belief system, how spirituality may relate to the presenting concern, and how spirituality may influence the counseling relationship. The ASERVIC spiritual competencies (2022) assert that clients' beliefs about spirituality and religion can be central to their worldview and thus clinicians should have knowledge of major world religions, spiritual systems, agnosticism, and atheism. Importantly, clients' spiritual identities often intersect in meaningful ways with other aspects of culture, such as race or ethnicity. For example, recent studies have found that Black clients in recovery were more likely to report the importance of spirituality than other racial groups (Kelly & Eddie, 2020) and Latino(a)(x) clients in addictions treatment were the most willing to incorporate spirituality into the counseling process (Diallo, Herold, Diallo, Marini, & Dominguez, 2021). Thus, rather than conceptualizing a client's spiritual identity in isolation, it should be considered in light of the client's other cultural identities to accurately conceptualize their worldview.

The third domain of the MSJCC is the *counseling relationship*. Clinicians should be aware of how their cultural identities (including their spiritual identities) and the clients' cultural identities will impact their unique therapeutic alliance. A clinician's spirituality may influence their personal values, and while this is perfectly acceptable, clinicians are expected to "be aware of your personal values and to monitor how your values are influencing your counseling work" (Herlihy & Corey, 2015, p. 198). Clinicians should utilize the skill of bracketing, or setting aside personal values in order to provide ethical clinical services to diverse clients (Kocet & Herlihy, 2014). For example, if a client in addiction counseling is seeking spiritual guidance within a particular religion, the clinician should help the client meet this goal by referring them to the appropriate religious leader, even if the clinician's personal values diverge from the identified religious tradition. Bracketing personal values can help ensure that clinicians create strong therapeutic alliances with clients of diverse religious and spiritual backgrounds and avoid the imposition of personal values (ACA, 2014, A.4.b). The ASERVIC spiritual competencies (2022) charge clinicians with evaluating the influence of their spiritual and/or religious beliefs and values on the counseling process.

Finally, the fourth domain of the MSJCC is *counseling and advocacy interventions*. This domain emphasizes the importance of employing interventions that are appropriate in light of the client's culture (including their spiritual cultural identity). There is a myriad of spiritually oriented interventions or approaches that may be helpful for clients in addiction counseling including experiential focusing, gratitude, forgiveness work, meditation, examining spiritual values, acts of service, exploring purpose, reflecting upon spiritual core beliefs, and contemplation. Young and Cashwell (2020) noted that in addition to specific psychospiritual interventions, "traditional counseling interventions can be adapted to be more spiritually sensitive" (p. 25). Determining which intervention to use and how it will be applied in session is contingent upon the client's spiritual and/or religious identity and the extent to which the intervention aligns with that identity. Moreover, the ASERVIC spiritual competencies (2022) assert that clinicians should collaboratively create goals with clients that are consistent with the clients' spiritual and/or religious identities and utilize spiritual and or religious interventions when appropriate. Therefore, a client in addiction counseling who self-identifies as an Evangelical Christian may find 12-Step Facilitation Therapy (Nowinski, Baker, & Carroll, 1995) and the work toward relying on a Higher Power (e.g., surrender) to be very congruent with their spiritual cultural identity. By applying the MSJCC (Ratts, et al., 2016), clinicians can ensure that they are honoring the spiritual and religious identities of diverse clients in addiction counseling and engaging in ethical clinical work.

Broaching

Another key element in addressing spiritual wellness in addiction counseling is broaching. Just like other facets of culture, clinicians are called to broach clients' spiritual identities in their clinical work. *Broaching* has been defined as a "consistent and ongoing attitude of openness with a genuine commitment by the clinician to continually invite the client to explore issues of diversity" (Day-Vines et al., 2007, p. 402). Rather than waiting for client initiation, it is important for clinicians to broach culture and the client's cultural identities (such as spirituality) in order to convey that culture is valued and all aspects of a client's culture are appropriate to discuss in counseling. Some clients may be hesitant to raise spiritual concerns in counseling thinking, "this is not an appropriate subject" especially when counseling occurs outside of faith-based treatment centers. However, clinicians can invite clients to talk about spirituality and/or religion by broaching this specific cultural identity. Broaching stems from a genuine curiosity to learn about the client and their worldview, thus it happens organically. For example, consider this hypothetical dialog between client and clinician in addiction counseling:

> CLINICIAN: It is nice to meet you Tara, I am glad you are here. I am sure you have a lot of thoughts and feelings about starting treatment here.
>
> CLIENT: Well, I've never been to counseling before…or any kind of treatment. I really have no idea what to expect in a facility like this…
>
> CLINICIAN: Well, I'd love to start by just getting to know you. What aspects of your identity or your culture are important for me to know?
>
> CLIENT: My identity? Well… I'm biracial…my mom is White and my dad is Latino. Is that what you want to know?
>
> CLINICIAN: Yes, that's it. Our cultural identities certainly include our race and ethnicity, like your biracial identity. Culture also includes age, gender, spirituality or religion, socioeconomic status, and sexual orientation – so I am curious about anything you'd like me to know about you as we get started.
>
> CLIENT: I see, well, I guess it's important that you know I am 22 years old. I am a female, I'm straight, and I'm Pentecostal.
>
> CLINICIAN: I appreciate you sharing that with me. I identify as a White, agnostic, heterosexual, female. We share some cultural identities and differ on others – I am wondering what comes up for you when you think about our work together?

CLIENT: I thought we were just going to jump into my alcohol and marijuana use... but it's nice to know a little bit about you. I guess I haven't ever met anyone who is agnostic before. Is it OK for me to talk about religion in here... you know, if it comes up?

CLINICIAN: Of course. The purpose of our time together is to help you meet your goals and examine your thoughts and feelings. All aspects of your identity are important to that process, including your spirituality.

CLIENT: Ok. I mean, I haven't been to church in years, but it's funny, I still call myself a Pentecostal.

CLINICIAN: Well, what does Pentecostal mean to you?

By broaching culture and Tara's unique cultural identities, the clinician communicated that these topics were both important and appropriate for counseling. Additionally, understanding the client's history with Christianity, and the Pentecostal denomination in particular, can help the clinician understand Tara's worldview more accurately and may prove to be a source of support during recovery.

ELEMENTS OF SPIRITUAL WELLNESS IN ADDICTION COUNSELING

There are many different ways in which clinicians can address spiritual wellness in addiction counseling. Below, you will find a description of some common elements, yet it is important for clinicians to consider the client's goals and spiritual identity in order to determine which approaches and interventions are most appropriate for the client. In addition, clinicians have the MSJCC, the ACA *Code of Ethics*, and the ASERVIC spiritual competencies to guide their integration of spiritual components into the counseling process.

Meaning-Making

Part of spiritual wellness in recovery is *making meaning* of one's experiences. Many clients will ask big existential questions during recovery like, "why did this happen to me?" or "why do I have a substance use disorder and my brother doesn't?" or "who am I when I'm not using?" or "Can I be forgiven?" In these times of questioning, regardless of a client's religious affiliation, they likely will explore their spirituality to find answers. Clients will search for meaning, clarify their values, and explore their beliefs. The process of making meaning out of an experience, like active addiction, is an important part of recovery and spirituality is a common vehicle for deriving meaning. Clinicians should be prepared to hold the space for clients who are doing this type of spiritual exploration with empathy, multicultural competence, and without imposing their own values. For example, read the hypothetical dialog between a client and clinician below:

CLIENT: I've been clean nine months today. I can honestly say, I never thought I'd be here.

CLINICIAN: It seemed like an insurmountable task to go this long without drinking.

CLIENT: Yes. I really didn't think it was possible. And at the beginning, I was so angry – I just kept asking, "why me?" and now, I am starting to see things a little bit differently.

CLINICIAN: How are you seeing things now?

CLIENT: Like there might have been a purpose to the last 10 years of drinking myself into oblivion. Like…maybe there was a reason for it all.

CLINICIAN: You are finding meaning in the experience.

CLIENT: Yah – like, I started reading the Bible again. I haven't picked it up in about 15 years, but it used to be important to me. I opened it right to the passage about Paul's thorn, and it really spoke to me.

CLINICIAN: What spoke to you?

CLIENT: Well, Paul…he was an apostle…has this "thorn in his flesh" and he asks God to take it away. He asked three times, but God didn't take it away. Instead, God said something like, "My grace is enough for you. I'll show my power through your weakness". And I thought, I've begged God to take away my addiction, but he hasn't. I think I will live the rest of my life with it. But, maybe he said "no" to me just like he said "no" to Paul….and maybe he is going to use it somehow.

CLINICIAN: So, your addiction, as hard as it is, could have a divine purpose.

CLIENT: Yes. I know it sounds crazy, but I guess I feel like it's my "thorn" and God isn't taking it away for a reason. Like, to teach me to depend on him….or maybe to show other people that they can get through hard times with God…I don't know… I'm not sure yet.

CLINICIAN: You have an energy in your voice when you talk about the purpose or meaning of your addiction that I haven't heard before.

CLIENT: Ha, I guess I do! I spend a lot of time thinking about it these days…like, how can this all be used for something good, you know?

In this dialog, the clinician uses reflections and open questions to create a space where the client can explore his spirituality (which in this instance expresses itself through the Christian faith tradition) and make meaning for himself. Meaning-making is an important part of recovery from a SUD and clients' spirituality often will be instrumental in this process.

12-Step Programs

Another spiritual element common in addiction counseling is participation in *12-Step programs*. The popularity of 12-Step fellowships cannot be overstated as Alcoholics Anonymous (AA) alone offers over 120,000 meetings spread across 180 countries (AA, 2022). Moreover, Senreich, Saint-Louis, Steen, and Cooper (2022) noted that newcomer membership increased in 2019, despite the COVID-19 pandemic, which forced 12-Step meetings to move online. 12-Step programs can provide structured support systems based upon spirituality for clients struggling with chemical addiction (e.g., AA, Narcotics Anonymous [NA] and Cocaine Anonymous [CA]) or behavioral addictions (Sex Addicts Anonymous [SAA], Gamblers Anonymous [GA], Food Addicts in Recovery Anonymous [FA]). Additionally, there are 12-Step groups for family members or friends supporting loved ones through addiction (e.g., Al-Anon, Nar-Anon, Gam-Anon, and S-Anon). The only requirement to attend a 12-Step program is the desire to stop the addictive behavior, and the fellowships are open to individuals of all genders, sexual orientations, socioeconomic statuses, and ages.

As the name suggests, 12-Step programs are built upon 12 steps or actions, which are perceived as essential for long-term recovery. Used as guideposts for members, the 12 steps involve admitting a powerlessness over one's life (step 1), making decision to turn one's life toward God (as understood by the individual; step 3), and taking responsibility for wrong-doings and making amends (step 8; AA, 2002). A basic premise of 12-Step programs is that the steps serve as a guide to incremental progress toward health and wholeness, rather than a recipe for perfection. It is important to note that submission to a higher power is of high importance within the 12-steps as seven of the 12 refer to God, a Higher Power, or spiritual awakening. In addition, many AA slogans reference God such as, "Let Go and Let God". "But for the grace of God go I", and "EGO is Edging God Out". The authors of the AA Big Book, after describing addiction, wrote: "There is a solution…we have had deep and effective spiritual experiences which have revolutionized our whole attitude toward life, toward our fellows and toward God's universe" (Alcoholics Anonymous, 2001, p. 25). According to 12-Step programs, the solution to addiction is a spiritual awakening that equips individuals toward long-term recovery.

Some clients may be hesitant to try a 12-Step program because of the emphasis on spirituality and spiritual themes. When discussing 12-Step programs with clients, it is important for clinicians to provide a menu of options that includes both peer support programs based on the 12 steps, and those that do not (such as SMART Recovery, Women for Sobriety, and Secular Organizations for Sobriety). Additionally, it is helpful to describe how non-religious individuals have made 12-Step programs work for them. Specifically, there is a chapter in the Big Book written to "We Agnostics" (Alcoholics Anonymous, 2001, p. 44). In this chapter, the authors write about the importance of admitting there is a higher power, yet specify that this higher power is what the individual understands it to be (e.g., God, another Deity, the universe, love, nature, or anything outside of the individual). When discussing 12-Step programs as a resource for clients, it is important to discuss the spiritual nature of the program and process what that might mean for the client.

Forgiveness

Forgiveness can be an important aspect of spiritual wellness for clients in addiction counseling. Oftentimes, clients with SUDs may have acted in ways contrary to their values and could benefit from forgiveness work directed toward the self. Additionally, addiction is strongly correlated with trauma (Najavits, 2002) and clients with trauma histories may benefit from forgiveness work directed toward someone else.

Before delving into the specifics of forgiveness-based clinical approaches, it is important to describe forgiveness. Noted as a collective concept recognized worldwide, forgiveness requires an internal, conscious decision to remove any ill will toward a situation, person, or event (Webb, Hirsch, & Toussaint, 2011, 2015). Worthington (2013a) posited that forgiveness is a complex process requiring a replacement of negative emotions with "positive, other-oriented emotions" (p. 17). Thus, forgiveness involves cognitions, emotions, and can be a complex, nuanced process that differs from one client to the next.

To address forgiveness work in counseling, the REACH model was developed to help clients replace negative emotions with positive or neutral emotions in order to achieve true forgiveness (Worthington, 2003). The REACH model of forgiveness often is used to facilitate the process of forgiving others, and it has received empirical support for promoting forgiveness across cultures (Lin et al., 2014; Wade, Hoyt, Kidwell, & Worthington, 2014). For example, when utilizing the REACH model with clients demonstrating both anxious and avoidant relationship attachment styles, researchers noted significant changes in revenge, rumination, benevolence, and empathy (Wade et al., 2018). Moreover, Worthington (2003) noted that processes associated with the model (e.g., thinking through, writing about, and emotionally processing the events) can provide relief and promote the decrease of depression, anxiety, anger, and sadness among clients.

For clients in addiction counseling who have been wronged (by a parent, a partner, a friend, a stranger, or another person, which may have occurred before or after substance initiation), the REACH model can help cultivate forgiveness for the perpetrator and thereby enhance spiritual wellness of the client. Worthington's (2003) forgiveness model involves five steps: (a) **r**ecall the hurt, (b) **e**mpathize, (c) **a**ltruistic gift of forgiveness, (d) **c**ommit publicly to forgive, and (e) **h**old on to forgiveness (the first letter of each step is reflected in the model's name, REACH; Worthington, 2003).

The first step of the REACH model, *recall the hurt*, presents an opportunity for clients to acknowledge the event or offense that hurt them within a nonjudgmental environment (Wade & Worthington, 2005). In recalling the hurt, clients can acknowledge the size of the wound and where they feel this wound within their physical body (e.g., behind their eyes, as a weight on their chest or shoulders) to analyze the experience objectively. Worthington (2003) discussed varying wound sizes, such as small "nickel wounds" like a client who felt disrespected by a comment made by a coworker, or a "five-hundred-dollar wound" which represents an event so large it changed the client's core way of being, like physical abuse from a parent.

The next step in the REACH model is to *empathize*. Worthington (2003) described empathy as a tri-level function: (1) understanding the other person's viewpoint on the situation, (2), recognizing the emotions of the other person, and (3) recognizing the other person's emotions while also feeling compassion for the person. Clinicians can facilitate a discussion with clients regarding how the perpetrator of the hurt might have viewed the scenario, what feelings may have occurred for the other person, and then follow up with how to care for the person who harmed the client. The last level of empathy is crucial, however, as true forgiveness cannot occur without compassion toward the offender. This level of forgiveness can be difficult to facilitate; thus, clinicians must approach this stage with utmost care. Worthington et al. (2000) said that attempting forgiveness without paying substantial attention to the client's cognitions and emotions around their experience of forgiveness will have little impact on forgiveness achievement. Consequently, the client and clinician may require multiple sessions exploring the size and depth of the wound as well as the emotions of both parties in the situation. When working through the empathizing stage, strategies to facilitate empathy include writing a letter to the offender, speaking about the situation to a trusted friend, writing a poem, or utilizing other creative arts to process the event from the viewpoint of the individual who caused the harm (Worthington, 2003).

The third step, the *altruistic gift of forgiveness*, is thought of as an "unselfish regard for another person" in which forgiveness is extended because it feels like the morally correct route to take (Worthington, 2003, p. 119). To forgive in this manner, the REACH model presents three parts of the altruistic gift of forgiveness: guilt, gratitude, and gift. This step may entail exploring a time in which the client wronged someone in the past (guilt), the emotions the client felt when they were forgiven by the person they wronged (gratitude), and what it would be like to extend forgiveness to the person who harmed the client (gift).

The next step is to *commit publicly to forgive*. A public commitment can entail writing a letter of forgiveness to the offender, verbalizing forgiveness, or signing a document crafted by the client. This public commitment to forgive can involve anything that provides the client with a concrete act to mark the event (Wade & Worthington, 2005). According to the

REACH model, upon completing the first four steps, forgiveness will eventually occur. However, various cues, interactions, or scenarios can re-trigger resentment in the client. Thus, the last step of the REACH model is to *hold on to forgiveness*. Worthington (2003) discussed several ways to hold on to forgiveness when resentment emerges such as revisiting the public commitment to forgive, seeking support from a trusted person, and making a choice not to ruminate on the negative thoughts and emotions triggered by the cue or stimulus causing resentment. The REACH model of forgiveness can be a helpful tool for clients in addiction counseling who have been wounded by another person.

Additionally, Worthington (2013b) described *six steps of self-forgiveness*, which also may be very useful in developing spiritual wellness among clients with addiction. These steps include: (a) receive divine forgiveness (which can include forgiveness from God, from nature, the Sacred, or humanity in general), (b) repair relationships (make amends with those who have been wronged), (c) rethink ruminations (eliminate or reduce mental obsession of the wrongdoing), (d) REACH emotional self-forgiveness (apply the REACH model to the self with the goal of both self-compassion and responsibility for actions), (e) rebuild self-acceptance (accept personal value despite mistakes), and (f) resolve to live virtuously (learn from mistakes and work toward living according to values; Worthington, 2013b). It is likely that clients in addiction counseling have both been hurt by others and have hurt others themselves, thus the forgiveness models created by Worthington can be a great intervention to foster spiritual wellness.

Although the REACH model presents steps to address forgiveness in a specific order, sizes of wounds, emotional experiences, and situations requiring forgiveness will vary by each client's individual experience. Therefore, applying forgiveness approaches, such as the the REACH model, requires a tailored approach specific to each client, as opposed to a prescribed checklist of items to accomplish. If clients begin to struggle with the initial steps of forgiveness and cannot access the emotions or understand the repercussions related to the event, Wade and Worthington (2005) noted that clinicians should avoid delving deeper into forgiveness methods until the client increases readiness. The authors suggested that clinicians ask clients about their readiness levels and broach topics of shame and guilt, prior to explicitly addressing events requiring forgiveness to avoid promoting false forgiveness (Wade & Worthington, 2005).

Notably, upon beginning forgiveness work, it is important to inform clients that this process will take time, with no guarantee of quick success. Complete forgiveness will not occur in one session, nor after one psychoeducational group on the topic. In fact, Worthington et al. (2000) discussed the concept of time and forgiveness, noting smaller time periods of application produced small to moderate changes in levels of forgiveness. The authors also noted the importance of applying the whole theory of the REACH model, and not simply utilizing interventions as interventions alone will be less effective (Worthington et al., 2000). Wade, Worthington, and Meyer (2005) echoed the importance of time when applying the REACH model, specifying six-to-eight-hour intervention groups produced more significant increases in forgiveness compared to shorter lengths or partial treatment.

CONSIDERATIONS FOR ADDRESSING CLIENT SPIRITUALITY

Ethical Considerations

Some clinicians fear having spiritual discussions with clients due to ethical concerns. For example, clinicians may be afraid of unintentionally imposing their values (ACA, 2014, A.4.b.), or working outside the boundaries of their competence (ACA, 2014, C.2.a). Yet there are ways that clinicians can ensure they are attending to clients' spiritual wellness in an ethical manner. First, clinicians always work within the client's frame of reference when discussing spirituality (just like other topics) without inserting their own beliefs or evaluations. Corey et al. (2003) noted, "There are many paths toward fulfilling spiritual needs, and it is not your role as a helper to prescribe any particular pathway" (p. 85). Thus, clinicians avoid imposing values by operating within the client's worldview and spiritual belief system. Second, when a client begins seeking answers to spiritual questions (e.g., What does this passage of scripture mean? How should I, as a Buddhist, behave in this situation?), the clinician can help connect clients to a spiritual director (Delaney, Forcehimes, Campbell, & Smith, 2009). Clinicians can clarify that they are ready to support the client in their exploration of spirituality, yet if they are seeking information related to theology, doctrine, specific religious beliefs, or religious guidance, a spiritual or religious leader in the community would be more appropriate. Specifically, the ACA *Code of Ethics* (2014) notes that clinicians "consider enlisting the support, understanding, and involvement of others (e.g., religious/spiritual/ community leaders, family members, friends) as positive resources, when appropriate, with client consent" (p. 4). In this way, clinicians work within their professional competence by differentiating between counseling and spiritual direction and referring clients to religious/ spiritual leaders when appropriate.

Spiritual Bypass

Another important consideration for addressing clients' spiritual wellness in addiction counseling is the risk of *spiritual bypass*. Spiritual bypass refers to the act of avoiding important, albeit difficult, psychological work, and personal problems by focusing solely on the spiritual plane (Cashwell, Bentley, & Yarborough, 2007; Welwood, 1984). Spiritual bypass may manifest in addiction counseling if a client says they do not need group counseling because they are praying about their addiction. Although prayer may be a useful tool and source of support for clients, if it is used as a means of avoiding necessary (and often painful or difficult) recovery work, it may be a form of spiritual bypass. Another example is a client who says they do not want to attend a 12-Step program because they have fasted and believe their addiction has been removed from their lives. Clinicians are not to dismiss or minimize clients' spiritual practices or beliefs, yet if spirituality is a means of circumventing necessary emotional or psychological work, it may be spiritual bypass.

If spiritual bypass is present, clinicians may consider utilizing Motivational Interviewing (MI; Miller & Rollnick, 2013) to help the client explore the spiritual bypass (Clarke, Giordano, Cashwell, & Lewis, 2013). MI is a communication style in which clinicians invite clients to work through ambivalence by exploring their own reasons for making a positive change (e.g., change talk) (Miller & Rollnick, 2013). The four processes of MI used to address ambivalence are: engaging, focusing, evoking, and planning (Miller & Rollnick, 2013). When applied to ambivalence around spiritual bypass, clinicians can use evoking techniques such as developing discrepancy, exploring goals and values, and asking questions that elicit change talk (e.g., "I wonder if there any downsides to relying only on prayer to help you overcome your alcohol addiction?") to draw out clients' own reasons for making a change. In the case of spiritual bypass, the positive change would be for clients to recognize the use of spirituality as a means of avoiding important psychological work and to reduce or eliminate this avoidance strategy.

Spiritual Struggle

Another important consideration for addressing spirituality in addictions counseling is for the wellness-based clinician to explore the extent to which *spiritual struggle* may be exacerbating or fueling the addictive behavior. Spiritual struggle is defined as "conflict or distress that center on religious or spiritual issues" and includes spiritual conflict with others (interpersonal), doubting or questioning spiritual beliefs (intrapersonal), or feeling anger toward or punished by a Higher Power (divine; Exline & Rose, 2013, p. 380). Spiritual struggle has been linked to distress and mental health issues (McConnell et al., 2006) and substance use (Stauner, Exline, Kusina, & Pargament, 2019). For example, among a large sample of undergraduates, researchers found significant, positive relationships between religious/spiritual struggles and problem drinking (Stauner et al., 2019). The relationship between addiction and spiritual struggle appears to be bidirectional in that spiritual struggle may increase one's likelihood of engaging in addictive behaviors (perhaps as a means to escape or cope with the struggle), while the engagement in addictive behaviors may increase one's likelihood of spiritual struggle (perhaps due to engaging in behaviors that are incongruent with one's spiritual values). Among adults in the United States who gambled in the past year, gambling scores significantly predicted six types of spiritual struggles and a significant correlation existed between gambling severity and religious and spiritual struggles (Grant Weinandy & Grubbs, 2021).

Therefore, it is imperative that clinicians assess the nature and expression of clients' spirituality, which could serve as a protective factor in recovery or a factor perpetuating the addictive behavior. In situations in which spiritual struggle is contributing to addictive behaviors, clinicians again can utilize MI to invite clients to move toward positive change (Miller & Rollnick, 2013). Giordano and Cashwell (2014) described how MI can be a useful tool for addressing spirituality in counseling, including spiritual struggle. Given that the primary aim of MI is to help clients become unstuck in their ambivalence (Miller & Rollnick, 2013), it can be applied to helping clients address spiritual struggle by inviting them to choose the path forward that is most congruent with their own value system (thereby avoiding the imposition of the clinician's values as prohibited by the ACA *Code of Ethics* [2014]). Addressing interpersonal, intrapersonal, or Divine struggles (Exline et al., 2014) in counseling can help clients strengthen the positive aspects of spirituality and decrease conflict that may be contributing to addictive behaviors. Thus, when addressing spiritual themes in counseling, it is important to consider whether the client's spiritual practices are aiding in the work of recovery or impeding the process.

CLIENT EXAMPLE

We know about several aspects of Eric's culture, namely that he is 35, biracial, male, heterosexual, lower socioeconomic status, and appears to be able-bodied. To accurately understand Eric's worldview, it is important to broach how he identifies regarding his spiritual cultural identity. One way to broach spirituality is to ask Eric to describe his thoughts and feelings about AA attendance. It seems as though he found value in the meetings he attended, yet also felt marginalized as the only person of color in the room. The clinician may ask specifically about the spiritual nature of AA, as in the dialog below:

> CLINICIAN: Tell me about your experience of AA. What was it like for you?
>
> ERIC: I don't know – I felt uncomfortable in a room of all middle-aged White men, but I guess it was OK overall.

CLINICIAN: What made it OK?

ERIC: Well, it was nice to know other people have problems with their drinking too.

CLINICIAN: It was validating to know you aren't the only one.

ERIC: Yes.

CLINICIAN: AA's program encourages reliance on a Higher Power in order to abstain from drinking. What does that bring up for you?

ERIC: A lot actually. My father's side of the family is very religious and I was brought up going to church. We were members of the only multiethnic church in town and I loved it when I was growing up… but then, things changed. When I started drinking and smoking in high school, I knew my church wouldn't like that, so I stopped going.

CLINICIAN: You didn't want your church community to know about your substance use.

ERIC: No, I knew they would just start throwing verses at me and telling me I was on the road to "eternal damnation". So, I sort of gave up on church…and a part of me thinks that God has been punishing me ever since.

CLINICIAN: What do you perceive as God's punishment?

ERIC: I don't know…maybe the miscarriages. I've had the thought that maybe if I was a better person and didn't drink and went to church, we would have had the babies.

CLINICIAN: That must be a very painful thought…to wonder if God is punishing you through miscarriages.

ERIC: (becomes tearful). I've never said it out loud before, but I can't help but wonder. I feel like God took one look at me and said, "He is no father. I won't give him any more children" (breaks into sobs). I feel like it's my fault.

Broaching the subject of Eric's spiritual identity revealed his past affiliation with Christianity and his current spiritual struggles. He is in the midst of existential meaning-making, of his life, his addiction, his relationship with God, and his wife's miscarriages. As Eric pursues long-term recovery, there likely will be numerous opportunities to engage and develop spiritual wellness. For example, the clinician may choose to explore Eric's core beliefs about himself, others, the future, and God to note any cognitive distortions or maladaptive beliefs. Additionally, Eric may benefit from self-forgiveness work following Worthington's (2013b) six steps. Eric feels immense guilt and shame and blames himself for his wife's miscarriages. Self-forgiveness and cognitive work may help him examine his beliefs, challenge distortions, and foster self-compassion coupled with responsibility for his actions.

REFERENCES

Alcoholics Anonymous (2001). *Alcoholics anonymous* (4th ed.). World Services.

Alcoholics Anonymous (2022). *Alcoholics anonymous.* Retrieved from https://www.aa.org

American Counseling Association (2014). *ACA code of ethics.* Retrieved from http://www.counseling.org/knowledge-center/ethics

Association for Spiritual, Ethical, and Religious Values in Counseling (2022). *Competencies for addressing spiritual and religious issues in counseling.* Retrieved from https://aservic.org/spiritual-and-religious-competencies/

Bell, J. S., Islam, M., Bobak, T., Ferrari, J. R., & Jason, L. A. (2022). Spiritual awakening in 12-step recovery: Impact among residential aftercare residents. *Spirituality in Clinical Practice.* Advanced Online Publication. https://doi.org/10.1037/scp0000296

Brown, D. R., Carney, J. S., Parish, M. S., & Klem, J. L. (2013). Assessing spirituality: The relationship between spirituality and mental health. *Journal of Spirituality in Mental Health, 15*, 107–122. https://doi.org/10.1080/19349637.2013.776442

Cashwell, C. S., Bentley, P. B., & Yarborough, J. P. (2007). The only way out is through: The peril of spiritual bypass. *Counseling & Values, 51*, 139–149. https://doi.org/10.1002/j.2161-007X.2007.tb00071.x

Chitwood, D. D., Weiss, M. L., & Leukefeld, C. G. (2008). A systemic review of recent literature on religiosity and substance use. *Journal of Drug Issues, 38*, 653–688.

Clarke, P. B., Giordano, A. L., Cashwell, C. S., & Lewis, T. F. (2013). The straight path to healing: Using Motivational Interviewing to address spiritual bypass. *Journal of Counseling & Development, 91*, 87–94.

Corey, G., Corey, M. S., & Callanan, P. (2003). *Issues & ethics in the helping professions* (6th ed). Brooks/Cole.

Day-Vines, N. L., Wood, S. M., Grothaus, T., Craigen, L., Holman, A., Dotson-Blake, K., & Douglass, M. J. (2007). Broaching the subjects of race, ethnicity, and culture during the counseling process. *Journal of Counseling & Development, 85*, 401–409.

Delaney, H. D., Forcehimes, A. A., Campbell, W. P., & Smith, B. W. (2009). Integrating spirituality into alcohol treatment. *Journal of Clinical Psychology, 65*, 185–198. https://doi.org/10.1002/jclp.20566

Diallo, A., Herold, M., Diallo, L., Marini, I., & Dominguez, A. (2021). Clients' willingness to incorporate religion or spirituality in counseling. *Rehabilitation Research, Policy and Education, 35*, 2–17.

Exline, J. J., Pargament, K. I., Grubbs, J. B., & Yali, A. M. (2014). The religious and spiritual struggles scale: Development and initial validation. *Psychology of Religion and Spirituality, 6*, 208–222. http://doi.org/10.1037/a0036465

Exline, J. J., & Rose, E. D. (2013). Religious and spiritual struggles. In R. F Paloutzian & C. L. Park (Eds.), *Handbook of the psychology of religion and spirituality* (2nd ed., pp. 380–398). Guilford Press.

Giordano, A. L. (2020). Bridging the great divide: Ethics of spiritually integrated counseling. In C. S. Cashwell & J. S. Young (Eds.), *Integrating spirituality and religion into counseling: A guide to competent practice* (3rd ed., pp. 31–52). American Counseling Association.

Giordano, A. L., & Cashwell, C. S. (2014). Entering the sacred: Using Motivational Interviewing to address spirituality in counseling. *Counseling & Values, 59*, 65–79. https://doi.org/10.1002/j.2161-007X.2014.00042.x

Giordano, A. L., Prosek, E. A., & Lankford, C. T. (2014). Predicting empathy: The role of religion and spirituality. *Journal of Professional Counseling: Practice, Theory, and Research, 41*, 53–66. https://doi.org/10.1080/15566382.2014.12033938

Grant Weinandy, J. T., & Grubbs, J. B. (2021). Gambling with God: The effect of gambling on religious and spiritual struggles. *Mental Health, Religion, & Culture, 24*, 437–449. https://doi.org/10.1080/13674676.2021.1878491

Gutierrez, D., Mason, N., Dorais, S., & Fox, J. (2021). Gradually sudden: Vital spiritual experiences for individuals in recovery from substance use disorders. *Spirituality in Clinical Practice, 8*, 16–29. https://doi.org/10.1037/scp0000218

Herlihy, B., & Corey, G. (2015). Managing value conflicts. In B. Herlihy & G. Corey (Eds.), *ACA ethical standards casebook* (7th ed., pp. 193–214). American Counseling Association.

Hodge, D. R. (2005). Spiritual lifemaps: A client-centered pictorial instrument for spiritual assessment, planning, and intervention. *Social Work, 50*, 77–87. https://doi.org/10.1093/sw/50.1.77

Hodge, D. R. (2015). *Spiritual assessment in social work and mental health practice.* Columbia University Press.

Howden, J. W. (1992). *Development and psychometric characteristics of the Spirituality Assessment Scale.* (Unpublished doctoral dissertation). Texas Women's University, Denton.

Kelly, J. F., & Eddie, D. (2020). The role of spirituality and religiousness in aiding recovery from alcohol and other drug problems: An investigation in a national U.S. sample. *Psychology of Religion and Spirituality, 12*, 116–123. https://doi.org/10.1037/rel0000295

Kocet, M. M., & Herlihy, B. J. (2014). Addressing value-based conflicts within the counseling relationship: A decision-making model. *Journal of Counseling & Development, 92*, 180–186

Lin, Y., Worthington, E. L., Griffin, B. J., Greer, C. L., Opare-Henaku, A., Lavelock, C. R., Hook, J. N., Yee Ho, M., & Muller, H. (2014). Efficacy of REACH forgiveness across cultures. *Journal of Clinical Psychology, 70*(9), 781–793. https://doi.org/10.1002/jclp.22073

McConnell, K. M., Pargament, K. I., Ellison, C. G., & Flannelly, K. J. (2006). Examining the links between spiritual struggles and symptoms of psychopathology in a national sample. *Journal of Clinical Psychology, 62*(12), 1469–1484. https://doi.org/10.1002/jclp.20325

McIntosh, D. N., Paulin, M. J., Silver, R. C., & Holman, E. A. (2011). The distinct roles of spirituality and religiosity in physical and mental health after collective trauma: A national longitudinal study of responses to the 9/11 attacks. *Journal of Behavioral Medicine, 34*, 497–507. https://doi.org/10.1007/s10865-011-9331-y

Miller, W. R., & Rollnick, S. (2013). *Motivational interviewing: Helping people change* (3rd ed.). Guilford Press.

Myers, J. E., Sweeney, T. J., & Witmer, J. M. (2000). The wheel of wellness counseling for wellness: A holistic model for treatment planning. *Journal of Counseling and Development, 78*, 251–267. https://doi.org/10.1002/j.1556-6676.2000.tb01906.x

Myers, J. E., & Williard, K. (2003). Integrating spirituality into clinician preparation: A developmental wellness approach. *Counseling & Values, 47*, 142–155. https://doi.org/10.1002/j.2161-007x.2003.tb00231.x

Najavits, L. M. (2002). *Seeking safety: A treatment manual for PTSD and substance use.* Guilford Press.

Nowinski, J., Baker, S., & Carroll, K. (1995). *Twelve step facilitation manual: A clinical research guide for therapists treating individuals with alcohol abuse and dependence.* National Institute on Alcohol Abuse and Alcoholism.

Ohrt, J. H., Clarke, P. B., & Conley, A. H. (2019). *Wellness counseling: A holistic approach to prevention and intervention.* American Counseling Association.

Pargament, K. I., & Abu-Raiya, H. (2007). A decade of research on the psychology of religion and coping: Things we assumed and lessons we learned. *Psyche & Logos, 28*, 742–766.

Pargament, K., Feuille, M., & Burdzy, D. (2011). The Brief RCOPE: Current psychometric status of a short measure of religious coping. *Religions, 2*, 51–76. http://doi.org/10.3390/rel2010051

Pew Research Center (2021). *About three-in-ten U.S. adults are now religiously unaffiliated.* Retrieved from https://www.pewresearch.org/religion/2021/12/14/about-three-in-ten-u-s-adults-are-now-religiously-unaffiliated/

Prochaska, J. O., Norcross, J. C., & DiClementi, C. C. (1995). *Changing for good: A revolutionary six-stage program for overcoming bad habits and moving your life positively forward.* New York: Avon Books.

Ratts, M. J., Singh, A. A., Nassar-McMillan, S., Butler, S. K., & McCullough, J. R. (2016). Multicultural and social justice counseling competencies: Guidelines for the counseling profession. *Journal of Multicultural Counseling & Development, 44*, 28–48.

Senreich, E., Saint-Louis, N., Steen, J. T., & Cooper, C. E. (2022). The experiences of 12-step program attendees transitioning to online meetings during the COVID-19 Pandemic. *Alcoholism treatment quarterly.* Advanced Online Publication. https://doi.org/10.1080/07347324.2022.2102456

Stauner, N., Exline, J. J., Kusina, J. R., & Pargament, K. I. (2019). Religious and spiritual struggles, religiousness, and alcohol problems among undergraduates. *Journal of Prevention & Intervention in the Community, 47*, 243–258. http://doi.org/10.1080/10852352.2019.1603678

Wade, N. G., Cornish, M. A., Tucker, J. R., Worthington, E. L., Jr., Sandage, S. J., & Rye, M. S. (2018). Promoting forgiveness: Characteristics of the treatment, the clients, and their interaction. *Journal of Counseling Psychology, 65*(3), 358–371. https://doi.org/10.1037/cou0000260

Wade, N. G., Hoyt, W. T., Kidwell, J. E. M., & Worthington, E. L. (2014). Efficacy of psychotherapeutic interventions to promote forgiveness: A meta analysis. *Journal of Consulting & Clinical Psychology, 82*, 154–170.

Wade, N. G. & Worthington, E. L. (2005). In search of a common core: A content analysis of interventions to promote forgiveness. *Psychotherapy: Theory, Research, Practice, Training, 42*(2), 160–177. https://doi.org/10.1037/0033-3204.42.2.160

Wade, N. G., Worthington, E. L., & Meyer, J. E. (2005). But do they work? A meta-analysis of group interventions to promote forgiveness. In E. L. Worthington (Ed.), *Handbook of forgiveness* (pp. 423–439). Taylor & Francis.

Webb, J. R., Hirsch, J. K., & Toussaint, L. (2011). Forgiveness and alcohol problems: A review of the literature and a call for intervention-based research. *Alcoholism Treatment Quarterly, 29,* 245–273. https://doi.org/10.1080/07347324.2011.585922

Webb, J. R., Hirsch, J. k., & Toussaint, L. (2015). Forgiveness as a positive psychotherapy for addiction and suicide: Theory, research, and practice. *Spirituality in Clinical Practice, 2*(1), 48–60. https://doi.org/10.1037/scp0000054

Welwood, J. (1984). Principles of inner work: Psychological and spiritual. *The Journal of Transpersonal Psychology, 16,* 63–73.

Wilt, J. A., Grubbs, J. B., Exline, J. J., & Pargament, K. I. (2016). Personality, religious, and spiritual struggles, and well being. *Psychology of Religion & Spirituality, 8,* 341–351. https://doi.org/10.1037/rel0000054

Witmer, J. M., & Sweeney, T. J. (1992). A holistic model for wellness and prevention over the lifespan. *Journal of Counseling & Development, 71,* 140–148. https://doi.org/10.1002/j.1556-6676.1992.tb02189.x

Worthington, E. L. (2000). Forgiveness usually takes time: A lesson learned by studying interventions to promote forgiveness. *Journal of Psychology and Theology, 28*(1), 3–20. https://doi.org/10.1177/009164710002800101

Worthington, E. L. (2003). *Forgiving and reconciling: Bridges to wholeness and hope.* InterVarsity Press.

Worthington, E. L. (2013a). *Forgiveness and reconciliation: Theory and application.* Routledge.

Worthington, E. L. (2013b). *Self-directed learning workbook: An intervention designed to promote self-forgiveness.* Virginia Commonwealth University.

Worthington, E. L., Jr., Sandage, S. J., & Berry, J. W. (2000). Group interventions to promote forgiveness: What researchers and clinicians ought to know. In M. E. McCullough, K. I. Pargament, & C. E. Thoresen (Eds.), *Forgiveness: Theory, research, and practice* (pp. 228–253). The Guilford Press.

Young, J. S., & Cashwell, C. S. (2020). Integrating spiritualty and religion into counseling: An introduction. In C. S. Cashwell & J. S. Young (Eds.), *Integrating spirituality and religion into counseling: A guide to competent practice* (3rd ed., pp. 3–30). American Counseling Association.

CHAPTER 10

EMOTIONAL WELLNESS: TURNING INWARDS TO EXPERIENCE HOLISTIC RECOVERY

INTRODUCTION

Our emotional lives are an irreplaceable and pivotal aspect of wellness. In some ways, the emotions we experience are the causal factors in our overall wellness. For example, when we are feeling sad, these emotions can easily trickle down into the other wellness dimensions making us feel spiritually hollow, triggering negative thoughts, de-motivating us from spending time with others (or causing us to interact negatively with others), and precipitating loss of interest in physical activity. The opposite can happen when experiencing pleasant emotions.

On the other hand, emotions are one of the best indicators of our wellness across dimensions (McKay, Wood, & Brantley, 2019). When we nurture wellness or are experiencing higher level of wellness in one or more dimensions, this is often reflected in how we feel. Take for example, a person whose daily wellness plan includes the following: wake up and exercise, consume a healthy breakfast, engage in work or meaningful activity during the day, and then participate in a social activity or hobby that induces flow in the evening. Following through on this plan could positively affect their emotional wellness. If we take care of ourselves, we tend to feel better and feel better about ourselves. When we attend to our wellness, our emotions (which can be like a window into our inner world) inform us of our needs, preferences, and "job performance" (how we're doing at taking care of ourselves).

EMOTIONAL INTELLIGENCE

What are emotions and how are they produced? From an emotional intelligence perspective, emotions are

> … organized responses, crossing the boundaries of many psychological subsystems, including the physiological, cognitive, motivational, and experiential systems. Emotions typically arise in response to an event, either internal or external, that has a positively or negatively valenced meaning for the individual.
>
> (Salovey & Mayer, 1990, p. 186)

The clinician can emphasize to clients that emotions, like each wellness dimension, are holistic in nature. Emotional intelligence entails being skilled at identifying emotions intrapersonally and within a social context for the purpose of refining cognitive processes such as decision-making and implementation (Salovey & Mayer, 1990).

Mayer and Salovey's Four Branch Model of Emotional Intelligence (1997) starts with noticing the emotion (via signs of emotions manifested physically, cognitively, and/or affectively), communicating of that emotion and one's needs, and applying emotions in the service of decision-making (Neubauer & Feudenthaler, 2005). Individuals with increased EI

DOI: 10.4324/9781003147954-10

capacity are able to drill down and identify specific emotions and make sense of them; in other words, comprehend why they might be feeling a certain way. Emotion regulation can sometimes be misconstrued as avoiding or suppressing negative emotions. However, similar to a mindfulness or Acceptance and Commitment Therapy philosophy, one is accepting of positive and negative emotions. This empowers the individual to discern which approach to the emotion ("engage" or "detach") will be most productive (Neubauer & Feudenthaler, 2005, p. 37). We wish to point out that we have omitted the social context aspects of EI which will be discussed more in the Connection Wellness chapter. However, it is worth noting that EI in one's social life allows the person to uncover the emotions conveyed in verbal and non-verbal communication with others and to mobilize this data toward positive personal and relational outcomes (Mayer, Caruso, & Salovey, 2016).

Individuals with substance use problems and disorders may face more challenges with emotion identification, emotion-informed meaning-making, and emotion regulation than those without these concerns. A meta-analysis of 95 studies involving 156,025 participants yielded several connections between the components of EI and the consumption of substances (Weiss et al., 2022). Problems with impulse control, acknowledging favorable and unfavorable feelings, the capacity to persevere toward goals when faced with one's feelings, difficulty mobilizing emotion regulation skills, and skillfulness at noticing and identifying feelings were related to substance use (Weiss et al., 2022).

TRAUMA AND EMOTIONAL WELLNESS

Of special consideration in the application of WBAC is the experience of trauma, which can markedly disrupt your clients' emotional wellness. Correlations between adverse childhood experiences (ACEs) and SUDs have been found in multiple studies (Leza, Siria, López-Goñi, & Fernandez-Montalvo, 2021). In one study, 36.6% of participants receiving SUD treatment also met the criteria for PTSD, whereas 10.2% of the control group met criteria for PTSD (Gielen, Havermans, Tekelenburg, & Jansen, 2012). Trauma symptoms and effects such as body dissociation (Price & Herting, 2013) and alexithymia ("… a deficit in emotion processing … characteristics include difficulty identifying and describing feelings as well as discriminating between feelings and physical sensations" [de Haan, van der Palen, Wijdeveld, Buitelaar, & De Jong, 2014, p. 137]) may pose a barrier to emotional wellness. Hence, trauma-informed approaches are vital to include during emotional wellness work and across the dimensions.

When embarking on activities and discussions of emotional wellness, which can be activating to clients, clinicians should equip clients with grounding skills to assist them if they dissociate or become flooded with emotions. Najavits (2017) noted three types of grounding: mental, physical, and soothing. A mental grounding example is the 3-2-1 exercise in which the client verbalizes three things they can see, hear, and touch, then two things they can see, hear, and touch, etc. (Baggerly, 2007). A second example is to "describe an activity in great detail" which entails the client elaborating on the step-by-step process of a daily endeavor such as getting ready for school or work (Najavits, 2017, p. 127). Another is a "safety statement" with the client verbalizing the following components: their name, a reminder that they are safe and in the present moment rather than the past, where they are currently located and the date. Instances of physical grounding include the client keeping a grounding object with them that they can touch if activated, "dig your heels into the floor" and say to oneself or aloud "… you're connected to the ground", and "run cool or warm water over your hands" (Najavits, 2017, p. 127). Soothing grounding can range from repeating a constructive or reassuring phrase from music or literature to "describe[ing] a place that you [the client] find soothing" (Najavits, 2017, p. 128).

INITIAL EMOTIONAL WELLNESS APPROACHES

The clinician will want to normalize for clients that it may take some time and practice before they feel more adept at identifying, labeling, and experiencing emotions. The metaphor I (Phil) have used and seen other clinicians use is that during periods of active use and even during times of abstinence or reduced use, their feelings may have been frozen. In early recovery, those feelings are only beginning to thaw out. Hence, clients may be feeling many ways ranging from numb to overwhelmed and flooded with feelings.

Inform your clients that to build this emotional wellness muscle, you'll be reflecting feeling frequently. This clinical skill will help the client both identify and make meaning of their feelings. You will also help increase their feelings vocabulary and ability to spot feelings when experienced. One way to do this is to frequently bring feelings into the conversation. For instance, at the beginning and at different points in a session, ask the client what they are feeling. Ensure that the client states a feeling word, rather than "good" or "bad", for example. Provide the client with a feelings chart (numerous ones can be found via the internet). *Convey to your clients that they will determine the rate and depth of feelings exploration* (Ford & Courtois, 2020; SAMHSA, 2020).

Clients may face barriers to emotional wellness and hold negative perceptions about feelings due to the following:

- Possibility that the client's caregivers did not model emotion processing, disregarded their feelings, or punished them for their feelings.
- The presence of co-occurring trauma and/or disorders.
- Clients with SUDs have anesthetized emotions via substance use. The longer their history of addictive substance use, the longer they have been without fully experiencing some emotions.
- Clients may face more emotional strife in their recovery than active addiction due to facing consequences that were eluded during active addiction.
- The clinician may have an emotion block or discomfort with their own and/or others' emotions (Ivey et al., 2005).

Defining and de-constructing the client's thoughts and feelings about feelings may be needed before venturing further into emotional wellness. Based on Leahy, Tirch, & Napolitano (2011), the clinician can invite the client to do a free writing exercise about emotions, inquiring, "what are the first things that come to mind when I say the word "emotions" or "feelings?"" You can also ask, "what do you like or appreciate about feelings and what do you dislike about feelings?" The clinician can select ideas that may contain myths and de-construct them with the client. This is similar to the "Thought Diary" from the Mental Wellness chapter in which the client identifies a more helpful thought about emotions or disputes the belief about emotions. Moreover, the client can also examine the pros and cons of adhering to the different myths. As another layer, you can encourage the client to explore where these myths came from with the following question: "What experiences and people in your life influenced these thoughts and feelings you have about emotions? How has the client's culture influenced their thoughts and feelings about emotions?" (Leahy et al., 2011).

The WBAC clinician should introduce EI as the pathway for increasing emotional wellness. As a part of this, the clinician should define emotions and why they are essential to our overall wellness. Refer to the Salovey and Mayer (1990) quote above for a definition of emotions. The clinician should then explain that emotions come into our awareness when one or more of our five senses relay information to the limbic system (part of the brain), which analyzes the emotion data and notifies the body on how to react (McKay et al., 2019). McKay et al. (2019) stated that emotions are signals that help you do the following: survive ("fight, flight, or freeze"), remember people and situations, cope with situations in your daily life, communicate with others, avoid pain, [and] seek pleasure" (p. 150).

CONNECTING EMOTIONAL WELLNESS TO HOLISTIC WELLNESS

During the intake session(s) and across each dimension, the clinician inquires about the effects of substance use and addictive behavior on wellness and vice versa. It is of paramount importance to do this during emotional wellness work because of the powerful connections between addictive behaviors and emotions. Key questions include:

- In what ways did your addictive behaviors help your emotional wellness?
- In what ways did these behaviors harm your emotional wellness?
- In what ways did the challenges you experienced with emotional wellness affect these behaviors?

An early activity to increase the client's comfort and skill with emotions is to ask the client to make a list of the emotions that have detracted the most from their wellness and recovery and a second part of the list that documents the emotions that have been most helpful in their wellness and recovery. The client should identify the specific wellness dimensions that were affected by different emotions and in what ways. This activity will also provide assessment information as it may become clear that some clients have difficulty identifying their emotions or using feeling words. Avoidance or discomfort with feelings may become apparent through this process and can be explored further.

The clinician may also request that the client create a list of thoughts and wellness activities across each wellness dimension that produce positive emotions. For instance, wellness thoughts can serve as mantras that can be repeated as needed to elicit positive emotions. The wellness activities list already developed by the client during the WBAC process can be incorporated or added here. A third option is to invite the client to list activities across the wellness dimensions that are helpful distractions when they are experiencing stress or distress. Additionally, the client can flag distractions that may be helpful in the short-term, but not desirable in the long term.

SETTING THE STAGE WITH SELF-MONITORING AND MINDFULNESS

Clients may be less effective at knowing when and how to implement emotion regulation strategies unless they have some sense of when and what emotions they are experiencing. Self-monitoring once again comes in handy as well as a mindfulness-based emotion intervention. Let's start with how to self-monitor emotions. Emotions are composed of four components (McKay & West, 2016). Those components include thoughts, feelings, sensations, and urges. As discussed in the Mental Wellness Chapter, thoughts are related to feelings and behaviors. Hence, when a thought crosses our mind, it can precipitate one or more feelings. Feelings are the words used to describe the affect, sensations reflect what we experience in our body such as heaviness in the chest, and "Urges are impulses to do something – or not to do something" (McKay & West, 2016, p. 20). McKay and West (2016) recommended charting these emotional elements over several days whenever a strong feeling(s) arise.

A translational skill described in the Mental Wellness chapter that can be applied to emotional wellness is urge surfing. Since an urge is an aspect of emotion, this same technique can be implemented with other emotions. McKay and West (2016) called the skill, emotion surfing, and note that it can be an antidote for emotion avoidance by showing the client that they can effectively encounter their feelings. The main difference with emotion surfing is that the client should observe and describe the thoughts, feelings, sensations, and urges that arise interspersed with identifying "where am I on the wave" (p. 57). A Subjective Units of Distress Score (SUDS) in which 1 is equivalent to "no distress", 5 represents "moderate distress", and 10 represents the "worst distress imaginable" (p. 34) allows clients to quantify "where am I on the wave". Similar to other evidence-based interventions such as Dialectical Behavior Therapy, Acceptance and Commitment Therapy, and Relapse Prevention, the client's job is to be an objective witness to their emotions (Leahy et al., 2011).

EMOTIONAL WELLNESS DECISION TREE

Participating in these initial emotional wellness activities positions the client to employ multiple options for coping. One theme of emotion work is that clients are empowered to navigate their emotions in a way that feels positive, meaningful, effective, and congruent for them. In WBAC, as the client increases their ability to ground themselves and observe their emotions, a set of reflection questions enables them to determine their next steps when challenging emotions are experienced. The WBAC clinician is shifting the client into an emotion management role where they are encouraged to make decisions about their responses to feelings. The self-reflection questions here represent a decision tree of sorts, enabling the client's discernment of the next steps. Upon awareness of a strong and painful emotion, clients can reflect on the following (Marlatt, Parks, & Witkiewitz, 2002; McKay & West, 2016; McKay et al., 2019):

- What is the emotion you are experiencing?
- Rate your distress level on the SUDs scale from 1 to 10.
- What triggered the emotion? Was it an internal or external trigger?
    - If an external trigger, do you want to address the situation at hand or remove yourself from the situation?
- Is the feeling partly or mostly due to a current need (Maslow's Hierarchy [1943]) or wellness need?
    - Basic needs: "air, food, water, shelter, and rest" (Hale, Ricotta, Freed, Smith, & Huang, 2019), physical or emotional safety.
    - Wellness needs examples: Mental stimulation, hope, social support, religious or spiritual, etc.

Emotional Wellness Decision Tree

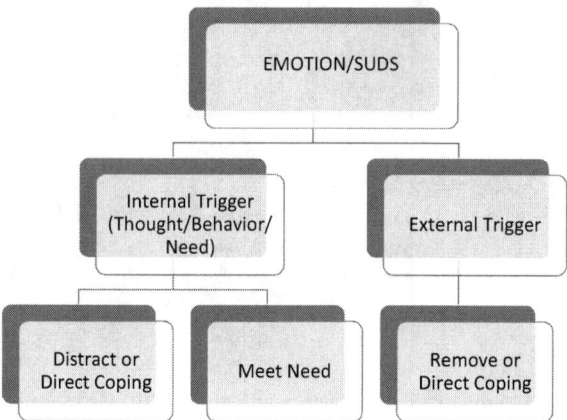

Figure 10.1 Emotional Wellness Decision Tree based on Marlatt, Parks, & Witkiewitz, 2002; McKay & West, 2016; McKay, Wood, & Brantley, 2019.

- If due to a current need, what can you do to fulfill that need at this time?
- If not primarily a current need, and emotions remain from the internal or external trigger, would it be most helpful to distract yourself or employ a skill to cope directly with the emotion (e.g., emotion surfing, cognitive-behavioral, emotional support, and expression).

Figure 10.1 contains a visual depiction of the emotional wellness decision tree. Each chapter in this book contains wellness techniques that can be implemented for distraction and/or coping. In the section below, we'll elaborate on emotional support and expression approaches.

EMOTIONAL SUPPORT AND EXPRESSION

One way to enhance emotional wellness is with support from helpful significant others. In the Connection chapter, you'll learn about different types of social support, one of which is emotional support. A friend, colleague, family member, etc. can be a listening ear allowing us to pause and examine our emotions, reduce a sense of isolation from some negative emotions, and revive our self-efficacy. This can be a constructive time for you to pause and reflect on a recent example of helpful and unhelpful support you have received when you talked with someone else to cope with painful feelings. It is true that the right social support for emotions holds the benefits listed above. The wrong social support may add to our distress. Consider asking the client about the qualities of helpful social supporters for emotions (Ohrt, Clarke, & Conley, 2019). These can include that the supporter has demonstrated themselves to be trustworthy, an effective listener, thoughtful provider of feedback (when feedback is requested), caring, etc. Clinicians should also inform clients that they can influence how helpful the supporter will be. Specifically, informing the listener of the type of support needed will allow them to be maximally supportive. For example, the client can request advice, encouragement, a sounding board with minimal advice, a brainstorming/problem-solving partner, a cheer-leader, a distractor, etc. It can be difficult to ascertain what one needs amid strong emotions. Hence, it may be easier for the client to know what they don't want. For instance, the client may apprise the listener that "I don't want to be told everything is ok".

If expressing emotions to someone else is not preferable or possible, it might benefit the client to use other outlets for emotional expression. As WBAC is strength-based, we first turn to the client to elicit avenues of emotional expression that have been helpful and not helpful and why. Additional forms of emotional expression that the client can experiment with include journaling and the creative arts. One caveat with emotional expression is that the client may need to establish boundaries on this skill because too much time processing emotions may be harmful (McKay & West, 2016). The client can rate their emotions before, during, and after an emotional expression activity using the SUDS scale to gauge its utility. The client may also want to set a timer on the expression activity so that they unpack the emotion in manageable portions (McKay et al., 2019). In line with WBAC's emphasis on balance, coupling emotional expression with a pleasing distraction activity may be an effec-tive succession of coping strategies.

In the final sections of this chapter, we'll examine three emotion-related constructs that merit consideration during counseling for emotional wellness with individuals in recovery: self-esteem, grief and loss, and hope.

SELF-ESTEEM

The experience of repeated relapses and wellness struggles can cloud one's view of self. On the one hand, shame entails feeling broken and bad as a person, and on the other hand, self-esteem involves feeling good about ourselves. Clients would do well to identify any well-ness challenges that have injured their self-esteem or resulted in shame. An adaptation of an experiential activity to address self-esteem allows clients to become aware of self-talk and behaviors that diminish or increase their self-esteem (Jacobs, 1994; Jacobs & Schimmel, 2013). The clinician holds one Styrofoam cup filled with water and uses Schiraldi's (2016) conceptualization of self-esteem to explain that this cup is full, (analogous to one's "core self") and that core self is "beautiful, lovable, and full of potential" (p. 34). The clinician then asks the client to identify (a) things they tell themselves, (b) things communicated to them by others overtly or covertly, (c) experiences, and (d) behaviors that detract from how they feel about themselves. Each time a self-esteem detractor is identified, the clinician asks about the size of the impact on their self-esteem [small, medium, or large]. The clinician then pours out water for each one as the client goes along, with small pours for small detractors and larger pours for larger detractors (Jacobs, 1994; Jacobs & Schimmel, 2013). Conversely, the clinician then asks about the same four categories that enhance the client's self-esteem and fills the cup back up accordingly.

During the debriefing of the activity, the clinician enlists the client in a brainstorm for ways to cope with self-esteem detractors and ways to call on and utilize self-esteem enhancers. According to Schiraldi (2016), growth (along with love and unconditional worth) is an element of self-esteem. Hence, reviewing the client's wellness progress and its implica-tions (as should be done throughout the WBAC process) is invaluable. Build in time to not only reflect on growth, but what this means for the client's self-esteem and how that growth benefits other dimensions of their well-being.

In later stages of recovery after the client has made progress, the client can take a deep dive (guided by the work of Carl Rogers) on the self-esteem enhancers and decipher which enhancers the client was seeking to please others and which ones were used to please themselves (Murdock, 2017). The client can then have increased awareness of what they want to engage in in their lives and why.

The person in recovery may have a difficult time filling the self-esteem cup. Maintaining a self-esteem journal compels the client to actively seek out things they like or value about themselves. Like many of the activities in this book, the process of self-esteem journaling alone can be therapeutic. The primary directions are to take five to ten minutes per day to write freely about something from their day that makes them feel positive about themselves. If nothing comes to mind from that particular day, the client can call to mind other aspects of themselves across the wellness dimensions that they value in themselves. A more structured approach entails using the dimensions as the guide for self-reflection. For example, the journaling session can center on writing about self-esteem-enhancing personal qualities from a particular wellness dimension.

GRIEF AND LOSS

Most mental health and addictions professionals have heard clients state that they cannot imagine living without their substance(s) of addiction, which sounds very much like what one would say about a loved one. The strength of the bond or attachment that develops between the person and the addictive behavior can be comparable to that of a relationship between two people (Luke, 2017). Furthermore, Luke (2017) noted that the addicted individual may experience more of a steadfast "relationship" with their substance or addictive behavior than another person. This is because it is possible that key people in their lives have not been dependable, whereas they can have faith in the substance to have its desired effect.

Furr, Johnson, and Goodall, (2015) identified 36 losses that could occur before active addiction, during active addiction, and upon receiving SUDs treatment. These losses included social status, economic status, educational status, relational loss, autonomy, meaning and purpose, career, and being the victim of abuse (physical, sexual, emotional). Furr and Hunsucker (2022) examined addiction recovery through several grief counseling lenses including William Worden's tasks of mourning listed below (2009):

Task 1: To Accept the Reality of the Loss

Task 2: To Process the Pain of Grief

Task 3: To Adjust to a World Without the Deceased

Task 4: To Find an Enduring Connection with the Deceased in the Midst of Embarking on a New Life (Worden, 2009, p. 39).

This model is edifying for clinicians using WBAC. One can extrapolate from Worden that it can be powerful to validate that there will be emotionally difficult parts of the recovery process. Specifically, major life changes involve gains and losses and the client may have also experienced additional losses that become activated in recovery. Hence, several helpful routes can be explored regarding grief and loss such as (a) losses the client anticipates if they are to make changes to their substance use, (b) losses the client has experienced in their life and/or related to their addiction that may impact their recovery, (c) losses that the client hopes can be resolved or recovered, and (d) potential gains from grieving the loss or change in addictive behavior.

One starting point is to ask the client to list the losses they anticipate if or when they choose to pursue wellness changes including substance use. The client should discuss the effect of these losses, losses the client hopes to recover, and potential gains from grieving these losses. As you ascertain that the client can cope with the emotional activation that can result from discussing profound grief experiences (which intersect with trauma), the client can also list life and/or addiction-related losses, how they may affect recovery, and possible coping skills (Furr, 2022). Furr (2022) advised that clinicians attend to appropriate pacing when de-constructing losses ensuring clients have coping skills and stabilization in their mental health and substance use. WBAC is not a trauma-focused approach so the focus would be on identifying the loss without fully describing what occurred and centering the dialog on the issues posed and how to address them.

You might consider administering Furr et al.'s (2015) "Experience of Loss in Addictions Inventory"; however, be aware that many of the losses presented in the inventory pertain to traumatic experiences rendering it important for the clinician to gauge timing and appropriateness for its use (Hunsucker & Furr, 2022). It is also important to discuss that some of these losses can be recovery related while others may not. Examples across the dimensions include loss of hobbies (mental wellness), loss of faith community (spiritual), loss of relationships from bridges burned, and anticipated relational loss to avoid substance-using peers (connection). Furthermore, Furr et al. (2015) mentioned Streifel and Servaty-Seib's (2009) highlighting of loss of the "clients' identity as an 'addict', giving-up ways of coping, and shifting their belief system and views of life" (p. 45). Identity and mental wellness transformations are also examined in the Culture, Context, Development, and Mental Wellness chapters, respectively.

Clients can write a letter to their addiction in order to attend to Worden's (2018) tasks of mourning. The substance or addictive behavior should be referred to using first-person language, with a sample opening phrase such as "Dear Alcohol, I know that we've been dating for several years, but I have written this letter to tell you that we can't see each other anymore" (Hagedorn, 2011, p. 115) or replacing "dating" with "close friends". Based on the work of Hagedorn (2011), the client writes one or more paragraphs on the following:

- What the client appreciates about the addiction.
- Ways in which the addiction has helped with life issues across each wellness dimension.
- Ways in which the addiction exerts control in the client's life, and what the addiction has taken from the client.

Furr and Hunsucker (2022) proposed additional prompts and de-briefing questions that can be integrated in the letter such as

- What qualities of the addictive behavior and the relationship/friendship will you miss the most?
- What are the advantages of breaking up or discontinuing the relationship/ friendship?
- What strategies will you implement if the relationship/friendship attempts to return?
- What strengths do you possess and will you cultivate in the absence of the relationship/friendship?
- What would you like to express in your goodbyes to the relationship/friendship?

The letter can be read aloud by the client during an individual session and de-briefing of the writing and reading experience should be conducted. Unique considerations exist for using this activity in group counseling. See Hagedorn (2011) for more information on facilitating this activity with counseling groups.

Furr (2022) defined Worden's internal adjustments and spiritual adjustments from Task 3 (2018) as an identity crisis ("who was I, who am I and who do I want to be") and an existential crisis ("what is this [life] for and what type of world am I living in"), respectively. Journaling or in-session inquiry into these topics can be worthwhile. For instance, using the wellness dimensions as a guide, the clinician can ask the client to journal about or discuss their vision for returning to and further discovering the person they want to be. What will they notice that lets them know they are feeling more positive and clearer about their identity? What constructive new thoughts and feelings would increasingly arise about themselves and the world? What parts of themselves would stand out even more? What parts of themselves would they like to restore? The client should attempt to note observable strides that would indicate progress (Hunsucker & Furr, 2022).

Harris and Winokuer (2016) also pointed out the relevance of rituals of grieving such as funerals. The client may need to grieve the loss of certain rituals tied to their addictive behavior. Clients may need to rid themselves of paraphernalia, contact information for sources of substances, etc. This can be an opportunity for grieving. The client throwing away a using device or their alcohol can be a time for the client to process (a) what they will miss, (b) what the most difficult changes will entail, (c) why they are parting ways with the addictive behavior, (d) what the elimination of these vessels for using represents and means to the person, (e) new rituals they hope to enact, and (f) what they are looking forward to in life without the substance or addictive behavior. Loved ones can be present for this ritual (provided that their presence and sharing are constructive) and share (a) what this "throwing away" of the addictive behavior means to them, (b) positive qualities/strengths this demonstrates about their loved one, (c) ways in which they will support their loved one, and (d) ways in which they hope their relationship with the loved one improves. This exercise addresses each of Worden's (2009) four tasks of mourning. Moreover, many aspects of this activity can still be used if the client chooses a harm reduction approach as it can provide a milestone of a changed relationship with their addictive behavior.

HOPE

A final critical emotional wellness component that is attended to in WBAC is hope. Research and clinical developments suggest that time spent discussing hope in counseling may be time well spent. Before we get to some of the hope techniques, let's define hope and examine the research base on hope in mental health, addiction, and counseling outcomes. Larsen et al. (2020) defined hope in psychotherapy as "the client's anticipation of meaningful change in the face of uncertainty. Client hope in psychotherapy is experienced in one or more of the following dimensions: relational (therapeutic and other), cognitive, emotional, temporal, behavioral, process, personal meaning, and spirituality" (p. 412). In this definition, you can hear the holistic nature of how these researchers have described the hope construct. Snyder (2000) theorized that hope consists of goals, pathways, and agency. Specifically, hope arises when a person has goals that they have a moderate (but not guaranteed) possibility of reaching in combination with ideas for how to reach the goal, and the belief that one can initiate progress and endure despite obstacles that may occur.

Lenz (2021) conducted a study on hope, resilience, and happiness in a youth population (middle and high school) and found that higher hope scores corresponded with fewer mental health symptoms. In a study of adolescents living in residential treatment, detention centers, and homeless shelters, participants with higher levels of hope (e.g., belief that positive events were imminent; Lippman et al., 2014) engaged in less alcohol, tobacco, and marijuana use over the past month (Brooks, Marshal, McCauley, Douaihy, & Miller, 2016). A study on adults living in recovery housing revealed that hope (agency and pathways) assessed four months prior is predictive of current depression and anxiety symptoms (May, Hunter, Ferrari, Noel, & Jason, 2015). Gutierrez, Dorais, and Goshorn (2020), discovered that the inverse relationship between the strides adults make in SUD recovery and their risk of relapse is partially mediated by hope. Based on their study, the researchers issued a powerful statement regarding the link between wellness and hope: "we suggest that helping professionals and addiction treatment professionals consider adopting a holistic approach to addiction recovery that includes factors associated with wellbeing and human flourishing, as opposed to focusing solely on the managing of behaviors" (p. 1954).

Hope approaches involve both "being" and "doing" aspects for the role of the clinician. Regarding "being", the clinician must accept the duality of the client's hopelessness and hope. A qualitative study of mental health professionals' hope-related work with clients illustrated the value of being able to sit with the client's thoughts and feelings of hopelessness (Larsen & Stege, 2010a). The illogicality of being a container for the client's hopelessness is that this paves the way for the client to experience hope and to create a constructive working relationship which also raises hope (Koehn & Cutcliffe, 2012).

Skills for Eliciting Hope

WBAC clinicians are adept at what Lopez et al. (2004) called "hope finding" (p. 390), identifying hope wherever it may reside. Hope finding can include the clinician's purposeful attending to the client's strengths and resources (Larsen & Stege, 2010a). One response option is to target your reflective listening skills on the hope that you're hearing; reflecting the hope you hear in the content or feelings from the client's comments. Based on wisdom from motivational interviewing, we know that clients will typically expound on the last thing the clinician said (Miller & Rollnick, 2013). Hence, if we reflect back the facets of hope we hear the client communicating, the client will likely engage in more dialog with you about hope. The reframe is a related skill in which the clinician listens for openings in the conversation to help clients see new possibilities and perspectives on challenges with which they are contending (Larsen & Stege, 2010a). Here are some examples below:

EXAMPLE 1:

CLIENT: This is my fourth time in treatment. I just keep messing up and ending up back here.

CLINICIAN: You've been persistent in your recovery journey. Seeking help if you need it.

EXAMPLE 2:

> *CLIENT:* I'm just not sure what I want to change about my wellness. There's so many direc-
> tions I could go in. In fact, I can never make decisions on anything. It's frustrating.
> *CLINICIAN:* You do know that you want to make a step forward and you have insight that
> decision-making is a challenge. You have several opportunities to choose from.

When finding hope, the clinician must use discretion; not overusing or misusing these skills in a manner that conveys that the client needs to be more optimistic or feel better.

You'll recall that hope is a holistic construct and hence can be explored from multiple directions. Larsen and Stege's (2010b) qualitative findings suggested that clinicians approached hope with clients along cognitive, behavioral, emotional, relational, and temporal dimensions. Thus, one thread for clinicians to pursue is to inquire about cognitions, behaviors, and relationships that could stimulate hope within the client. Larsen and Stege (2010b) elucidated how this is done in the behavioral domain stating, "Inviting clients to discuss hopeful actions was based on the premise that clients are likely to feel better about themselves and their circumstances when they behave in ways that they perceive as hopeful" (p. 300). The following are prompts across the wellness dimensions that can stimulate hope (Koehn, O'Neill, & Sherry, 2012; Larsen & Stege, 2010b):

- Tell me about a thought/feeling/experience/interaction you have had related to your recovery or wellness plan that makes you feel hopeful.
- What thoughts/feelings/experiences/interactions make you feel less hopeful or hopeless about being able to achieve your harm reduction/abstinence/wellness plan goals?
- If you do experience lapses or relapses in your wellness plan, what are some things you can think/feel/do that may bring hope?
- What thoughts/feelings/experiences/interactions have occurred since our last session that have made you feel hopeful about your life and/or wellness plan?

Koehn et al. (2012) developed a technique called the hope log; a weekly record of occurrences that increase or decrease hope. The hope log includes columns in which the client rates how hopeful they were feeling from 1 to 10 before and after the occurrence. Two key process questions from Koehn et al. (2012) that empower the client and maintain a focus on strengths and the relationship between wellness and substance use are the following (p. 445):

- "What are some of the things you are doing (or what are some of the personal qualities you have) that play a part in these hope fostering events occurring?"
- "How are your hope levels connected to your desire to use or not use substances?"

Hope collage is an activity that calls on the client to depict "people, places, or things" that they hope to gain through their holistic recovery and/or that make them feel hopeful about their holistic recovery (Koehn et al., 2012, p. 449; Larsen, Edey, & Lemay, 2007). The clinician should have a poster board for the collage, pictures and magazines from which words and images can be found, and other art supplies accessible to compose the collage. The authors recommend allotting clients 20–30 minutes to ponder and pick the facets of their collage. They also recommend stressing to clients that the goal of the activity is to promote insights and is not related to the artfulness of the collage.

The verbal de-constructing of the collage is an indispensable conclusion to this activity. The clinician can pose prompts such as (Koehn et al., 2012, p. 445): "What does hope mean to me? What is it about these images that inspire hope? How do I see change in my life happening, and what resources are needed? What is my role in promoting change?" The collage can also be transformed into a concrete resource by asking the client to identify how and when they can use the collage (Koehn et al., 2012).

Explorations of self-esteem, grief and loss, and hope provide the WBAC clinician with a roadmap for navigating and promoting emotional wellness among clients. We now turn to the case of Eric to see how strategies from this chapter might apply in the case.

CLIENT EXAMPLE

Although Eric was willing to enter addictions counseling and sought abstinence as his substance use goal, he made several statements indicating doubts about success and lower self-efficacy about being successful with his wellness plan longitudinally. The clinician recognized that attending to hope could attenuate some of these potentially relapse-inducing feelings.

> CLINICIAN: You mentioned some self-doubt that this treatment process will work. I can hear that it means a lot to you to live out your wellness plan goals. Tell me about the hope you do feel for this process regardless of whether it's big or small [Reframe of client's fears and using solution-focused type assumption question to elicit hope/begin hope discussion].
>
> ERIC: I have noticed that I did feel more hope after coming here for the first session. I felt like me taking the step to actually come to counseling gives me hope because counseling is some form of action. And I feel like Kelly and Lia maybe feel more hopeful since I've come to counseling and that gives me hope.
>
> CLINICIAN: Seeking counseling has been this ripple effect of hope; seeing progress and how that has instilled hope in your family [Reflection of hope expressed by the client which may facilitate further elaboration].
>
> As sessions progressed, the clinician recognized that Eric possessed strengths in the feelings dimension per his ability to experience feelings (becoming tearful when talking about his daughter). His emotional wellness challenges seemed to center on in-the-moment emotion identification, making sense of his emotions, and emotion management. The WBAC clinician wanted to facilitate client insight into the roots of these challenges.
>
> CLINICIAN: What did you observe and learn about feelings from your family?
>
> ERIC: My mom was sad a lot. That was hard to watch. She never talked about how she was feeling, but I could see it. My dad, at the time, didn't talk much about how he was feeling. Well... actually.... he would look very stressed out and angry, especially if I was misbehaving or some issue was happening at work or with mom.
>
> CLINICIAN: How did your dad cope with those feelings?
>
> ERIC: I still don't really know. I just know that he would leave the house a lot if he was stressed. I assume he was meeting up with friends or maybe other women. He didn't drink much or use any drugs, from what I remember.

CLINICIAN: It sounds like your experience at a young age was that feelings are negative; they're associated with problems and that feelings are to be kept to yourself and dealt with on your own [Reflection synthesizing the client's observational learning about feelings].

ERIC: Yes.

CLINICIAN: Experiences with emotions when we're growing up can still affect us in adulthood. What messages from your youth about emotions do you still carry with you today and how have they affected your wellness and substance use? [Helping the client make connections between his past experiences with emotions and current beliefs and responses to emotions].

ERIC: I guess they didn't leave me much to carry. I didn't learn how to talk about or deal with emotions. I'm scared of emotions.

CLINICIAN: Afraid of emotions [Underlining this feeling; encouraging the client to elaborate]. How does your drinking and wellness fit into this?

ERIC: That's how I chose to deal. Drinking. It was an escape. Like my dad running off when he was pissed. I have shit I've been dealing with over the years and I have tried to handle it my own way.

CLINICIAN: Drinking was the best option you could find to cope. A way to escape from feeling. I want to pause a moment and honor that in spite of not having family role models for managing feelings, in our sessions, you have demonstrated courage to sit with this topic and insight about your feelings. You have been able to pinpoint and make meaning of several of your feelings [Reframing emotion wellness problems as a strength].

Note how in the last segment here that the clinician underscored client insight into his relationship between drinking and feeling. Additionally, the clinician applied strengths-building by denoting a positive quality in the client and his emotional wellness skills with the goal of fostering the use of these skills and strengths.

CONCLUSION

Eliciting positive emotions and the necessary matriculation through painful emotions is a major part of emotional wellness for persons with SUDs and related concerns. We believe that a large part of the therapeutic value we provide clients is in facilitating meaningful experiences and skills from which the client may be deficient. WBAC places a premium on helping clients build these skills in a way that supports the recovery process.

REFERENCES

Baggerly, J. (Director). (2007). *Disaster mental health and crisis stabilization for children* [Video/DVD]. Microtraining Associates. Retrieved from https://video.alexanderstreet.com/watch/disaster-mental-health-and-crisis-stabilizationfor-children

Brooks, M. J., Marshal, M. P., McCauley, H. L., Douaihy, A., & Miller, E. (2016). The relationship between hope and adolescent likelihood to endorse substance use behaviors in a sample of marginalized youth. *Substance Use & Misuse, 51*(13), 1815–1819. https://doi.org/10.1080/1 0826084.2016.1197268 de Haan, H. A., van der Palen, J., Wijdeveld, T. G., Buitelaar, J. K., & De Jong, C. A. (2014). Alexithymia in patients with substance use disorders: State or trait? *Psychiatry Research, 216*(1), 137–145. https://doi.org/10.1016/j.psychres.2013.12.047

Ford, J. D., & Courtois, C. A. (2020). *Treating complex traumatic stress disorders in adults: Scientific foundations and therapeutic models* (2nd ed.). Guilford Press.

Furr, S. R. (2022). Is addiction a loss to grieve? In S. R. Furr & K. Hunsucker, (Eds.), *Grief work in addictions counseling* (pp. 1–17). Routledge.

Furr, S. R., & Hunsucker, K. (2022). Counseling activities to address grief and substance use. In S. R. Furr & K. Hunsucker (Eds.), *Grief work in addictions counseling* (pp. 274–285). Routledge.

Furr, S. R., Johnson, W. D., & Goodall, C. S. (2015). Grief and recovery: The prevalence of grief and loss in substance abuse treatment. *Journal of Addictions & Offender Counseling, 36*(1), 43–56. https://doi.org/10.1002/j.2161-1874.2015.00034.x

Gielen, N., Havermans, R., Tekelenburg, M., & Jansen, A. (2012). Prevalence of post-traumatic stress disorder among patients with substance use disorder: It is higher than clinicians think it is. *European Journal of Psychotraumatology, 3*(1), 17734. https://doi.org/10.3402/ejpt.v3i0.17734

Gutierrez, D., Dorais, S., & Goshorn, J. R. (2020). Recovery as life transformation: Examining the relationships between recovery, hope, and relapse. *Substance Use & Misuse, 55*(12), 1949–1957. https://doi.org/10.1080/10826084.2020.1781181

Hagedorn, W. B. (2011). Using therapeutic letters to navigate resistance and ambivalence: Experiential implications for group counseling. *Journal of Addictions & Offender Counseling, 31*(2), 108–126. https://doi.org/10.1002/j.2161-1874.2011.tb00071.x

Hale, A. J., Ricotta, D. N., Freed, J., Smith, C. C., & Huang, G. C. (2019). Adapting Maslow's hierarchy of needs as a framework for resident wellness. *Teaching and Learning in Medicine, 31*(1), 109–118. https://doi.org/10.1080/10401334.2018.1456928

Harris, D. L., & Winokuer, H. R. (2016). *Principles and practice of grief counseling* (2nd ed.). Springer Publishing Company.

Ivey, A. E., Ivey, M. B., Myers, J. E., & Sweeney, T. J. (2005). *Developmental counseling and therapy: Promoting wellness over the lifespan.* Houghton Mifflin/Lahaska.

Jacobs, E. (1994). *Impact therapy.* Psychological Assessment Resources.

Jacobs, E., & Schimmel, C., Impact therapy (2013). *Impact therapy shield, filter, cups.* [Video]. YouTube. Retrieved from https://www.youtube.com/watch?v=zFAdsG2Azg0

Koehn, C., & Cutcliffe, J. R. (2012). The inspiration of hope in substance abuse counseling. *The Journal of Humanistic Counseling, 51*(1), 78–98. https://doi.org/10.1002/j.21611939.2012.00007.x

Koehn, C., O'Neill, L., & Sherry, J. (2012). Hope-focused interventions in substance abuse counselling. *International Journal of Mental Health and Addiction, 10*, 441–452.

Larsen, D., Edey, W., & Lemay, L. (2007). Understanding the role of hope in counselling: Exploring the intentional uses of hope. *Counselling Psychology Quarterly, 20*(4), 401–416. https://doi.org/10.1080/09515070701690036

Larsen, D. J., & Stege, R. (2010a). Hope-focused practices during early psychotherapy sessions: Part I: Implicit approaches. *Journal of Psychotherapy Integration, 20*(3), 271–292. https://doi.org/10.1037/a0020820

Larsen, D. J., & Stege, R. (2010b). Hope-focused practices during early psychotherapy sessions: Part 2: Explicit approaches. *Journal of Psychotherapy Integration, 20*(3), 293–311. https://doi.org/10.1037/a0020821

Larsen, D. J., Whelton, W. J., Rogers, T., McElheran, J., Herth, K., Tremblay, J., Green, J., Dushinski, K., Schalk, K., Chamodraka, M., & Domene, J. (2020). Multidimensional hope in counseling and psychotherapy scale. *Journal of Psychotherapy Integration, 30*(3), 407–422. https://doi.org/10.1037/int0000198

Leahy, R. L., Tirch, D., & Napolitano, L. A. (2011). *Emotion regulation in psychotherapy: A practitioner's guide.* Guilford Press.

Lenz, A. S. (2021). Evidence for relationships between hope, resilience, and mental health among youth. *Journal of Counseling & Development, 99*(1), 96–103. https://doi.org/10.1002/jcad.12357

Leza, L., Siria, S., López-Goñi, J. J., & Fernandez-Montalvo, J. (2021). Adverse childhood experiences (ACEs) and substance use disorder (SUD): A scoping review. *Drug and Alcohol Dependence, 221*, 108563. https://doi.org/10.1016/j.drugalcdep.2021.108563

Lippman, L. H., Moore, K. A., Guzman, L., Ryberg, R., McIntosh, H., Ramos, M. F., & Kuhfeld, M. (2014). *Flourishing children: Defining and testing indicators of positive development. Springer briefs in well-being and quality of life research.* https://doi.org/10.1007/97894-017-8607-2

Lopez, S. J., Snyder, C. R., Magyar-Moe, J. L., Edwards, L. M., Pedrotti, J. T., Janowski, K., Turner, J. L., & Pressgrove, C. (2004). Strategies for accentuating hope. In P. A. Linley & S. Joseph (Eds.), *Positive psychology in practice* (pp. 388–404). John Wiley & Sons, Inc.

Luke, C. (2017, September 27). *Addiction as a relational disorder: A neuro-informed treatment perspective.* NAADAC recorded webinar. Retrieved from https://www.naadac.org/addiction-as-relational-disorder-webinar

Marlatt, G. A., Parks, G. A., & Witkiewitz, K. (2002) *Clinical guidelines for implementing relapse prevention therapy.* University of Washington.

Maslow, A. H. (1943). A theory of human motivation. *Psychological Review, 50*(4), 370–396. https://doi.org/10.1037/h0054346

May, E. M., Hunter, B. A., Ferrari, J., Noel, N., & Jason, L. A. (2015). Hope and abstinence self-efficacy: Positive predictors of negative affect in substance abuse recovery. *Community Mental Health Journal, 51,* 695–700.

Mayer, J. D., Caruso, D. R., & Salovey, P. (2016). The ability model of emotional intelligence: Principles and updates. *Emotion Review, 8*(4), 290–300. https://doi.org/10.1177/1754073916639667

Mayer, J. D. & Salovey, P. (1997). What is emotional intelligence? In P. Salovey and D. Sluyter (Eds.), *Emotional development and emotional intelligence: Educational implications* (pp. 3–31). Basic Books.

McKay, M., & West, A. (2016). *Emotion efficacy therapy: A brief, exposure-based treatment for emotion regulation integrating ACT and DBT.* Context Press/New Harbinger Publications.

McKay, M., Wood, J. C., & Brantley, J. (2019). *The dialectical behavior therapy skills workbook: Practical DBT exercises for learning mindfulness, interpersonal effectiveness, emotion regulation, and distress tolerance* (2nd ed.). New Harbinger Publications.

Miller, W. R., & Rollnick, S. (2013). *Motivational interviewing: Helping people change* (3rd ed.). Guilford Press.

Murdock, N. L. (2017). *Theories of counseling and psychotherapy: A case approach* (4th ed.). Pearson.

Najavits, L. M. (2017). *Recovery from trauma, addiction, or both: Strategies for finding your best self.* Guilford Press.

Neubauer, A. C., & Feudenthaler, H. H. (2005). Models of emotional intelligence. In R. Schulze & R. D. Roberts (Eds.), *Emotional intelligence: An international handbook.* Hogrefe & Huber Publishers.

Ohrt, J. H., Clarke, P. B., & Conley, A. H. (2019). *Wellness counseling: A holistic approach to prevention and intervention.* American Counseling Association.

Price, C. J., & Herting, J. R. (2013). Changes in post traumatic stress symptoms among women in substance use disorder treatment: The mediating role of bodily dissociation and emotion regulation. *Substance Abuse: Research and Treatment, 7,* 147–153. https://doi.org/10.4137/SART.S12426

Salovey, P., & Mayer, J. D. (1990). Emotional intelligence. *Imagination, Cognition and Personality, 9*(3), 185–211.

Schiraldi, G. R. (2016). *The self-esteem workbook* (2nd ed.). New Harbinger Publications.

Snyder, C. R. (2000). Hypothesis: There is hope. In C. R. Snyder (Ed.), *Handbook of hope: Theory, measures, and applications* (pp. 3–21). Academic Press.

Streifel, C., & Servaty-Seib, H. L. (2009). Recovering from alcohol and other drug dependency: Loss and spirituality in a 12-step context. *Alcoholism Treatment Quarterly, 27*(2), 184–198. https://doi.org/10.1080/07347320902785558

Substance Abuse and Mental Health Services Administration (SAMHSA) (2020). *Substance use disorder treatment for people with co-occurring disorders. Treatment improvement protocol (TIP) series, No. 42. SAMHSA publication no. PEP20-02-01-004.* Substance Abuse and Mental Health Services Administration.

Weiss, N. H., Kiefer, R., Goncharenko, S., Raudales, A. M., Forkus, S. R., Schick, M. R., & Contractor, A. A. (2022). Emotion regulation and substance use: A meta-analysis. *Drug and Alcohol Dependence, 230,* 109131. https://doi.org/10.1016/j.drugalcdep.2021.109131

Worden, J. W. (2009). *Grief counseling and grief therapy: A handbook for the mental health practitioner* (4th ed.). Springer.

CHAPTER 11

CONNECTION WELLNESS: ENHANCING RECOVERY THROUGH RELATIONSHIPS

INTRODUCTION

It is well-known among addictions professionals that the disease or process of addiction takes an enormous toll on intimate relationships. One can see the devastation through ruined marriages, intimate partner violence, angry words that leave long-term resentments, and physical, emotional, and/or sexual abuse. Websites with statistics on the "costs of addiction" display economic indicators, with recent estimates in the billions of dollars of lost revenues per year (e.g., worker absenteeism due to intoxication). However, these estimates do not consider the loss of relationships, connections, friends, and family. If dollar estimates included these losses, that number would indeed be incalculable. Put simply, social context, ranging from social isolation and ostracism to social competence and support, has a profound impact on the trajectory and stability of substance use disorders (Pomrenze, Paliarin, & Maiya, 2022).

The relationship between social connection and addiction, however, is bidirectional (Pomrenze et al., 2022). Interpersonal problems can be present either before an addiction starts or as a result. Whatever the direction of influence, problems with wellness connection either leads to addiction or exacerbates addiction problems already present. Enhancing client connection wellness is a key element to successful recovery.

In this chapter, we place a spotlight on connection wellness as a domain of overall holistic wellness and its relation to substance addiction. We start by defining connection wellness and explore its impact on addiction (and vice versa). We then examine interpersonal based triggers for relapse, followed by how WBAC clinicians can strengthen connection and reduce relapse. The chapter concludes with an examination of how connection wellness, and thereby recovery, can be enhanced in the case of Eric.

DEFINING CONNECTION WELLNESS

Ohrt, Clarke, and Conley (2018) defined connection wellness as "the experience of interacting with or forming relationships with others through the use of interpersonal skills and resources resulting in increased well-being" (p. 138). Connection wellness is a key pillar of overall wellness and healthy human functioning. By "connection", we are talking about people having social support, supporting others, and minimizing isolation. Each of these components of connection wellness will be explored in this chapter.

Probably one of the earliest theorists who stressed the importance of social relationships and mental health was Alfred Adler. For Adler, individuals were considered healthy if they successfully met the three tasks of life: work, friendship, and love.[1] Notice how for each of these tasks, relationships are needed for success. In work, most occupations involve successfully navigating relationships with co-workers, associates, management, and so forth. Friendship refers to platonic relationships and love refers to intimate relationships. Adler

DOI: 10.4324/9781003147954-11

believed that individuals who pursue these tasks with an attitude of cooperation are happier and more successful.

Adler proposed another concept that implies connection as the *key* to mental health: Social interest. Social interest generally refers to "community feeling", cooperation with others, and having a genuine concern for others and the "common good". In other words, individuals with high social interest move through life with a positive attitude and approach problems from a cooperative, common-sense perspective (Ansbacher, 1991). In contrast, those with low social interest operate according to their own private logic and move through life with a more isolated, selfish perspective. Dreikurs (1990), a colleague of Adler's, believed that addiction resulted from low social interest where children were pampered and ill pre-pared for the tasks of life. Almost every mental health problem Adler discussed usually had low social interest at its core and needing improvement.

Connection wellness, it seems, has a substantial theoretical backing, starting with Adler's view on the importance of social relationships, cooperation, and having a healthy attitude toward society. These concepts are central to mental health. Sweeney's (2019) contemporary book on Adlerian counseling and psychotherapy discusses Adler's ideas within the frame-work of Wellness theory; indeed, the natural confluence of Adlerian and Wellness theories rests on the combined view that connection is vital to living a well lived life.

Empirical research supports the positive relationship between connection and mental health. Haslam and colleagues (2022) noted how healthy, interpersonal connections promote a sense of purpose, support, and social confidence, all important implications for mental health. The key components to connection wellness include limiting isolation, enhancing social support, and strengthening social skills, all of which contribute to both physical and mental well-being. We will say much more about these components in the sections that follow.

THE RELATIONSHIP BETWEEN ADDICTION AND CONNECTION WELLNESS

In probably no greater area of mental and behavioral health is connection more important than addiction. Isolation tends to embolden addictive behavior; connection is the antidote to isolation and, the less isolated, the less likely one will engage in substance use behavior. Indeed, there is a well-documented connection between isolation stress and addiction (Hanlon, Shannon, & Porrino, 2019). Based on neuroimaging data, Hanlon et al. found that those with cocaine use disorder have a higher response to "social exclusion" compared to a control group. This means that social exclusion (i.e., isolation) and its associated stress create a heightened response in the brain regions associated modulators of substance use behavior – emotion reg-ulation, urges, arousal, and perception of physical discomfort. Addiction professionals have long known that isolation and addiction go hand in hand. We now have neurological evidence that supports this general observation. Whether isolation causes or is exacerbated by addiction, there appear to be clear changes in the brain when one experiences this social stress, such that emotions become dysregulated, and cravings and arousal for drugs increases.

Bacon and Engerman (2018) also found that social stress contributes to substance use. In their study, college student drinkers who were in an ostracized treatment condition expe-rienced lower mood and less sense of belonging compared to students in a control condi-tion. The ostracized group also tended to consume more alcohol. Being ostracized from a group, whether that be a family, peer group, or other organization, seems to impact one's psychology such that they feel less control over their lives and like they do not fit in. Turning to alcohol and or other drugs to cope may be a way to deal with these feelings. In animal models, persistent, succinct periods of social defeat stress (SDS) or protracted social isolation in adolescence unmistakably leads to escalations in substance use (Pomrenze et al., 2022).

Nakken (1996) discussed the addictive cycle and relationship processes that occur when one is consumed by drug use. For Nakken, the addictive process is the "out-of-control and aimless searching for wholeness, happiness, and peace through a *relationship with an object or event*" [p. 2, emphasis added]. In other words, a person in the throes of addiction will seek to substitute healthy human connections with a relationship to an object, in this case drugs. Nakken further proposed three stages in the development of the addictive personality.[2] In all three stages, internal change, lifestyle change, and life breakdown, personal and intimate relationship becomes increasingly troubled, and the person develops a totally consuming dependence on drugs.

Interpersonal-Based Relapse Triggers

Isolation

Research findings strongly support the notion that social isolation is associated with increased substance use (Pomrenze et al., 2022). Metaphorically speaking, isolation is addiction's best friend. When one is isolated from others, the addictive process as outlined by Nakken (1996) can take a firm hold; attempts at recovery work against the addictive process. An isolated person finds themselves in an addiction mindset, which can spiral out of control leading to relapse and continued use. This is because there is no human support system in the client's life that can help them counter negative thinking or provide an alternative way to live. The cognitive-behavioral model of addiction and substance use (Liese & Beck, 2022) helps us understand that after an activating event (internal or external trigger), anticipatory thoughts (e.g., if I take a hit, my pain will go away) can take hold which leads to craving. At this point, the client has a choice: They can either abstain or give themself permission to use. An isolated individual, without sufficient social supports and coping resources, will almost always choose the path to continued use.

Limited Social Support

The importance of social support to overall wellness cannot be overstated. As Ohrt et al. (2019) noted, social support can be lifesaving! Aside from benefits to mental and physical health (Ohrt et al., 2019; Segrin, McNelis, & Swiatkowski, 2016), social support has been found to relate positively to self-efficacy connected to one's abstinence (Stevens, Jason, Ram, & Light, 2015). Self-efficacy, a term coined by Albert Bandura (1977), refers to the belief and expectation that one can overcome obstacles through coping behavior and sustained effort. Thus, the higher the social support, the greater one's self-efficacy that they can be successful in recovery (note that this finding was correlational; the relationship works the other way as well, namely, that the higher the self-efficacy, the greater the social support). Naturally, an isolated person will have limited to no social support. However, one does not need to be completely isolated to experience deficits in social support. For example, a person with cocaine use disorder may continue to have non-using peers (and thus not be isolated), but experience little social support – family may "disown" the person, non-using friends are too busy and can't provide the support needed, and/or the individual cannot afford social support activity such as group therapy. Such limited support becomes a serious trigger for substance use and relapse. Moos, Fenn, Billings, and Moos (1988–1989) found that, compared to non-problem drinkers, clients who struggled with alcohol use disorder had significantly fewer social resources. More recently, Panebianco, Gallupe, and Colozzi (2016) set out to study the differences between support systems of substance free versus participants who relapsed. The authors found that the substance free participants had more robust, varied, and reciprocal social support networks compared to relapsed participants.

The Panebianco et al. (2016) finding deserves additional attention. Social support works both ways (Ohrt et al., 2019). Individuals tend to think that those struggling with addiction need strong social support to aid in their recovery, which of course is the case, but the opposite is also important, that clients be supportive of others in their life. One example of this is volunteerism; several studies have found negative relationships between service activities and alcohol consumption among college students (Crawford, Novak, & Jayasekare 2019; i.e., the more one serves others, the less one tends to drink). Clients who have limited social networks and do not engage in the human community by giving back are at risk for continued substance use.

Challenging Relationships

Whereas positive social relationships are rewarding, relationship challenges, such as constant fighting, aggression, or stonewalling, are distressing and enhance sensitivity to reinforcing substances, encourage the search for drugs, and fosters the consumption of drugs (Pomrenze et al., 2022). In other words, challenging and difficult relationships can be a significant relapse trigger. Challenging relationships create considerable stress in one's life, as the client navigates several difficult emotions such as contempt, shame, guilt, anger, fear, and jealousy. Such negative emotions can set out a cascade of psychological, social, and biological reactions that greatly increase the potential for relapse. We advocate that all WBAC clinicians assess for challenging relationships among clients struggling with addiction. Helping the client form more positive bonds with others becomes an imperative part of the treatment plan.

CONNECTION WELLNESS IN RECOVERY

Although recovery is a unique experience for every client, almost all will have to address issues with connection. As such, promoting connection wellness becomes an integral part of the recovery strategy. In the sections below, we outline specific WBAC strategies that can help clients heal hurt relationships and form more preferred social relations that do not involve the use of drugs.

Assessing for Isolation, Emotional Intelligence, Social Strengths, and Deficits

The first step in helping clients strengthen connection wellness is to assess for social strengths and deficits within the client's life. The WBAC clinician can look for "red flags" that suggest connection wellness is not optimal. Common red flags can include poor work relationships (being fired or on probation), poor relationship judgment, strained family relations, limited or no peers/friends, and couple or martial difficulties. In some cases, the presenting clinical issue will be relationship difficulties; however, after further exploration, substance use problems come to the surface. I (TFL) recall counseling a marital couple whose presenting issue was that they argued too much, especially after work hours. After helping the couple with basic communication skills, I explored what a "typical day" looked like for them. I learned that after dinner both would have a "few drinks". When explored further, I was surprised that a "few drinks" meant more like five or six. In addition, almost all arguments between the couple occurred during this drinking period. The couple was encouraged to strengthen their connection by doing things together without alcohol. Structured activities included taking a walk together, watching a movie, and having conversations that included their hopes and dreams.

In addition to looking for red flags, Ohrt et al. (2019) noted that there are a bevy of formal assessments to help WBAC clinicians evaluate connection wellness. A full overview is beyond the scope of this chapter; however, these instruments can elaborate on the client's level of social skills, extent of loneliness and isolation, existing social support (or lack thereof), and evidence of and extent of social conflict (Ohrt et al., 2019). One such scale is the *Social Skills Inventory* (SSI; Riggio & Carney, 2003), which assesses six social skills that are thought to undergird social competence through full length (90 items) or brief (30 items) versions (Mindgarden.com, 2022): emotional expressivity, emotional sensitivity, emotional control, social expressivity, social sensitivity, and social control. The SSI provides scores in both the social and emotional competence domains; that is, clients receive feedback on how well they send, receive, and manage both social and emotional messages (Mindgarden.com, 2022).

The *UCLA Loneliness Scale* (Russell, 1996), currently in its third version, is a popular 20-item measure that assesses how detached and lonely one is from others (SPARQtools, 2022). The 20 items cover several elements of loneliness including meaning in relationships, isolation from others, and being part of a group (SPARQtools). This would be an excellent measure to include to determine if loneliness and isolation play a prominent role in one's addiction lifestyle.

The *Multidimensional Scale of Perceived Social Support* (MSPSS; Zimet, Powell, Farley, Werkman, & Berkoff, 1990) is a brief 12-item instrument designed to assess subjective levels of social support. Three sources of social support make up subcomponents of the scale: family, friends, and significant other (Zimet et al., 1990). The MSPSS has demonstrated psychometric rigor across different groups, including women, adolescents, pediatric residents, and undergraduate students (Zimet et al., 1990). The SSI, UCLA Loneliness Scale, and the MSPSS are some commonly used formal assessments the WBAC clinician can access to evaluate connection wellness. These instruments are psychometrically sound and brief, allowing clinicians the advantage of gaining insights into connection wellness and being time efficient in the process.

Informally, connection wellness can be evaluated via the intake/clinical interview, or the wellness assessment as outlined in Chapter 4. Exploring the client's past and current social life, their perception of social support, and how they believe alcohol and/or drugs have impacted their connection to others can be helpful. Exploring past social relationships, such as those within the elementary, middle, and high school environment can help determine if connection problems were evident before substance use or if substance use led to connection problems. Often, both scenarios are at play. When asking about social relationships, WBAC clinicians also keep an eye open to the quality of these relationships and if the client feels supported within them. Questions such as, "Do you feel supported in your current social relationships?" and "Tell me about the quality of your social life" can help assess for this.

Once the clinician has a general sense of the level of social support, further questioning can help clients get more focused and specific about their connection wellness related to skills, obstacles, hopes and fears. See Table 11.1 for a review of probing questions to accomplish these goals.

An excellent informal tool for relationship assessment is the Adlerian lifestyle assessment (ALA). The ALA is a semi-structured inventory that the clinician uses within the first sessions

Table 11.1 Probing Questions to Help Further Assess Connection Wellness, Impacts of Substance Use and Other Dimensions of Wellness

Questions to Assess Connection Wellness	Why Ask It?	Questions to Assess Impact on Substance Use	Impact on Other Dimensions of Wellness
Who is in your social circle?	To broadly assess social relationships	How has your social circle impacted your substance use?	How has your social circle impacted other dimensions of wellness?
Name one person in your life you feel supported by. In what ways do they support you?	To assess for instances of social support	How has this person impacted your substance use?	How has this person impacted other dimensions of wellness?
What is the biggest factor or problem resulting in your connection wellness being lower than you liked?	To assess obstacles to greater connection wellness	How has this factor or problem impacted your substance use?	How has this factor or problem impacted other dimensions of wellness?
Who in your inner or outer circle do you want to feel more supported by or have an improved relationship with?	To assess obstacles individuals who can provide more social support	How would feeling more supported from someone in your inner circle impact substance use?	How would feeling more supported from someone in your inner circle impact other domains of wellness?
With whom in your inner circle do you have the most conflict/ strain with? How has this affected you?	To assess and process conflicts or obstacles within one's connection wellness	How has this relationship impacted your substance use?	How has this relationship impacted your other domains of wellness?
What specifically occurred that led the conflict to reach its peak?	To assess and process conflicts or obstacles within one's connection wellness	What about this conflict connects with substance use?	What about this conflict connects with the other domains of wellness?
What has gotten in the way of you improving relationships or getting the social life or social support that you want?	To assess obstacles to connection wellness	How have these obstacles to a better social life impacted your substance use?	How have these obstacles to a better social life impacted the other domains of wellness?

(Continued)

Table 11.1 (Continued)

Questions to Assess Connection Wellness	Why Ask It?	Questions to Assess Impact on Substance Use	Impact on Other Dimensions of Wellness
What type of social support do you want more of?	To assess the type of social support for which the client is looking	How would having more of the social support you want impact substance use?	How would having more of the social support you want impact the domains of wellness?
What is getting in the way of asking for more social support?	To assess obstacles to asking for social support	How does not asking for social support impact your substance use?	How does not asking for social support impact the other dimensions of wellness?

Sample questions from Ohrt, J. H., Clarke, P. B., & Conley, A. H. (2019). *Wellness counseling: A holistic approach to prevention and Intervention:* American Counseling Association (pp. 148–150).

with a client. The ALA is relationship focused, inquiring about early family experiences including parent-child relations, sibling-sibling relations, early recollections, and past and current social experiences (e.g., school and work). The ALA focuses on both past and current family and peer relationships to assess the client's "movement in life"; that is, does the client move toward others in the spirit of social interest, or away from others toward isolation. After using the ALA, clinicians can get a strong sense of the client's social ability, basic mistakes in social living, and whether problems in living, such as addiction, are related in any way to the client's social environment. According to Adlerian theory, there is a connection between social interest and psychopathology and/or behavioral problems. For excellent resources on how to conduct the ALA, consult Sweeney (2019), and for using the ALA specifically with addiction, see Lewis (2023). Table 11.2 provides several sample questions from the ALA.

The WBAC clinician must get a solid understanding of how wellness connection relates to addiction (Ohrt et al., 2019). Improving one can improve the other. That is, clients who mitigate or stop using substances will have better relationships and support within their social groups and family. Conversely, clients who work to improve their social support will feel more confident and motivated in their recovery. The scaling question as outlined by Ohrt et al. (2019) is a useful tool to assess for social support. After helping clients define what connection wellness means to them, ask, "On a scale from 1 (minimal perceived social support) to 10 (maximum perceived social support), rate your level of connection wellness". Assume the client responds with a "4". Follow-up with the question, "What makes it a 4 and not a 2?" Asking why it is not a lower number allows the client to acknowledge some connection wellness is evident, which can be built upon. A second follow-up question can be, "What would it take to increase that to a 5 or 6?" Avoid going too high in this second question. For example, asking what it would take to get to a ten would be too big of a jump for clients and feel overwhelming. Small incremental steps to improve connection wellness works best.

Improving Social Support

With addiction, concerns arise over how clients can procure social support when so many relationships have been damaged due to the substance use. Many clients may feel defeated

Table 11.2 Sample Questions/Probes from an Adlerian Lifestyle Assessment to Evaluate Relationship and Connection Health and Wellness

Sample Questions to Assess Parent-Child Relations	Sample Questions to Assess Sibling-Sibling Relations	Sample Questions to Assess Early Recollections	Sample Questions to Assess Past and Current Social Experiences
How did your parents relate to their children?	How did you get along with your siblings?	Please list five to six early recollections of your childhood. Describe the scene and be as specific as possible.	How did you get along with your peers during your elementary years?
Who received the most attention from your parents? The least?	Who fought with whom? Who played together? Who cared for and protected whom?	What sticks out for you're the most in your recollection(s)?	What teachers did you like/dislike in elementary school? Why?
Describe your mother and father.	Who was the most like you (sibling)? In what respect? Least like you? In what respect?	What emotion do you experience when you recount your recollection?	Describe your relationships with peers in high school.
Who was more ambitious for the children?	How would you perceive your role in the family growing up?	What is the most vivid part?	How were your relationships with teachers in high school?
Were there any additional parental figures or adult role models as a child?	Did you or your siblings experience any childhood sicknesses, surgeries, or accidents?		Describe your current relationships with friends, co-workers, and significant others?

Questions based on Manaster and Corsini (1982) and Maniacci (1999).

in this area, with pain, resentment, and lost friendships as the addiction takes over their lives. Gottman and Silver (2015) outlined the "four horsemen of the apocalypse" that, if evident, can doom intimate relationships – criticism (a total, negative opinion of another's character), contempt (negative, disrespectful thoughts and actions towards a partner), defensiveness (blaming a partner disguised as defending your position), and stonewalling (zoning out and removing oneself from the other). One can only imagine how addiction leads to and/or exacerbates these negative relationship dynamics. In WBAC, improving social support as a conduit for connection wellness should be a top priority, as the rewards of healthy relationships can shield against the "rewards" from addictive behavior (Pomrenze et al., 2022). Here are some strategies for increasing social support.

1. *Psychoeducation.* Educating clients on the importance of building positive, healthy human relationships, and how these can bolster one's social support system, can go a long way in helping clients successfully navigate their recovery. Educating clients on the four horsemen, for example, can help them identity these toxic patterns as well as their "antidotes" (Gottman, 2010). For example, the antidote to

criticism is what Gottman and Gottman (2015) call the "softened start up". Instead of approaching one's partner going from 0 to 60 in a few seconds, couples are encouraged to approach each other gently, communicating their feelings, what their feelings relate to, and what they need in the moment (Gottman & Gottman, 2015). The antidote for contempt is building a culture of appreciation (Gottman, 2010). For defensiveness, it is taking responsibility instead of blaming the other person (Gottman, 2010). Finally, the antidote to stonewalling is physiological self-soothing (Gottman, 2010). Because relationship stress can release cortisol and other stress hormones, individuals can become physiologically flooded, making it much more difficult to have calm, respectful conversations. Self-soothing can be activities such as removing oneself from the room, taking a walk, deep breathing, or mediation, ideally for 20 minutes (Gottman & Silver, 2015). After one has calmed down, the discussion and problem solving can resume. Healthy communication patterns, exploring ways to increase one's social network, and teaching social skills can also be a part of psychoeducation.

2. *Encourage mutual help group attendance.* In our experiences, mutual support groups are a critical component to recovery. When I (TFL) teach graduate students in substance use disorders (SUD) counseling, I often share Stephanie Brown's (1995) perspective on the "triadic relationship" when working with addictions: The counselor, the client, and AA (or whichever group the client is attending). The implication is that mutual help groups can be a complementary component of addictions counseling and need not conflict with the counselor's clinical agenda. Helping clients work through a particularly difficult step, for example, can be valuable clinical work that helps the client get unstuck on their road to recovery.

Twelve-step groups are one of the main methods that counselors can use to help clients avoid isolation and improve social support. Indeed, a key reason why these groups are helpful to so many is because they connect clients with others who are going through or have gone through similar struggles. As such, mutual groups provide an important boost to connection wellness. Camaraderie, support, and fellowship are encouraged as attendees share their experiences and explore their struggles with like-minded individuals. We can't think of a better way to help clients get out of the pit of isolation and kick start enhanced social support than mutual help groups.

Some clients may be reticent about attending mutual help group meetings. Specific hesitancies can run the gamut , from legitimate concerns to outright myths. For example, a client juggling many responsibilities from work to childcare may have a bona fide concern that time to attend meetings is limited. On the other hand, some may feel that meetings are covered in secrecy and that only "losers" go to "those" meetings. It is important for the WBAC counselor to listen for and be aware of how the client perceives mutual help meetings. We have found that psychoeducation can be helpful to clarify misunderstandings and provide examples of clients who have had successful experiences. In addition, it may take attending a few different meetings (at different locations) to find the right fit.

Although 12-step philosophy is similar across all groups, meetings can differ in tone, atmosphere, and commitment. Clients sometimes avoid attending based on a one-time negative experience. If clients felt uncomfortable in a first meeting, WBAC clinicians can encourage them to "shop around" as not all fellowships are the same. When clients find the right fit, mutual help meetings can provide the social support to enhance and strengthen their connection wellness. Keep in mind that there are several types of mutual help groups. For example, traditional groups such as AA and NA, focus on the 12 steps and incorporate spirituality into their recovery philosophy. Other groups, such as SMART recovery, are more secular in nature, do not rely on a classic 12-step model, and instead focus on triggers, thinking errors, and cognitive-behavioral activities to strengthen recovery. Other mutual help groups are geared for family members who live with an individual struggling with addiction (e.g., Al-Anon, Al-Ateen; see Chapter 9 for more on mutual help groups).

3. *Individual, couples, and/or family counseling focused on connection wellness.* Counseling can be an important avenue for enhancing social support. With the aid of an empathic counselor, clients begin to unravel their isolation and feel supported in their recovery journey. Based on common factors research, the therapeutic alliance is one of the largest contributors to successful client outcomes (Hubble, Duncan, Miller, & Wampold, 2010). We surmise that a large reason for this is because of the social support the alliance engenders.

  The client's closest social relationships come from intimate partners and family members. Couple and family counseling can help repair animosities, repair cut off relationships, and improve poor communication among struggling familial interactions. Addiction becomes a "family problem" based on unhelpful generational patterns, poor family structures, or cutoff emotional issues that serve to maintain the addiction. Psychoeducation can point out flawed family dynamics, encouraging more prosocial interactions that increase connection wellness across the entire family network. Members struggling with addiction can gain understanding and empathy for how their behavior has impacted others. Social support activities and skills can be taught to non-using members to support their loved one's recovery.

  Issues related to trauma and the family need to be addressed in a delicate and appropriate manner. Although not a trauma-based approach, WBAC clinicians are sensitive to trauma issues and understand the profound impact they can have on family dynamics and behavior, including the development of addiction. Indeed, numerous authors have pointed out the link between childhood trauma and PTSD and substance addiction (Cabanis, Outadi, & Choi, 2021; Mergler et al., 2018). The combined effects of childhood trauma and PTSD are particularly devastating, leading to higher levels of anxiety, depression, suicidal ideation, earlier age of first substance use, higher levels of marijuana use, and more lifetime drug overdoses compared to those having no experiences of childhood trauma or PTSD (Mergler et al., 2018). WBAC clinicians should always assess for experiences of trauma and their connection to substance use behavior. Clients should be given the time and space to share and process these experiences when they are ready. WBAC is also well-suited as a preventative approach to ensure someone who has experienced a traumatic event, but has not yet developed an addiction, has the support in the various wellness dimensions to mitigate negative impacts of the trauma. For example, exploring with clients ways to enhance body, mind, spiritual, and connection wellness can be a buffer against turning to drugs to soothe internal and/or external pain.

4. *Giving to others and learning how to ask for support.* According to Ohrt et al. (2019), "One of the most therapeutic actions that a client can take that potentially fosters multiple wellness domains, including connection, is to give to others" (p. 151). Giving can take many forms, including volunteering of time, providing social support, or

simply being present to someone who is struggling. Giving confers numerous wellness benefits including feeling good about oneself, increased self-regard, enhanced relationships, and finding a purpose in life (Ohrt et al., 2019). Giving is part and parcel of 12-step mutual help groups, discussed above. For those who attend AA long enough, for example, opportunities open where one can become a sponsor for another. Sponsors give their time, wisdom, and advice to newer members who may be struggling to remain abstinent. I (TFL) recall one client who embraced the sponsor role and found that it changed his life for the better by strengthening his own recovery.

With addiction, clients may have such a negative self-concept that they can't possibly believe that they have anything to offer. WBAC clinicians can encourage the client to give by brainstorming ideas or even practicing giving in session (e.g., giving a complement; role playing). Another way to encourage giving is for the client to join a SUD counseling group. Although not unique to WBAC, group therapy, by its very nature, encourages altruism, one of 11 key "therapeutic factors" that account for its clinical effectiveness (Yalom & Leszcz, 2020). Group therapy is a natural venue where clients help each other by listening, offering hope, and being supportive. In this sense, group therapy is a win-win proposition; the client not only receives help from others but also gains by giving time, attention, and support to other group members (Yalom & Leszcz, 2020).

Besides engaging in kind and generous acts, giving to others helps clients get out of their own minds (Ohrt et al., 2019). As noted, substance use thrives when one is isolated. That is, in an isolated state, one's mind tends to ruminate on addiction and negative thinking where nothing else matters but the next high. Shifting to a giving mindset interrupts this addiction process and promotes all the other touted benefits.

Whereas giving has many advantages, this intervention would be contraindicated for clients who over-involve themselves with others to the neglect of their own wants and needs (Ohrt et al., 2019). We have worked with clients who have taken drastic steps to make sure others are cared for, only to neglect their own health and needs to remain substance free. Over-involvement is sometimes called "enmeshment" or "co-dependency"; however, these instances usually involve the non-using spouse/partner, family members, or partner. We will turn to these topics in Chapter 12 on family wellness.

Another way to enhance social support is to encourage clients to ask for support. As noted, the self-concept of clients with substance use disorders can hit rock bottom, perpetuating the irrational belief that they do not deserve help. Societal messages contribute to negative schemas that they are unlovable, beyond help, and unworthy of healing and wellness. WBAC clinicians challenge these irrational thoughts, often through CBT methods, to help clients explore their falsity and engage in behaviors that directly contradict the notion that they are not worthy of assistance. Keeping the broader goal of enhanced connection wellness in mind, WBAC clinicians can offer homework assignments where clients are instructed to ask loved ones, friends, or fellow clients for help. Role playing these interactions and addressing underlying fears can be beneficial with these interventions. For example, one suggestion is to think of asking for help as an experiment (Bernhard, 2011). Bernhard recommends four steps in asking for help

1. *Get clarity on what you need help with and make a list.* The client may need help with groceries, dropping kids off to school, or transportation to an appointment.
2. *Who in the client's life could offer help?* List friends and relatives who helped, even if it was some time in the past.

3. *Who would be a good match for various tasks?* Clients should consider who in their life is approachable and would be more amendable to helping. Considerations can include time availability, comfort level with the person, their strengths, and so forth.

4. *Choose one item from your list and reach out to a person who can most likely help.* Bernhard (2011) suggested to be direct. As such, asking, "can you please take me to an appointment, as I am not in a condition to drive at the moment" would be better than, "I wish there was someone who could take me to the appointment".

Asking for help can be practiced in session as well, such as role playing the client asking the clinician for help during the session.

You might be thinking that with the ever-increasing move toward videoconferencing and online platforms to hold meetings, clients would have an abundance of options for increasing social support. However, it appears that in person social support compared to videoconferencing is perceived as having more advantages for those struggling with addiction. For example, Barrett and Murphy (2021) found that face to face 12-step meetings were perceived as being more supportive and effective compared to meetings through videoconferencing. Of course, this study only examined 12-step meetings, but the implication is that there is something powerful about having people present in one's life on the road to recovery. This would be important for WBAC clinicians to keep in mind. When helping clients find ways to increase social support, explore both online and in person options. Both have advantages, with in person support being the ideal method to help clients recover.

Improving Social Skills

Strengthening social support becomes more challenging if clients struggle with basic social skills needed to develop and maintain social relationships and enhance connection wellness (Ohrt et al., 2019). Social skills deficits can manifest for any number of reasons, including mental health issues, neurodevelopmental disorders (e.g., autism spectrum), personality characteristics, and lack of parenting role models (Ohrt et al., 2019). But what are examples of socials skills that successfully help individuals navigate through social experiences of life? As noted in the introduction to this chapter, the Adlerian concept of social interest is a good place to start. To have strong social interest, one must have a genuine concern for others, a belief in the common good, and using "common sense" to resolve interpersonal difficulties rather than "private logic". In other words, the person adopts a useful, rational approach to social problem solving that takes into consideration other viewpoints rather than operating from internal cognitive distortions which are often flawed. Other key social skills include empathy, listening skills, evoking likes/dislikes, reading and responding appropriately to emotions, showing compassion, and affirming positive attributes of others.

Within addiction, social skills may atrophy due to the client's increasing isolation, finding it progressively more difficult to procure the social support needed to help them with the tasks of recovery. In other cases, social skills deficits may proceed and lead to the development of addiction. Indeed, social skills deficits seem to be a strong risk factor for a wide range of psychological difficulties (Segrin et al., 2016), including substance use (Mahdi & Karimi, 2012). "There are few individual variables that are as consequential to well-being as social skills ..." (Segrin et al., 2016, p. 122).

Building social skills may begin with formal and/or informal assessments as noted above, and then exploring ways clients can improve in this area. Clients can practice social skills in the safety of the clinician's office such as affirming strengths of others, reflective listening (to show empathy), assertiveness skills, asking for what they want, and reading emotions with the clinician. Let's take building assertiveness skills as an example. Assume a client struggling with cocaine addiction has a difficult time saying "no" to his buddies when going out. Although the client does not really want to use, he ends up doing so to please his friends. The client can build his assertiveness skills by speaking directly to the clinician who role plays one of his friends. The clinician can pretend to tempt the client and then instruct him to respond back in an assertive manner. The client, for example, might practice by calmly saying "no, I don't feel like using tonight" and sticking to that answer. If the clinician persists in tempting him even more, the client can increase his voice and intensity to "No! I do not feel like using tonight!" The clinician can then check in with the client to process being more assertive. Initially, the client may be uncomfortable with greater assertiveness; however, with time and practice, their increased confidence, as well as improved social skills, will spill over into other areas of their lives and recovery.

Clinician and client can then process these activities and reflect on how social skills can improve one's connection wellness. Group counseling provides a powerful venue to work on socials skills, as feedback comes from not only the clinician but also group members. The therapy group serves as a microcosm of one's social life, and thus deficits and problems in this area tend to get replayed in the group format (Yalom & Leszcz, 2020). In SUD counseling groups, members have "seen it all" and know all the tricks and manipulations one uses when problematically using drugs (Brooks & McHenry, 2015). Feedback, if properly managed, can help clients become aware of their impact on others and at the same time practice new social skills in the here and now of the group.

New social skills learning can be strengthened by giving clients homework assignments. For example, clients who struggle with assertiveness may be encouraged to ask loved ones for what they need, such as space, time alone, or to have a conversation. Family members, if feasible, should have "buy-in" and further encourage the client to practice. As with in-session practice, clients can be encouraged to journal and/or reflect on the consequences of using new skills, how they improve their connection wellness, and how making these healthier connections can mitigate their substance use. Journal prompt examples could be as follows

1. In what ways have improving your social skills impacted the other wellness domains?
2. What have been some positive consequences of using these new social skills? What have been some unexpected consequences?
3. How have your improved social skills impacted your connection wellness? Overall wellness?
4. What other areas would you like to improve in terms of social skills and connection wellness?

In summary, connection wellness and addiction appear to be bidirectional; problems in connecting with others can lead to addiction and addiction can lead to and exacerbate connection problems. Several interpersonal triggers for relapse were reviewed, and a bevy of interventions were highlighted to reduce isolation, enhance social support, and improve social skills. Let's now assess how connection wellness concepts can be utilized in the clinical case of Eric.

CLIENT EXAMPLE

In the case of Eric, connection wellness would be an important component to focus on as part of an overall holistic WBAC approach. For the WBAC clinician, one of the first steps to accomplish this would be to evaluate his connection wellness via formal and/or informal assessments. Because the clinician speculated that Eric was lacking in social support and seemed somewhat isolated in his life, he decided to administer a general intake questionnaire, MSPSS, the UCLA Loneliness Scale, and the ALA. The MSPSS confirmed that Eric was struggling with social support, especially in the areas of family and significant other. The UCLA Loneliness scale corroborated the clinician's hunch that Eric was also feeling isolated in his life.

From the intake and ALA, we gain some clarification on Eric's upbringing and how this contributed to his current social life. Eric grew up with a lot of tension and negative emotion in the home, with significant stressors leading to constant arguing between his parents. His substance use has created a strained relationship with his wife, Kelly, and he has a history of poor relations with his father.

Enhancing Eric's connection wellness should include interventions that strengthen his social support, reduce his feeling of isolation and loneliness, and improve family relations, especially with his wife and father. In addition, the clinician noticed that stress has been a consistent theme throughout Eric's life, and this often creates tension in his current relationships.

The first intervention is to encourage Eric to attend a mutual support group. Although Eric tried this before, he only attended for a brief time and noted that he would be open to continuing if he found the right home fellowship. Because of some potential resistance, the clinician should provide psychoeducation on the benefits of mutual help meetings, clarify any misunderstandings, and encourage Eric to "shop around" until he finds one that is a fit. The social support of these meetings, in addition to how they can address Eric's increasing isolation, could be important steps in not only stopping substance use but also enhancing connection wellness. Al-anon, a 12-step mutual help group for family members of individuals with alcohol use disorders, may be a consideration for Kelly, who is also struggling with a sense of isolation and limited social support.

Another intervention to address connection wellness is couples counseling. In couples counseling, the WBAC clinician can help Eric and Kelly strengthen their communication and minimize the four horsemen. Instead of showing contempt, for example, the couple can practice showing mutual appreciation and taking responsibility for their actions and feelings. The couple can practice the "softened start up" exercise when they have disagreements where one partner shares how they feel, about what, and what they need from their partner moving forward (Gottman & Gottman, 2015). For example, in a recent argument about Eric's drinking, Kelly could say, "I feel angry … when you drink after telling me you won't … and I need a commitment from you to our family". Eric also would benefit from strategies to heal his relationship with his father. He holds strong resentments for how he was raised, and this has created somewhat of a cutoff in this relationship. Exploring these issues with Eric and his father and providing an outlet for Eric to voice these concerns could lead to an increase in social support for Eric.

Finally, the WBAC clinician should encourage Eric to find a network of non-drinking friends that he can hang out with on a casual basis. AA is a clear avenue for this, but consideration should be given to other community resources and activities that might be available. Firmly establishing himself in such groups can provide the additional social support and friendship he needs to strengthen connection wellness and successfully navigate his recovery.

NOTES

1   Adlerian theorists have proposed additional tasks over the years, but these three were Adler's original.
2   In this case, the addictive personality emerges from the addictive process, rather than being present before drug use.

REFERENCES

Ansbacher, H. L. (1991). The concept of social interest. Individual Psychology: *Journal of Adlerian Theory, Research, & Practice, 47*, 28–46.

Bacon, A. K., & Engerman, B. (2018). Excluded, then inebriated: A preliminary investigation into the role of ostracism on alcohol consumption. *Addictive Behaviors Reports, 8*, 25–32.

Bandura, A. (1977). Self-efficacy: Toward a unifying theory of behavior change. *Psychological Review, 84*, 191–215.

Barrett, A. K., & Murphy, M. M. (2021). Feeling supported in addiction recovery: Comparing face-to-face and videoconferencing 12-step meetings. *Western Journal of Communication, 85*, 123–146.

Bernhard, T. (2011, June 16). How to ask for help: Learn to communicate skillfully with others so you can get the help you need. *Psychology Today*. Retrieved from https://www.psychologyto-day.com/us/blog/turning-straw-gold/201106/how-ask-help

Brooks, F., & McHenry, B. (2015). *A contemporary approach to substance abuse and addiction counseling* (2nd ed.). American Counseling Association.

Brown, S. (1995). A developmental model of alcoholism and recovery. In I. D. Yalom (General Ed.), *Treating alcoholism* (pp. 27–53). Jossey-Bass.

Cabanis, M., Outadi, A., & Choi, F. (2021). Early childhood trauma, substance use and complex concurrent disorders among adolescents. *Current Opinion in Psychiatry, 34*, 393–399.

Crawford, L. A., Novak, K. B., & Jayasekare, R. R. (2019). Volunteerism, alcohol beliefs, and first-year college students' drinking behaviors: Implications for prevention. *The Journal of Primary Prevention, 404*, 429–448.

Dreikurs, R. (1990). Drug addiction and its individual psychological treatment. *Individual Psychology, 46*, 208–216.

Gottman, J. M. (2010). *Stop the four horsemen with their antidotes*. The Gottman Institute, Inc.

Gottman, J. M., & Gottman, J. S. (2015). *The ten principles of effective couples therapy: What science tells us and beyond*. PESI.

Gottman, J. M., & Silver, N. (2015). The *seven principles of making marriage work: A practical guide from the country's foremost relationship expert* (Revised Edition). Harmony.

Hanlon, C. A., Shannon, E. E., & Porrino, L. J. (2019). Brain activity associated with social exclusion overlaps with drug-related frontal-striatal circuitry in cocaine users: A pilot study. *Neurobiology of Stress, 10*, ArtID: 100137. https://doi.org/10.1016/j.ynstr.2018.10.005.

Haslam, S. A., Haslam, C., Cruwys, T., Jetten, J., Bentley, S. V., Fong, P., & Steffens, N. K. (2022). Social identity makes group-based social connections possible: Implications for loneliness and mental health. *Current Opinion in Psychology, 43*, 161–165.

Hubble, M. A., Duncan, B. L., Miller, S. D., & Wampold, B. E. (2010). In B. L. Duncan, S. D. Miller, B. E. Wampold, & M. A. Hubble (Eds.), *The heart and soul of change: Delivering what works in therapy* (2nd ed. Chapter 1, pp. 23–47). American Psychological Association.

Lewis, T. F. (2023). *Substance abuse and addiction treatment: Practical application of counseling theory* (2nd ed.). Cognella.

Liese, B. S., & Beck, A. T. (2022). *Cognitive-behavioral therapy of addictive disorders*. Guildford.

Mahdi, R. M., & Karimi, N. (2012). The relationship between self-efficacy, impulsiveness, and social skills with substance abuse. *Journal of Iranian Psychologists, 8*, 73–82.

Manaster, G. J., & Corsini, R. J. (1982). *Individual psychology: Theory and practice*. Adler School.

Maniacci, M. P. (1999). Clinical therapy. In R. E. Watts & J. Carlson (Eds.), *Interventions and strategies in counseling and psychotherapy* (pp. 63–65). Accelerated Development.

Mergler, M., Driessen, M., Havemann-Reinecke, U., Wedekind, D., Ludecke, Ohlmeier, M., Chodzinski, C., Teuniben, S., Kemper, U., Renner, W., & Schafer, I. (2018). Differential relationships of PTSD and childhood trauma with the course of substance use disorders. *Journal of Substance Abuse Treatment, 93*, 57–63.

Mindgarden.com. (2022). *Social skills inventory.* Retrieved from https://www.mindgarden.com/144-social-skills-inventory#horizontalTab3

Moos, R. H., Fenn, C. B., Billings, A. G., & Moos, B. S. (1988–1989). Assessing life stressors and social resources: Applications to alcoholic patients. *Journal of Substance Abuse, 1*(2), 135–152.

Nakken, C. (1996). *The addictive personality: Understanding the addictive process and compulsive behavior.* Hazelden.

Ohrt, J. H., Clarke, P. B., & Conley, A. H. (2019). *Wellness counseling: A holistic approach to prevention and intervention.* American Counseling Association.

Panebianco, D., Gallupe, O., & Colozzi, I. (2016). Personal support networks, social capital, and risk of relapse among individuals treated for substance use issues. *International Journal of Drug Policy, 27*, 146–153.

Pomrenze, M. B., Paliarin, F., & Maiya, R. (2022). Friend of the dev: Negative social influences driving substance use disorders. *Frontiers in Behavioral Neuroscience, 16*, ArtID: 836996. http://doi.org.ezproxy.lib.ndsu.nodak.edu/10.3389/fnbeh.2022.836996.

Riggio, R. E., & Carney, D. C. (2003). *Social skills inventory manual* (2nd ed.). Mind Garden, Inc.

Russell, D. (1996). The UCLA loneliness scale (Version 3): Reliability, validity, and factor structure. *Journal of Personality Assessment, 66*, 20–40. https://doi.org/10.1207/s15327752jpa6601_2.

Segrin, C., McNelis, M., & Swiatkowski, P. (2016). Social skills, social support, and psychological distress: A test of the social skills deficit vulnerability model. *Human Communication Research, 42*, 122–137.

SPARQtools (2022). UCLA loneliness scale (version 3). Stanford University. Retrieved from https://sparqtools.org/mobility-measure/ucla-loneliness-scale-version-3/

Stevens, E., Jason, L. A., Ram, D., & Light, J. (2015). Investigating social support and network relationships in substance use disorder recovery. Substance Abuse, 36, 396–399.

Sweeney, T. J. (2019). *Adlerian counseling and psychotherapy: A practitioner's approach* (6th ed.). Routledge.

Yalom, I., & Leszcz, M. (2020). *The theory and practice of group psychotherapy* (6th ed.). Basic Books.

Zimet, G. D., Powell, S. Z., Farley, G. K., Werkman, S., & Berkoff, K. A. (1990). Psychometric characteristics of the multidimensional scale of perceived social support. *Journal of Personality, 55*, 610–617. https://doi.org/10.1080/00223891.1990.9674095.

CHAPTER 12

ELEVATING FAMILY WELLNESS IN ADDICTIONS COUNSELING

INTRODUCTION

It would be fair to say that substance misuse and overdose have reached epidemic proportions in the United States. Consider the fact that from 2018 to 2019, drug deaths increased by 5%, and are four times as high since 1999 (CDC, 2020). Among families, Merikangas et al. (1998) found an eight-fold increase in drug addiction among children of parents with drug addiction across a broad range of substances. The fallout from addiction in the family can be devastating, including negative impacts on children, financial issues, problems with trust, and increases in stress (Ranieris, 2022). Some families will continue to struggle with addiction issues, sometimes for generations, while others will find a healing path and change patterns that support a substance free life and all its benefits. Family counseling is but one mode to help families break destructive patterns and find healing in their recovery journey.

Family therapies look beyond the identified client to see how the family system, structure, or emotional functioning is sub-optimal and may even be maintaining the substance use behavior. From this view, addiction is not considered an individual problem, but a family problem. From a WBAC lens, families possess their own wellness identity (norms and habits, what they prioritize, what they may disregard) and levels of wellness balance and imbalance. One family member's substance use and wellness challenges can affect the balance of the family system just as the wellness identity and balance of the family system can affect the client with substance use concerns. We often think that addiction only impacts the individual; however, addiction can impact siblings, parents, grandparents, and even family friends (Lambert, Unterberg, & Riggio, 2018). Gladding (2019) noted that substance misuse behaviors permeate into other significant relationships and impact all who encounters the struggling member. This causes family members of those in recovery to become disconnected from their own wellness. Once the family becomes aware of their wellness priorities, strengths, and struggles such as unhealthy patterns, structures, or emotions, they will be in a better place to support and encourage one another. A common refrain we hear is that a client can be helped individually, but if they go right back into a dysfunctional system (i.e., family), the system, through homeostasis, will resist change and promote continued substance use. Although we have successfully worked with many clients on an individual basis, not paying attention to the family wellness dynamics can lead to less-than-optimal outcomes.

In this chapter, we explore some traits and qualities of families with SUDs that can manifest and then explore common family counseling modalities and theories that can be useful when working with addiction in the family. Following this general overview of family approaches, we will review the WBAC approach to family counseling which draws on traditional theories and incorporates family wellness concepts into the family counseling process. The chapter ends with a family counseling intervention demonstrated with the case of Eric.

DOI: 10.4324/9781003147954-12

DEFINING "FAMILY"

Before we dive deeper into this topic, let's review what exactly we mean by "family". Today, many alternative family lifestyles have evolved (Gladding, 2019). The most common family forms include the *nuclear family* (husband and wife with child/children), *the single-parent family* (including one biological or adoptive parent who is responsible for childcare), and *the blended family* (two people marry and at least one of them was previously married with a child/children; Gladding, 2019). In addition to types of families, conceptualizations of family differ across cultures. For example, among European-American families, the nuclear system is what defines family. Among African American groups, family not only includes the nuclear group but also extended relatives such as grandparents, aunts, uncles, and even close friends. Some people choose to distinguish between their biological or adoptive family and their *chosen family* (i.e., group of people one has embraced, loved, regardless of marriage or ancestry – such as close friends). As you can see, the concept of family is beautifully diverse, with culture having a large impact on how a client perceives one's family. The WBAC clinician is always sensitive to how the family defines itself and tailors interventions that are culturally appropriate.

WHAT IS FAMILY COUNSELING?

Family counseling is a mode of therapy where a clinician meets with one or more members of a family to help them function better as a unit or system. Family counselors may work with the entire family or one member of the family; it is not essential (although certainly ideal) to have every family member attend. Thus, family counseling has more to do with the perspective the clinician takes (e.g., systems, structural, or strategic thinking), rather than the number of people present in therapy (Gladding, 2019). The family counselor knows, for example, that change in one unit of the system will spur change in the entire system. There are several common terms that are used in family counseling. Let's turn to these next.

Common Terminology

Systems

The family unit is thought to be a system of persons in which all members impact each other in a recursive fashion (Gladding, 2019). "Systems thinking" refers to clinicians who adopt a systems approach to their work. A key hallmark of systems thinking is the nature of causality. That is, instead of adopting a linear cause/effect approach, family counselors understand the circular causality within a family system. This is because family interactions can be notoriously complex – saying A causes B is too simplistic for a complex system. In a family system, A may cause B, but B also causes A, which can then lead to C, which feeds back to influencing A. This recursive influence is the hallmark of the systems process. A person might say, "my spouse nags at me all day and that is why I drink". However, the family therapist using a systems perspective would look at all causal factors and how each influences the other to influence the drinking.

Homeostasis

Homeostasis is when a system acts in such a way to maintain certain behaviors and the status quo. In other words, systems generally resist change unless there is intervention to help them in the process. Homeostasis is deeply connected to communication patterns called feedback loops (Gladding, 2019). Feedback loops can either encourage change in the system or keep things the same (Gladding). For example, positive feedback loops encourage change and move toward growth, whereas negative feedback loops occur when families sabotage a member's recovery and return the family toward continued addiction.

Using addiction as a foundation, an example of a positive feedback loop is when an adolescent in the family sincerely tries to stop using, and this behavior is strongly supported by the parents. The teenager is provided the resources needed to remain abstinent from drug use, thus building trust and respect among other family members. An example of a negative feedback loop would be where a father decides to stop excessive drinking. However, the father's drinking covered up dysfunctional communication and other issues within the family. A alcohol free father means these dysfunctional patterns would come to the surface, which would be too much for other family members to bear. As such, the children act out and the spouse/partner becomes defiant to "drive" the father back to drinking and thus continue the pattern of secrecy. In this case, the family operates to maintain the status quo, even though it is not in their best interest.

Roles

All members of a family adopt certain roles, whether addiction is present or not. However, there are specific roles within families in which addiction is present that can serve to maintain the substance use behavior and hide family problems. The purpose of family roles is to distract from the ravages of addiction within the family unit. In addition to the person with a SUD, here are some common roles (Wegscheider, 1981).[1]

1. *Family hero.* The family hero is usually a child that can do no wrong. They are successful in sports, school, and almost anything they try. Their message to the world is, "see, look at me and how successful I am, our family can't be that bad".

2. *Scapegoat.* The scapegoat is considered the "problem child" and tends to act out to divert attention from the substance use in the family. If energy and time are directed toward the scapegoat's shenanigans, less time is given to the embarrassing family secret of addiction.

3. *Lost child.* The lost child is reclusive and quiet, not causing any stir within the family. They may feel depressed and withdrawn. The thinking goes like this, "If I can just be quiet, and not draw any new, bad attention to the family, I will be helping them".

4. *Mascot.* Often the youngest child, the mascot is the silly person of the group, and uses humor as a distraction from the serious issues related to the addiction in the family.

5. *Family manager.* The family manager, typically the spouse/partner without a SUD, protects the person with a SUD from facing consequences of use. For example, they may call into work for their spouse/partner, clean up messes around the house, or avoid social gatherings so as not to expose the family secret of addiction.

I (TFL) have found these roles useful when working with families struggling with addiction. Many members clearly identify with one or more roles. Once a family understands the purpose of the different roles, and how they maintain substance use behavior, empathy is developed and greater motivation toward resolving the "real" issue – severe substance use within the family – occurs. The WBAC clinician can then transform these roles to relate to wellness dimensions. For example, the family could be asked, "who in the family can take leadership in the role of building "mental wellness?"

Rules

As with roles, all families have rules by which they operate. Rules can be spoken, but they are often unspoken within families in which addiction is present. Many rules revolve around not speaking about the issue, such as "substance use is not to be discussed at any time". This is because if the issue is not talked about, it doesn't happen (Vertava Health, 2016). Another rule might be, "Don't feel or you will get hurt" (Vertava Health). The emotional pain of watching a loved one destroy their life or be in a good mood one moment but hateful the next can be emotionally draining. Family members learn to suppress their feelings because it is too painful to confront the issue. Rules can be useful or not useful; family counselors can help families discard toxic rules and identify agreed-upon rules that support recovery, enhance wellness, and respect all parties involved.

Boundaries

Boundaries refer to the "physical and psychological factors that separate people from one another and organize them" (Gladding, 2019, p. 294). Three types of boundaries include clear, rigid, and diffuse (Gladding, 2019). Clear boundaries occur when family members maintain healthy communication patterns and do not get too caught up in another member's life. They can freely give and receive information and advice without becoming overly emotional in the process. They can not only interact with each other but also maintain individuality. Rigid boundaries occur when family members are cut off from each other or are inflexible in their interactions. The net effect of rigid boundaries is lack of communication, which can preclude understanding and empathy. The final boundary type is diffuse boundaries. Here, there is little separation between family members, such that they become overly emotional with each other and lose their individuality or autonomy (Gladding, 2019). In Gestalt therapy, this process is called confluence and is characterized by a loss of the sense of self.

Problematic boundaries can show up within families in which addiction is present, leading to ever increasing substance use problems. For example, with rigid boundaries, substance use may fill a void for the lack of closeness, connection, and emotional stability within the family. Boundaries that are too diffuse can encourage adolescent substance use because of the limited structure in place to monitor behavior. Families need to become aware of these unhealthy patterns along with strategies to promote clear boundaries to increase their family wellness.

Codependency

Codependency is a relationship dynamic where one member (stereotypically the spouse/partner without a SUD) becomes over involved with another member (stereotypically the spouse/partner with a SUD) such that the partner with the SUD does not experience any consequences for their substance use. This pattern is typically seen in a family system. A hallmark of codependency is that the member without a SUD loses a sense of self, throwing all their energy into taking care of the addicted family member. According to Doweiko and Evans (2019), this fills the codependent member with meaning and addresses internal emptiness and low self-esteem. A codependent person thrives on feeling like they are sorely needed, and thus recovery or abstinence is discouraged because it would take away their life meaning (Doweiko & Evans, 2019). Closely aligned with codependency is enabling, where the codependent member will engage in behaviors that excuse the substance use. For example, a spouse/partner may call into work for the member with a SUD who is hung over from a night of heavy drinking. This absolves the member with a SUD of any substance-related consequences.

Codependency is an excellent example of inappropriate boundaries (Doweiko & Evans, 2019), discussed above. The boundary in this case is too diffuse, where the codependent member blends self-identity with that of the member with a SUD. Their life is tied up in making others happy.

Common Characteristics of Families with SUDs

No two families are alike. However, across the broad spectrum of families, there are some common characteristics that affect the initiation, maintenance, and relapse of substances. Factors that lead to *initiation of use* include exposure to drugs, permissive (or rigid) parental oversight, family disconnection, and households where both parents need to work and make ends meet (thus having less time to supervise children/adolescents; Mathew, Regmi, & Lama, 2018). Factors that serve to *maintain drug use* include modeling of drug use behavior, association of cues to substance use, poor-quality relations with family members, especially the parent-child bond, and family attitude toward drug-taking behavior (Mathew et al., 2018). Factors associated with *poorer recovery* include communication difficulties, boundary issues, absence of family warmth, and parental non-involvement (Dodgen & Shea, 2000; Mathew et al., 2018, as cited in Mathew et al., 2018).

As one can see, the quality of family relationships, communication patterns, and interactions seem to play a large role in the initiation, maintenance, and recovery aspects of substance use. Families that tend to show warmth between members, with clear, consistent communication patterns, expectations, and boundaries seem to be better able to weather the inevitable storms that families go through. At the risk of oversimplifying, much of family counseling is helping families to establish healthier modes of interaction – communicating more effectively, establishing clear boundaries, and finding ways to support each other. Families battling addiction usually struggle in these areas.

Common Family Counseling Theories

Family counseling lends itself well to addressing psychological and behavioral problems that have complex etiologies, such as addiction. Family counseling is a viable option to work with clients, as its aim is to not only help the identified client but also adjust the surrounding social environment to encourage abstinence, recovery, and mental health instead of addiction. Although there are several approaches to working with families in which addiction is present, some of the most common are the Bowen family systems approach, structural family therapy, and multisystemic therapy. Our purpose here is to briefly review each of these family counseling models as a foundation from which WBAC family wellness can be integrated into family work. A brief review of each follows below.

Bowen Family Systems Approach

One of the most well-known family therapies is the Bowen family systems approach developed by Murray Bowen. Although not specifically designed for addiction issues, the approach is useful across a range of psychological and behavioral problems families may be experiencing. Bowenian theory, also known as "systems theory", is *intergenerational*, meaning that Bowen believed that psychological and behavioral problems, unless resolved, will repeat themselves and pass down from generation to generation. From this view, family patterns and experiences, even from previous generations, can have a profound impact on the behavior of the current generation. It is remarkable to us how relevant this is to addiction. With many clients, a simple examination of their family's history will often show signs of substance use behavior up to two or three generations previous.

One way that systems therapists examine intergenerational patterns is through the genogram. A genogram is a schematic family tree that illustrates members of the family and how they relate to each other. Within the genogram, medical, behavioral, and/or psychological issues can be highlighted as well as relationship dynamics such as cut offs between members, abuse, or distant relationships (GenPro, n.d.). From the genogram, intergenerational patterns can be pointed out to clients so they can see how they are "replaying" the common issues within the family in the present moment. In most cases, going back two to three generations is enough to provide a wealth of information.

Another important concept from systems theory is *differentiation of self*. Differentiation refers to a separation between one's emotional and intellectual self (Lewis, 2023). In essence, differentiation is the ability to remain calm during emotional turmoil, and at the same time rationally relate to people in the system (Bowen, 1978). Another way to think of differentiation is to be closely connected to one's family *and* be able to individuate and show autonomy in the world – a balance of individuality and togetherness (Gladding, 2019).

Undifferentiation, also called "fusion" (Bowen, 1978), is where the emotional and intellectual selves are combined such that the individual is primarily dominated by automatic emotional responses, without the intellectual capacity to balance out reactions to stress. In undifferentiated families, members may manifest psychological and behavioral problems (Gladding, 2019), especially when under duress. For example, when members of a family have a significant, emotionally charged argument, an undifferentiated person may become emotionally overwhelmed and be unable to bring any intellectual capacity to the situation. To handle such intense emotions, they might turn to drugs to cope. From a systems perspective, a goal of therapy would be to strengthen the family member's differentiation of self by learning healthier coping mechanisms, better communication of needs, and finding activities to enhance self-esteem. In most families in which addiction is present, all members could benefit from strengthening differentiation.

Structural Family Therapy

Structural family therapy is a well-suited approach for working with addiction issues. Developed by Salvador Minuchin, structural family therapy places emphasis on practicable family structures that create stability and can weather family crises (Juhnke & Hagedorn, 2006). Family structures can be useful or problematic. According to Taibbi (2011), healthy family structures begin with the parental subsystem. Parents who are on the same page regarding most family issues, communicate well, have good parenting skills, provide caring and structure, and appreciate the nuances and abilities of their child/children promote healthier family functioning (Taibbi, 2011). Of course, the parental subsystem is not the only structure within a family; the sibling subsystem may have their own challenges as well. According to Juhnke and Hagedorn, if all subsystems within the family are taught healthy patterns of relating and communicating, the overall family system is strengthened.

Another aspect of structural family therapy is to assess for unhelpful power hierarchies that may serve to maintain substance use behavior. For example, within families in which addiction is present, the substance using parent may be disengaged from the other parent, while the non-using parent fuses with the child/children for social and emotional support (Taibbi, 2011). This pathological structure leads to continued disengagement in the parental/marital dyad and places undue pressure on the children to provide emotional support to the non-using parent. The result is continued substance use by one parent, increasing distance in the parental/marital dyad, and potential behavioral and mental health problems among the children. In structural family therapy, adjusting the power structure so that both parents are on the same page and involved equally with the children would begin the process of healing (Taibbi, 2011). From this adjustment, addiction issues can be addressed from a healthy family structure instead of family chaos.

Multisystemic Therapy

Multisystemic family therapy (MST) is an intensive community-based program where treatment providers can have access to families multiple times a week. Session locations are flexible in that families can meet where they feel most relaxed, including their own home (Miller, Forcehimes, & Zweben, 2019). MST is generally geared toward reducing adolescent mental health and substance use problems through working with the family and other community resources. Interventions are behavioral in nature and target risky delinquent behavior, including substance use (Miller et al., 2019). MST also focuses on preventative efforts by helping teenagers learn educational, vocational, and positive peer social skills to reduce the chances of relapse (Miller et al., 2019). Empirical research supports MST as a family-based addiction treatment. In a meta-analysis examining the effectiveness of MST, van der Stouwe, Asscher, Stams, Dekovic, and van der Laan (2014) found significant treatment effects across a range of delinquent behaviors, including substance misuse. Although MST focuses on adolescent behavioral issues, it is considered a family intervention and thus attention is paid to the entire family dynamic. Schaeffer, Swenson, and Powell (2021) found that MST significantly reduced parental substance use and child neglect compared to a general community treatment among families who were under Child Protective Services.

WBAC could be an excellent adjunct to MST. For example, in addition to assessing dysfunctional behaviors and teaching behavioral skills, adolescents could learn about the dimensions of wellness and activities they could engage in to enhance their body, mind, spirit, and connection wellness. Family engagement could reinforce pro-wellness behaviors such as improving nutrition, exercising (or movement) as a family, and strengthening family connections. Family improvement in one area of wellness can spill over to others. We will say much more about how WBAC can be infused into family counseling and interventions to promote family wellness in the sections that follow.

BACKGROUND ON THE WBAC FAMILY COUNSELING APPROACH

The concepts and theories of family therapy reviewed above can serve as a foundation from which the WBAC family approach operates. However, the WBAC family approach differs by placing a premium on exploring wellness within the family as an avenue to heal addictions.

Most addictions treatment programs integrate family counseling into their treatment process. Some programs may utilize as few as one family session while others may offer multiple supports and sessions for families. The WBAC family counseling approach can be adapted within the time frame allotted by the treatment provider. WBAC is founded on the notion of lifestyle balance – clients finding their ideal balance of attending to each dimension of their wellness. Family rules, roles, and boundaries are implemented to achieve or preserve homeostasis and can increase or decrease individual and family wellness. Families also have their own wellness identity. Some families stress certain facets of wellness (e.g., physical wellness activities such as sports or spiritual wellness activities such as retreats, camps, attending services, time in prayer) while devoting less attention to other facets of wellness (cognitive stimulation activities, school, and career development [mental wellness] or addressing family members' emotional lives).

The family resilience (FR) model is integrated into WBAC. The prominence of strengths in this model aligns with that in WBAC. Families who thoughtfully grapple with their issues (which necessitates utilizing the family's capital) can attain family wellness (Walsh, 1996, 2002). Walsh (1996, 2002) endorses *belief systems*, *organizational patterns*, and *communication processes* as paramount to family wellness. Belief systems entail the family having a collective viewpoint that begets favorable change from unfavorable problems. This includes a prolapse mentality (issues that arise are opportunities for learning) on family stressors such that they can be edifying and improve the wellness of the family. Organizational patterns refer to the family working in partnership, implementing helpful rules, roles, and boundaries, utilizing resources such as friends, and maximizing the fiscal advancement of the family. Finally, communication processes involve creating a constructive emotional tone in the family via listening skills and "problem-solving" skills (Walsh, 2002).

Belief systems and in particular, organizational patterns, and communication processes are integrated into the dimensions of wellness to inform the family wellness approach. Family mental wellness, for instance, pertains to the family building in rules, roles, boundaries, and resources that enhance each member and the family unit's cognitive experience, mindset, and level of mental stimulation. See Figure 12.1 for the concepts that comprise family wellness in each dimension.

INTERVENTIONS FOR ADDRESSING FAMILY DURING INDIVIDUAL SESSIONS

The beginnings of family work in WBAC with adolescent and adult clients may start with the individual. You may have multiple entry points for exploring family with your individual client: one method of beginning family work with individual clients is to ask about the client's relationship with each family member, seeking strengths and challenges in their relationship and ways in which that particular family relationship enhances or diminishes their dimension-specific and overall wellness. Handout 12.1 displays a chart to document this exploration with the client. In an example of an adult client living with his parents, the client notes a strength of his relationship with his mother is the fun that they have together which enhances his physical and mental wellness. A challenge is that they do not talk about serious matters, and he does not feel comfortable sharing emotions and stressors in his life with his mother as she rarely talks about emotions or invites him to talk about stressors. This has negatively impacted the client's emotional wellness via the emotional social support he desires.

Family Wellness Dimensions

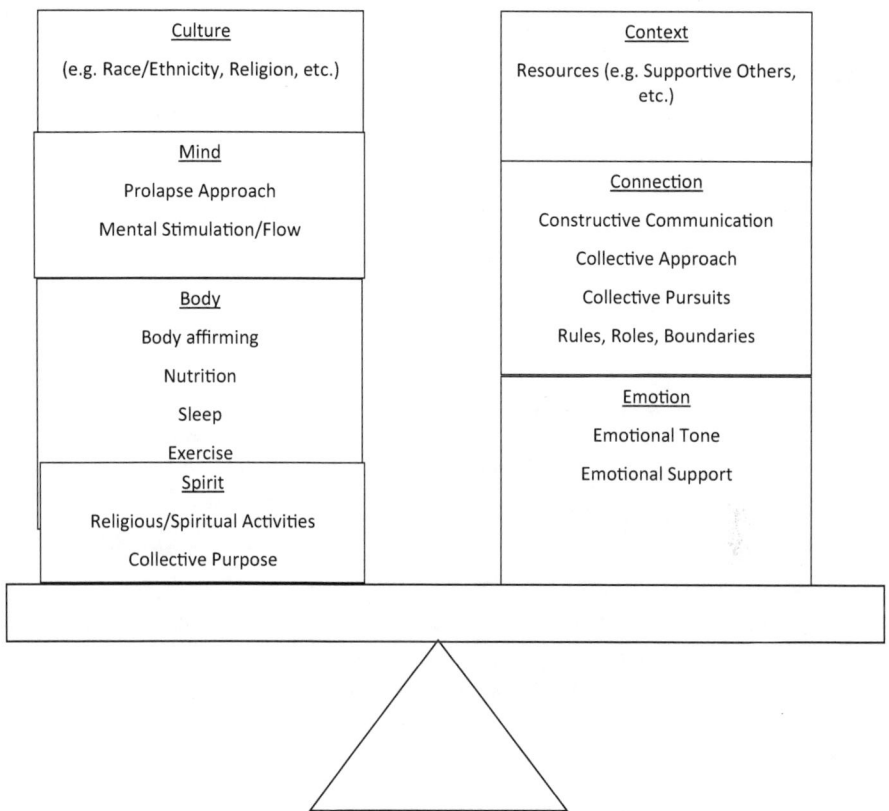

Figure 12.1 Family Wellness Dimensions based on Walsh (1996, 2002)

This also affects his self-esteem because of his belief that his mother may judge him negatively if he shares emotions and vulnerability.

Individual counseling related to family also offers the clinician the chance to provide information on the different family roles, as noted earlier. Make sure to clarify for the client that individuals can fall into multiple roles and to leave space for the client to identify family roles they relate to that were not mentioned by the clinician and may be unique to the client's culture. Explore what it was like for the client living in those roles as they grew up. Elicit specific examples of behaviors that frequently arose from living in the roles they identified.

A powerful exercise can be to help the client examine how growing up in those roles affects their wellness in their current life across the dimensions (pros and cons). You can then affirm the client for their self-awareness and willingness to process these roles and encourage them to take the next key step: take time to reflect on what aspects of these roles they want to hold onto as part of who they are and/or how they act and what aspects of those roles they want to release from themselves or incorporate with more intentionality. For example, someone who identifies the role of mascot may decide that they want to maintain much of

Handout 12.1 The Impact of Family Relationships on Wellness

Relationship With _____			`
Strengths of the Relationship	Wellness Impact	Challenges in the Relationship	Wellness Impact

the aspects of humor they cultivated to preserve homeostasis in their family as it feels like a talent of theirs, yet they want to eliminate their use of humor to hide from painful feelings or using humor to make fun of others to increase their own self-esteem. It can be helpful to create two four-column charts (one on the front of a page and one on the back of a page) to list out the thought processes (column 1), behaviors (column 2), and emotions (column 3) they experience when aligned with that role along with the situations that trigger them enacting that role behavior (column 4). On the other side, list out new thoughts, behaviors, and emotions they would like to experience instead and if there are specific situations in which these behaviors are appropriate. Help the client consider giving this revised role a name that is a better fit. For example, instead of "mascot", a new role name could be "considerate/reflective humorist".

Assist the client in envisioning the impact of making these desired changes on their wellness and assess wellness changes over time as the client implements these new parts of themselves. The grief and loss skills and techniques discussed in Chapter 10 are also important to infuse in conjunction with the client deciding to let go of certain roles. The client may experience feelings of grief and loss from releasing parts of themselves or behaviors they have engaged in for many years, even if these roles brought stress into their lives.

SETTING THE STAGE FOR FAMILY SESSIONS

Individual Session with the Identified Client

Family sessions can require a high expenditure of psychological energy on the part of your client, even more so than individual or group counseling sessions. The client is no longer in the cozy comfort of being able to share their innermost thoughts in privacy alone with the clinician. Now, family members (some who they may perceive as supportive and hold a positive relationship and others who they fear they have burned bridges with) will be gathered in one room. The client may already feel ashamed that the family is having to gather related to their challenges with addiction or possibly angry that they have been scapegoated given global problems in the family.

The clinician needs to check in with their client about their thoughts and feelings about having a family session. What are their greatest concerns? What potential benefits do they perceive? What interactions do they fear occurring during the family session? Do they have any requests of you regarding how you'll manage the family session (Mittelman, Epstein, & Pierzchala, 2003). The clinician should also provide information on what the family session(s) will entail and allot time for the client to ask questions and air concerns. Of utmost importance, the client and clinician need to determine who will attend the family sessions.

For adolescents, the significant others in the household should all attend (unless the clinician becomes aware of reasons for a member of the household not to attend). Further, if there are close others in the adolescent's life that spend time with them and provide caregiving and/or hold a powerful influence on them, they might be considered to attend as well. Make clear to your client that family members do not have to be blood relatives; rather they can be significant others who the client considers family. For adult clients, all household members should attend. If the client has no family members in the area, these meetings can possibly take place via HIPAA-compliant telemental health platforms. If the client is estranged from family, they are encouraged to identify at least one supportive person that could attend (e.g., someone from their faith community, an advocate from their homeless shelter, and a non-substance-using and supportive friend).

Family Session One

After introductions are made during the first family session, you should clarify the reason(s)/purpose of the family sessions. Frame the purpose of the session as a critical opportunity to provide support for the client, to grow in their relationships, and to deepen their own individual wellness which will benefit themselves, the client, and the family. The family should then come together to create rules for the family session – guidelines that need to be in place for them to have a productive discussion. You can offer examples like respectful communication and provide a description of what this can look like.

You will begin to get an assessment of the family's communication patterns simply from this exercise. It might also be helpful for the clinician to establish the importance of listening to each other and that many times the clinician will ask family members to talk directly to each other (Edwards, 1997) to encourage effective listening behavior. You can ask a listening family member to paraphrase back to the other family member what they heard the speaking family member saying. The use of "I-Messages" is also promoted by the clinician (Burr, 1990 as cited in Erford, Eaves, Bryant, & Young, 2010; McKay, Fanning, & Paleg, 2006). Specifically, family members express, "I feel _____ (feeling) when you _____ (behavior) because _____ (consequence)" (Erford et al., 2010, p. 28) instead of employing language with accusations and partiality, lacking in accountability such as "you make me feel _____" and "you need to change _____" and "you always _____ (opinion)" (Erford et al., 2010; McKay et al., 2006).

Family Strengths

It can be powerful for the client to hear their family members' motivations for attending the family session as it opens. The clinician can elicit this by asking family members to share why it was important for them to be here. The clinician should provide psychoeducation on the wellness model of addiction. Listen carefully for indications that family members hold different perceptions of the client's addiction than the client. In particular, be aware of family member moral model beliefs about addiction (that the client's addiction is due to the client's lack of inner strength to control their use or that they hold inferior morals or their addiction boils down to patterns of regretful choices). Such beliefs can be challenged with more compassionate, alternative perspectives (e.g., addiction is a disease concept; psychological issues being primary to addiction).

Family members and support persons being present for sessions allows the clinician to obtain collateral information on the client's strengths which builds relationships and sense of support between the client and their support persons and increases the client's confidence and awareness of strengths. You can kick off this part of the family session by reiterating that WBAC is a strengths-based approach given that building upon strengths can be a more effective pathway to change than over focusing on other facets. Then ask each attendee to identify strengths they have noticed in the client. They can offer specific examples that illustrate that strength if they would like. Invite family members to share additional strengths that fall specifically within the wellness dimensions. Encourage each person to speak directly to the client. Allow the client to share how it is for them to hear these strengths articulated by their loved ones. Be sure to write down what you hear so that you and the client can discuss them in future sessions, including how these strengths can facilitate their wellness and recovery and ways to build the strengths into the wellness plan, if the client so chooses.

Client and family members are also directed by the clinician to disclose concerns about what could detract from the client's wellness and recovery based on their awareness of the client's past wellness and substance use struggles. You might preface this discussion by guiding each family member to start with language such as "I am concerned about ...." and the concerns should be grounded in objective observations rather than opinion that can risk representing judgment. The clinician can redirect, as needed, the client and family members when this occurs. A client might state, for instance,

> I am concerned that in the past, when I have tried to cut down on my alcohol use, my husband will still bring over his drinking buddies who I'm also friends with and makes it difficult and, quite frankly, embarrassing not to drink with.

A conversation can then ensue to navigate how to handle this with the clinician providing coaching on listening and problem-solving skills while reinforcing the client and family members when they successfully utilize these skills. A family member, for instance, might state that

> I am concerned about my brothers' friends. He has been a very loyal friend in the past and I'm worried that he will not be willing to part ways with some of his using associates. Last time he ended up in treatment was because of a relapse with friends.

These discussions allow the client and family to dip their toe into practicing having difficult conversations. The clinician will again gain assessment information and can begin imparting some of the helpful communication skills described in Chapter 11 (connection wellness).

The client then should be prompted to share what aspects of their wellness plan they would like support from by their loved ones. The client can be informed about this in advance of the session so they can begin formulating ideas of what to request. Here are some examples of support that clients can request:

- Accountability for the wellness plan. For instance, checking in weekly about progress or challenges.
- Partnering for exercise.
- Teaching them to cook or preparing an occasional healthy meal for the client.
- Joining them in working on their own wellness plan.
- Reiterating that they are someone who can be contacted for emotional support.

The strategies listed above are some of the suggested topics if you only have limited time (e.g., one session) at your treatment site for interaction with the family. However, if your client is an adolescent and/or you can have multiple sessions with your adult clients and their families, the subsequent sections will detail additional family approaches.

Family Sessions Two and Beyond

Identifying Family Member Models of Addiction

Most family components of addiction treatment programs involve providing information on addiction to increase empathy for their loved one, empower families who perceive they have a dearth of knowledge about addiction, and to address any incorrect beliefs about addiction. Additionally, in WBAC, the clinician explores the family members' personal models of addiction and how they have influenced their interactions with their loved one with a SUD (Clarke & Scholl, 2022). The five-dimension wellness model is presented and the clinician explains the role of each dimension of wellness as a cause or contributor to addiction. This includes elucidating how mental (e.g., brain disease facets of addiction, the effect of addiction on thinking), body (e.g., imbalances in sleep, body image, exercise, nutrition), spirit (e.g., lack of meaning in life or spiritual conflict), emotion (e.g., effect of trauma, emotion regulation difficulties, stress management), connection (e.g., stress with close others, social skills issues, substance-using peers), developmental (e.g., adjusting to one's current stage in life), and contextual wellness (e.g., negative peer influences at school, pandemic stress, prevalence of drugs in the neighborhood, work or financial stress; Clarke & Scholl, 2022; Thombs & Osborn, 2013, 2019) may lead to addiction.

One common model of addiction that often shows up in family counseling, and one of which clinicians should be aware, is the moral model of addiction. This model entails the perception that the client's addictive use of the substance or behavior is within their control and results from repeated ineffective choices (Alderson, 2020; Cavaiola & Smith, 2020). This model also attributes the addiction to the identified client's personal make-up or integrity and can include inadequate self-control in the face of triggers. Emphasize that for different individuals, specific dimensions factor more heavily into their addiction and recovery than others and yet a holistic perspective is important because most or all wellness dimensions are associated with the development of addiction and the road to recovery (Clarke & Scholl, 2022).

To deepen this process, the clinician can have each family member (including the identified client) complete a rank order activity in which they rank the wellness dimensions they believe are most strongly correlated with their loved one's addiction from most to least cor-related (Clarke & Scholl, 2022). The identified client can share their rankings first followed by the family members. As each family member shares, ask them and the identified client to note how their view of their loved one's addiction may have affected their interactions with them. Secondly, ask family members and the client to reflect on how any discrepancies between their models of addiction have played out in their relationship, for better or worse. Help the client and family envision what their relationships would look like if they were "on the same page" about their perspectives on the client's addiction and took a holistic or comprehensive view of the etiology and effects of addiction. What are the implications of learning about information on addiction and their loved one's addiction of which they were unaware?

For instance, a family member who strongly values physical wellness may view the cli-ent's lack of physical activity, nutrition, and self-care throughout much of their life as the primary reason for their addiction. On the other hand, the client perceives that a sense of meaninglessness (spiritual) and brain disease (mental wellness) were most implicated. The family member might acknowledge that because of their view they tended to make negative comments about the client and their struggles with physical wellness and correspondingly espouse some of the moral model tenets such as the client is "lazy" and "unmotivated". As the family member witnesses the client in tears and expressing the hurt this has caused, the family member vows to be more supportive. The clinician then prompts both to discuss what that support could look like.

Be sure to address the moral model of addiction if it arises as middle to high on the client's or family member's rankings as assent of this model can be harmful (Clarke & Scholl, 2022). Whereas it is possible that believing in this model can be helpful, such as improving life choices and exerting more thoughtful control over aspects of their lives, clients who believe in this model are likely to feel othered, ashamed, and discouraged. These feelings can be exacerbated when family members sanction/validate the moral model regarding their loved one's addiction. Offer space for the client to discuss how (if at all) moral model beliefs of the family have impacted them. The clinician should also deliver information on the myths and harmful effects of the moral model.

Family Goal Setting

The clinician should build in time throughout family counseling sessions to incorporate dis-cussions of family wellness in greater depth. You should provide a definition and proposed components of family wellness (see Table 12.1). Family wellness can be defined as the result of family support, collective pursuits and purpose, utilization of resources and management of stressors across mind, body, spirit, emotion, and connection wellness in the family (Cran-dall et al., 2020; Duncan, Garrison, & Killian, 2021; Hernandez, 2013; Sixbey, 2005; Walsh, 1996, 2002). The clinician conveys that the family is an interconnected unit; thus, the inter-actions and events in the family affect each member as well as the family as a whole (see "sys-tems" discussion above). Family wellness counseling will seek to support the family member receiving treatment and also strengthen the family which can further facilitate the wellness of each family member (Hernandez, 2013). Launch the family members' participation in the conversation by asking each to share how they would define family wellness or what family wellness means to them, including the primary components they believe comprise family wellness. Consider incorporating follow up prompts such as "what experience(s) have you had that highlighted the importance of these components of family wellness?"

Table 12.1 Family Wellness Dimension Descriptions

Family Wellness (Ohrt, Clarke, & Conley, 2019; Walsh, 1996, 2002)

Mental	Family supports constructive beliefs (self, other; world)	Family creates environment of mental stimulation (e.g. engage in regular flow activities)	Family encourages shared problem-solving	Family facilitates mental growth via supportive challenging	Family fosters intrinsic motivation for physical wellness (helping family members discover their own personal joy in wellness activities)
Physical	Active lifestyle is promoted	Self-care is promoted (e.g. sleep and personal hygiene)	Family messages and actions promote healthy body image	Healthy Nutrition is modeled and practiced	
Spiritual	Family facilitates opportunities for members to identify meaning and purpose	Family members derive meaning via their involvement in the family	Family facilitates opportunities for members to cultivate religious or spiritual beliefs and practices while supporting members who do not share those beliefs or practices	Family provides opportunities for spiritual development such as faith communities, linking to information and resources	
Emotional	Models, practices, and imparts emotion regulation skills	Creates an environment that is accepting of emotions	Creates an environment conducive to sharing emotions as desired	A warm emotional tone pervades, as opposed to one of anxiety, allowing relational health and development	
Connection	Family members model and practice social skills such as active listening, assertiveness	Family members ask each other for what they need and extend support to help each other related to emotions, tasks, etc.	Family members support appropriate building of relationships external to the immediate family	Family members provide opportunities for socialization and assist in meaning making of these experiences	

It can be beneficial to involve family members in assessing the family and sharing those outcomes with each other (Edwards, 1997). Prompt each family member to rank order the facets of their family wellness from strongest to weakest. They can add or eliminate elements from this model if they seem to not fit with their perception of family wellness. Invite each member to share one or two examples of positive family wellness that have occurred in their family and one or two examples of family wellness struggles or instances that illustrate lower family wellness. Additionally, clinicians can explore the "making meaning in adversity" (Sixbey, 2005) or prolapse factor of FR by asking if past stressors have occurred for the family that the members feel the family navigated effectively overall. Elicit specific steps and family wellness strengths that were drawn upon by the family members and unit that can be attributed to favorably addressing the stressor. Allow space for family members to respond to each other after hearing each family member share.

The WBAC clinician then facilitates further interaction among the family to determine two to three family wellness goals. You can kick off this discussion by directing the family to process themes they noticed from the members about areas where there is stronger and weaker wellness. The family can be asked about additional behaviors that struck them about high family wellness examples, family wellness struggles, and instances of FR. The family then decides upon their wellness goals. They also develop objectives for how they can accomplish these goals. The formation of objectives should be grounded in "We-statements" (Burr, 1990) in lieu of "you need to" statements. The conversation alone provides the clinician with assessment information on family communication. Pay attention to who leads the discussion, who talks the least, which parties in the family collaborate, how any conflict is managed, who appears engaged, who appears disengaged, and nonverbal communication (e.g., body language conveying disconnection from the family; Edwards, 1997). When information saturation has been reached about the relating that occurs among the family members, you should increase your activity level or directiveness by interrupting unhelpful patterns and guiding the family members back to the rules it agreed upon, listening skills, "I" messages", etc.

Once the family wellness goals and action steps have been identified, each family member notes at least one contribution (with action steps) per family wellness goal that they will endeavor towards in order to make the family goals a reality. Request that the family members maintain a watchful eye for even the smallest signs of progress and any efforts made by themselves, family members, and the unit as a whole (O'Hanlon & Weiner-Davis, 2003). Ensure that you inquire about identified progress at each family session. The remainder of the format for an individual wellness plan can be used for the family wellness plan. Figure 12.2 contains a sample wellness goal and individual contribution section for each wellness dimension.

FAMILY WELLNESS PLAN

Family Wellness Goal **(Connection)**: increase connection wellness, specifically constructive communication

- Subgoal: Use the listening skills introduced in counseling if a disagreement or difficult topic arises.
  - Action Step 1: Identify common areas of disagreement or patterns of topics that cause tension.

- Action Step 2: Practice the listening skills in counseling and at home, starting by using them in non-conflict conversations.
- Action Step 3: Discuss effectiveness of the skills in counseling and ways to improve.

Individual Contribution: identify areas in which I may contribute to conflicts.

- Action Step 1: In session, ask for family feedback for ways I contribute to conflict.
- Action Step 2: Practice responding to feedback without anger using deep breathing and listening skills.

Family Wellness Goal **(Physical Wellness)**: increase physical wellness via improved nutrition.

- Subgoal: Cook one nutritious family meal together per week and freezing leftovers that can be eaten in the days following.
  - Action Step 1: Set aside a time to schedule out the days this will occur over the next two months.
  - Action Step 2: Set ground rules for cooking that will be written down and hung up in the kitchen.

Individual Contribution: To not takeover the meal (I will assist rather than be the team leader for the cooking) and will monitor that I am doing the same number of tasks as my other family members.

- Action Step 1: Identify a role I can play in the cooking (e.g. support) to be discussed with family.
- Action Step 2: Use my knowledge of cooking to provide meal ideas and assist with the shopping.

Family Wellness Goal **(Emotional Wellness)**: learn ways to support each other emotionally and the type of emotional support that each family member values.

- Subgoal: able to describe each family member's preferences for emotional support and family member reports of increased emotional support on 1–10 scale.
  - Action Step 1: Explore and identify via family counseling the preferred ways that each member likes to receive support.
  - Action Step 2: Read and discuss information provided by counselor defining emotional support and different ways it can be provided.

Individual Contribution: start my own individual counseling (within the next month) to address emotional triggers.

- Action Step 1: Stick with therapist/therapy for at least five sessions. I have gone to therapy before but I stopped going when we explored more of my feelings and past experiences.
- Action Step 2: Identify in therapy ways I can support myself emotionally and be more supportive of family members.

Family Wellness Goal **(Spiritual Wellness):** increase clarity about our individual and family values in order to reduce the frequency of arguments about decisions.

- Subgoal: Hold a family meeting in the next two weeks to discuss what we value as a family and what brings meaning to each individual member.
  - Action Step 1: Identifying rules and decisions that represent our values.
  - Action Step 2: Ensuring each family member shares at least 1 thing that brings them meaning and 1 way the family can support this.
  - Action Step 3: Each family member is to use the active listening skills during the family meeting (using paraphrases, not jumping in while a member is still talking, "I language", etc.)

Individual Contribution: identify at least 3 values to seek support in fulfilling and 3 values that my husband and I wish to impart to our family.

- Action Step 1: Meet with my husband prior to the family meeting to gain consensus on the values we want to instill in the family.
- Action Step 2: Spend at least 20 minutes reflecting and writing down in a journal what brings or could bring more meaning to my life and how my family can support that.

Family Wellness Goal **(Mental Wellness):** work on developing constructive family beliefs.

- Subgoal: Shift from blaming family and identified client for family problems to a prolapse approach (what can be learned) and ways to support a prolapse approach for each member.
  - Action Step 1: Invite the identified client to share ways in which they have felt blamed and scapegoated by the family related to their addiction.
  - Action Step 2: Identifying non-constructive family beliefs and possible origins of these beliefs that feed blaming each other.

- Action Step 3: Develop and write down family mantras reflecting constructive beliefs including challenges the family has successfully navigated.

Individual Contribution (Identified Client): open up to my family on at least one occasion during a counseling session and at least once outside of session about the ways our beliefs have affected me as well as the role I seek in making positive change in our family's beliefs.

- Action Step 1: The thought of sharing ways in which I have been scapegoated by my family with my family makes me nervous. So I will practice disclosing these thoughts to my close friend.
- Action Step 2: In individual counseling, I will reflect on how past trauma our family has faced has affected my individual and our family's mental wellness.
- Action Step 3: I will identify ways I contribute to negative belief patterns in the family.
- Action Step 4: I will journal about how my recovery may positively affect my individual and family's mental wellness.

Figure 12.2 Example Family Wellness Plan.

Individual Family Member Wellness Plans

Family members may not be fully aware of the impact of the presence of addiction in the family on their personal wellness. The importance of this topic has been evidenced by researchers studying "caregiver burden" for loved ones of persons with SUDs (Russell, D'Aniello, Tambling, & Stekler, 2022). For example, substance-related incarceration, frequency of supervised withdrawal management, and decreased social support were linked with caregiver burden (Soares, Ferreira, & Pereira, 2016). Take a moment and reflect on factors that could detract from the wellness of the caregivers and family members of your client with addiction concerns. Some of these may include

- Obtaining and paying for treatment (Russell et al., 2022)
- Stigma (Russell et al., 2022)
- Frequent worry about person with SUD's safety
- Efforts to ensure safety and wellness for person with SUD
- Stress-inducing/tense interactions/communications with the person with SUD
- Role stress – from adopting a difficult family role to safeguard homeostasis
- Coping with consequences resulting from the person's use such as incarceration (Soares et al., 2016).

A former clinical supervisor of mine (Phil) opened my eyes further to what family members experience. The supervisor explained how if a family member with an SUD ends up in the hospital because of their use (for example, crashing their car, falling off a ladder, etc.), they may have been unconscious at some point and unaware of what occurred. However, for non-using family members, the story can be quite different; a family member can be highly aware of what transpires if they find their family member with an SUD unconscious, have to take them to the hospital, and be with them as they recover from their serious injuries. These experiences can cause significant anxiety and trauma for the loved one.

Thus, if family members can attend their own sessions without the client, the clinician can facilitate the family member's ventilation about aspects of relating to their loved one with a SUD, caregiving, and experiences that have been most difficult and stressful (Russell et al., 2022). Inquire about what has been the hardest for family members. Then link these experiences to the wellness model, discussing the impact of these challenges on the dimensions of wellness. You should also process what stronger areas of wellness have helped them sustain themselves and flourish at times in the face of these strains. See Chapter 3 for how to form the wellness plan.

Inform the family members that attending to their own wellness will be essential since the wellness and recovery of their loved one with addiction cannot be guaranteed. Further, the wellness of individual family members and the family as a whole may increase the likelihood of positive wellness and recovery outcomes and at the very least, bolster the family members' wellness so that they individually and collectively have increased capacity to support their loved one with an SUD.

In the next section, we will talk about family rules and boundaries that can be discussed in individual and family counseling when an SUD is present. These strategies can be used individually and with family members attending family programming sessions without the client.

Boundaries

One unique consideration when assisting family members with developing their individual wellness plans is to discuss, promote, and encourage healthy boundaries. Explain that "boundaries are usually physical as well as psychological barriers that exist both within families and with the outside world. Each individual family member may have their own physical or emotional boundary or comfort zone" (Cavaiola et al., 2022, np). Moreover, boundaries help people protect their wellness by ensuring they interact with others in a way that is congruent for them and ensure that one does not enable a loved one's substance use.

Others may try to cross boundaries the family member has set, and the family member may try to cross boundaries others have set, all of which can result in decreases in well-being. However, boundaries should also be adaptable in instances when changing the boundary would be constructive for oneself and others. Provide examples of the types of boundaries such as the following:

Diffuse Boundary Example 1. "More times than I can count, I have set aside time for myself to engage in _____ wellness activity but completely dropped those plans to address _____ issue for my adult loved one in recovery despite promises to myself that I would no longer constantly put their needs ahead of mine".

Diffuse Boundary Example 2. *"I don't really have a curfew or many rules on who my teenage son can spend time with."*

Rigid Boundary Example 1. *"Years ago, my husband and I agreed not to talk about topic _____. It's become problematic though because we need to address this issue as it's gotten worse over time, but we have chosen to avoid it.*

Rigid Boundary Example 2. *"When everyone gets home from school or work, each person goes to their own space in the house and does something by themselves. My parents do not want us to bother them.*

Clear Boundary Example 1. *"We have daily 'family time' rules when we spend time together as a family without our phones. However, there are times when different members do need some alone time, and we allow for that on occasion when needed".*

One approach to examining spoken and unspoken boundaries is to process how the family members respond to each other. During family programming when the client is not present, family members can examine how they respond to their loved one with an SUD. The family can identify difficult interactions or arguments that recur and reflect on the following prompt: "When my loved one does or says X, I tend to respond by saying or doing Y". Another avenue for journeying into boundaries is to examine them across the wellness dimensions for the family. Claudia Black (2019) noted that boundaries span the wellness spectrum. For instance, emotional ("strong emotions should always be shared regardless of consequence"), spiritual ("we always pray together and seek the guidance of religious text to resolve family conflicts or stressors"), body ("my parents are always in my room, digging through my things"), connection ("our family typically communicates by yelling if there is a problem", mental ("as a family, if a problem arises, we collectively assume that the worst possible outcome will happen and we each shut down").

Rather than positioning family members as codependent or enabling, WBAC family work entails the clinician exploring the implications of these boundaries on their individual and family wellness beginning with evaluating whether the boundary is clear, rigid, or diffuse. Family members then reflect on ways different boundaries are helpful and/or harmful to their wellness. With an objective eye, the family member determines if each boundary is constructive or destructive as well as how it may impact their and the client's wellness. The WBAC clinician then requests the client ascertain options for ways they could respond, revise, or discard boundaries that could benefit their wellness and the client's wellness and recovery in the long-term. The word "long-term" is critical here as the wellness-enhancing response will at times not feel pleasant in the moment or be more challenging to implement.

Rules

Rules inform us on what to do and how to be (Black, 1981). Direct clients to first identify explicit rules they have set in the home. This will add clarity to the definition of rules. Families may talk about rules such as curfew, bedtime, substance use, use of social media, screen time, chores, etc. You can then ask about implicit rules in the home. Examples of these include "Mom rather than Dad is the only person to set rules for the home", "the teen boys can go on dates, but the teen girls cannot", "the favorite child in the home does not have to adhere to all the rules like the other children". An extension of the rules concept are *assumptions* and *values* that the family holds such as a family that celebrates academic success and intellectual activity involvement, while minimally recognizing athletic achievement (valuing mental wellness). For a family member who is skilled at physical endeavors and lacks success in academics, they may experience a scapegoat role or feel distanced from the family. Similar to work with family boundaries, the family discusses wellness pros and cons of their rules and values and options for revising, discarding, and/or adding rules or values.

Progress

Similar to WBAC individual sessions, the clinician should ask each family member about any small indication of family wellness progress at subsequent family sessions. Normalize that wellness changes can be challenging and take time but encourage family members to stay attentive to any signs of progress. You'll need to check in on the impact of rules and boundary changes, individual wellness plans, family wellness goals and objectives, and so forth. The central WBAC questions can always be incorporated as they are designed to evaluate progress and barriers while increasing the client and family's motivation towards their own wellness recovery.

- How are the changes you noticed impacting your individual wellness and your family's wellness?
- How has attending to your own wellness plan been helpful to you and your family?
- In what ways have the rules and boundaries shifts you've made affected your wellness?
- What have been the biggest challenges thus far?
- What have been the biggest barriers you have faced thus far?
- What individual and family strengths can be brought to bear to address this wellness goal or barrier?

CLIENT EXAMPLE OF FAMILY WELLNESS COUNSELING

Family Roles

Eric and his counselor explored the influence of his family of origin experiences on repeated behaviors or roles in his life. Eric recognized through counseling that he at times was in "lost child" and "scapegoat" roles. Eric recalled his siblings receiving more attention because of their successes in school and sports as well as their outgoing nature. Eric performed well in school and his activities but did not receive the same level of acknowledgment from his parents. Eric felt mostly "lost" when it came to his relationship with his father. He did perceive himself as having a unique relationship with his mother and that he could cheer her up during her periods of depression. But his insecurities and desire to fit in resulted in him engaging in behaviors that got him in trouble such as skipping school, talking back to teachers, and substance misuse.

Eric's counselor noted that he seems to vacillate between "lost child" and "scapegoat" behaviors when he becomes overwhelmed as an adult citing examples of him shifting from being meaningfully involved in the family and figuratively disappearing. He also tends to be less present when feeling depressed or acting out, both leading to and because of his drinking. Eric was able to identify thoughts, feelings, and emotions when he is in both roles. For example, he journaled about cognitions such as "Nobody gets me and how much I have to carry in this family", "My daughter cares much more about her mom and her friends than me", "I'm not going to say anything about _____ because my wife has enough stress on her plate". These thoughts result in feelings of loneliness and affect his sense of purpose (spiritual wellness), mood (emotional wellness), and sense of closeness with others (connection wellness).

Family Sessions

The client, client's spouse Kelly, their daughter Lia, and client's father John attended family sessions. The emotional tone of the family appeared distanced with Lia sitting close to her mother and a serious demeanor exhibited by the family. The family engaged in the counseling, although primarily following the counselor's lead with minimal emotions expressed. The family landed on goals related to communication (connection wellness), emotional wellness, and contextual wellness. Lia, with prompting from the counselor, shared her concerns with communication and why she sought for the family to address this.

> CLINICIAN: Lia, would you be willing to say more about what you mean by communication as your family wellness goal?
>
> LIA: We don't talk much about things. When I told Dad I think he drinks too much, he kinda shut down that conversation. Mom and Dad seem to not talk to each other a lot.
>
> CLINICIAN: You're wanting more open lines of talking among all of your family members.
>
> LIA: Yeah.
>
> CLINICIAN: Tell me more about what you've noticed that lets you know that your family doesn't talk much about things.
>
> KELLY: Lia is not being fully accurate about ....
>
> CLINICIAN: Sorry to interrupt, mom, but let's go ahead and hear Lia's thoughts on this.
>
> LIA: Mom makes a face when she is upset at Dad. And I know she's mad, but she doesn't say anything to him. Dad sometimes stays to himself or on his phone or the TV. Me and grandpa are pretty close. We'll play chess together.
>
> CLINICIAN: Tell me about a time when the family communicated well?
>
> LIA: If we do fun things, we talk more. Sometimes Mom, Dad, and Grandpa will all come to my game. In the car on the way home, everyone is excited and talking. Sometimes Dad and I will make a pizza and we'll all eat together and talk about what we did that day.
>
> CLINICIAN: When you have these special shared moments, everyone talks more, and everyone feels better.

Later, in a couples' session with Eric and Kelly only, Kelly disclosed about attempting to shield Lia from Eric's drinking in different ways and didn't realize that this had resulted in her overtly and covertly communicating that Lia should not talk about this in depth. Hearing their daughter's perspective on how they interact forced the couple to open up about their marital concerns.

> ERIC: After the first miscarriage, I feel like we were able to talk about the sadness and the feelings. But things got numb for us after the second and third miscarriage. It hurt and we both didn't know how to be there for each other. The drinking helped.

KELLY: And I took the drinking as a "slap in the face" to me. I wanted him to be there for me. I'm learning more through this counseling how this affected him too. I think as dad came to live with us, we grew apart even more because we were both now caregivers for our daughter and dad. No time for us.

ERIC: And you (clinician) and I have talked about this quite a bit – but like, both Kelly and I didn't have great role models for communication with how our parents were. I still, in my mind, am having a hard time with the idea of being the bigger person and trying to communicate with dad when he never gave much effort to spend time with me.

The communication challenges also extended to a lack of clarity and consistency with rules for their daughter. They viewed her as responsible and hence did not formally set many rules. Over time, Lia had increasingly pushed boundaries by spending less time on schoolwork and extracurricular activities and more time with friends and not following through with consequences if she got in trouble. The WBAC clinician helped Eric and his wife develop rules and rewards and how to discuss these with Lia. The family, using the wellness model, also identified family activities that seemed to bolster conversation and set a minimum number of family wellness activities to engage in per week.

During a later session, the clinician examined progress.

CLINICIAN: What progress have you observed since our last family session two weeks ago. I want to hear about it, even if it seems small.

JOHN: I see Eric and Kelly being better parents. Better than his mom and I.

I feel like we are doing more things as a family. Eric being in treatment – it's been good for him.

KELLY: And Eric and I are really sticking to the rules with Lia. She wasn't allowed to go over to a friend's house as a consequence and Lia tried to go to me and convince me to let her go, but I stayed strong.

CLINICIAN: Eric – what does it mean to hear this and how (if at all have these positive changes affected your wellness and recovery)?

ERIC: Dad – it means a lot to hear you say that. I always knew I was good with work stuff but felt like I could be a better father and husband. With Kelly's support, I feel like I'm getting better at both. And doing our weekly family fun date has been awesome. I do feel more of that connection wellness and less irritable (emotion wellness). I feel like an edge has come off some of my stress and cravings.

CONCLUSION

As you can see, couples and family counseling is a necessary element of WBAC. Families are a significant part of the client's context and impact their intrapersonal experience as well. If the clinician can mobilize the family towards supporting the client's wellness plan, the client will have a higher likelihood of meeting their wellness recovery goals. WBAC provides a chance for families to build cohesion (Walsh, 1996, 2002). This is accomplished via the members all pursuing individual and family wellness goals. WBAC is also a holistic approach for supporting the family members and loved ones so that they attend to their own wellness.

Handout 12.2   Family Wellness Plan

Family Wellness Plan
Family Wellness Goal (Dimension _____):
- Subgoal:
  - Action Step 1:
  - Action Step 2:
  - Action Step 3:

Individual Contribution:
- Action Step 1:
- Action Step 2:
- Action Step 3:

NOTE

1   Although Wegscheider focused on families in which alcohol use disorders are present, it is our opinion that these roles are important across many different substances within the family.

REFERENCES

Alderson, K. G. (2020). *Addictions counseling today: Substances and addictive behaviors.* Sage.

Black, C. (1981). *It will never happen to me: Growing up with addiction as youngsters, adolescents, adults.* Central Recovery Press.

Black, C. (2019). *Family strategies: Practical tools for professionals treating families impacted by addiction.* Central Recovery Press.

Bowen, M. (1978). *Family therapy in clinical practice.* Jason Aronson.

Burr, W. R. (1990). Beyond I-statements in family communication. *Family Relations, 39*(3), 266–273.

Cavaiola, A., Giordano, A. L., & Golubovic, N. (2022). *Addiction counseling: A practical approach.* Springer.

Cavaiola, A. A., & Smith, M. (2020). *A comprehensive guide to addiction theory and counseling techniques.* Routledge.

Center for Disease Control, National Center for Health Statistics (2020). *Wide-ranging online data for epidemiologic research (WONDER).* Retrieved from http://wonder.cdc.gov

Clarke, P. B., & Scholl, M. B. (2022). Integrating the models of addiction into humanistic counseling for individuals with substance use disorders. *The Journal of Humanistic Counseling, 61*(1), 2–17. https://doi.org/10.1002/johc.12171

Crandall, A., Weiss-Laxer, N. S., Broadbent, E., Holmes, E. K., Magnusson, B. M., Okano, L., Berge, J. M., Barnes, M. D., Hanson, C. L., Jones, B. L., & Novilla, L. B. (2020). The family health scale: Reliability and validity of a short- and long-form. *Frontiers in Public Health, 8,* 587125. https://doi.org/10.3389/fpubh.2020.587125

Dodgen, C. E., & Shea, W. M. (2000). *Substance use disorders: Assessment and treatment.* Academic Press.

Doweiko, H. E., & Evans, A. L. (2019). *Concepts of chemical dependency.* Cengage.

Duncan, J. M., Garrison, M. E., & Killian, T. S. (2021). Measuring family resilience: Evaluating the Walsh family resilience questionnaire. *The Family Journal, 29*(1), 80–85. https://doi.org/10.1177/1066480720956641

Edwards, J. T. (1997). *Working with families: Guidelines and techniques* (4th ed.). Foundation Place.

Erford, B. T., Eaves, S. H., Bryant, E. M., & Young, K. A. (2010). *35 techniques every counselor should know*. Merrill.

GenPro (n.d.). What is a genogram? Retrieved from https://genopro.com/articles/what-is-a- genogram/

Gladding, S. T. (2019*). Family therapy: History, theory, practice*. Pearson.

Hernandez, J. L. (2013). *Family wellness skills: Quick assessment and practical interventions for the mental health professional*. W. W. Norton and Company.

Juhnke, G. A., & Hagedorn, W. B. (2006). *Counseling addicted families. An integrated assessment and treatment model*. Routledge.

Lambert, S. F., Unterberg, H., & Riggio, M. (2018). *Family systems theory*. In P. S. Lassiter & J. R. Culbreth (Eds.), *Theory and practice of addiction counseling* (pp. 177–198). Sage.

Lewis, T. F. (2023). *Substance abuse and addiction counseling. Practical application of counseling theory*. Cognella.

Mathew, K. J., Regmi, B., & Lama, L. D. (2018). Role of family in addictive disorders. *International Journal of Psychosocial Rehabilitation, 22*(1) 65–75.

McKay, M., Fanning, P., & Paleg, K. (2006). *Couple skills: Making your relationship work* (2nd ed.). New Harbinger Publications.

Merikangas, K. R., Stolar, M., Stevens, D. E., Goulet, J., Preisig, M. A., Fenton, B., Zhang, H., O'Malley, S. S., & Rounsaville, B. J. (1998). Familial transmission of substance use disorders. *Archives of General Psychiatry, 55*, 973–979. https://doi.org/10.1001/archpsyc.55.11.973

Miller, W. R., Forcehimes, A. A., & Zweben, A. (2019). *Treating addiction: A guide for professionals* (2nd ed.). Guilford.

Mittelman, M. S., Epstein, C., & Pierzchala, A. (2003). *Counseling the Alzheimer's caregiver: A resource for health care professionals*. AMA Press.

O'Hanlon, B., & Weiner-Davis, M. (2003). *In search of solutions: A new direction in psychotherapy* (2nd ed.). W. W. Norton and Company.

Ohrt, J. H., Clarke, P. B., & Conley, A. H. (2019). *Wellness counseling: A holistic approach to prevention and intervention*. American Counseling Association.

Ranieris, J. N. (2022). The 6 most serious side effects of drug addiction on family members. *Discovery Institute*. Retrieved from https://www.discoverynj.org/the-most-serious-effects-of-drug-addiction-on-family-members/

Russell, B. S., D'Aniello, C., Tambling, R. R., & Stekler, N. (2022). Internalized stigma and caregiver burden among parents of young adults with substance use disorders. *Family Relations*. https://doi.org/10.1111/fare.12782

Schaeffer, C. M., Swensen, C. C., & Powell, J. S. (2021). Multisystemic therapy – Building stronger families (MST-BSF): Substance misuse, child neglect, and parenting outcomes from an 18-month randomized effectiveness trial. *Child Abuse & Neglect, 122*, ArtID: 105379. https://doi.org/ezproxy.lib.ndsu.nodak.edu/10.1016/j.chiabu.2021.105379

Sixbey, M. T. (2005). *Development of the family resilience assessment scale to identify family resilience constructs* [Doctoral dissertation, University of Florida]. ProQuest Dissertations & Theses Global.

Soares, A. J., Ferreira, G., & Graça Pereira, M. (2016). Depression, distress, burden and social support in caregivers of active versus abstinent addicts. *Addiction Research & Theory, 24*(6), 483–489. https://doi.org/10.3109/16066359.2016.1173681

Taibbi, R. (2011). *Families in crisis: Strategies for defusing, defining, and problem-solving*. Pesi Seminars.

Thombs, D. L., & Osborn, C. J. (2013). *Introduction to addictive behaviors* (4th ed.). Guilford Press.

Thombs, D. L., & Osborn, C. J. (2019). *Introduction to addictive behaviors* (5th ed.). Guilford Press.

van der Stouwe, T., Asscher, J. J., Stams, G. J. J. M., Dekovic, M., & van der Laan, P. H. (2014). The effectiveness of multisystemic therapy (MST): A meta-analysis. *Clinical Psychology Review, 34*, 468–481.

Vertava Health (2022). *The four rules in an addicted home*. Retrieved from https://vertavahealth.com/blog/the-four-rules-in-an-addicted- home/

Walsh, F. (1996). The concept of family resilience: Crisis and challenge. *Family Process, 35*(3), 261–281. https://doi.org/10.1111/j.1545-5300.1996.00261.x

Walsh, F. (2002). A family resilience framework: Innovative practice applications. *Family Relations, 51*(2), 130–137. https://doi.org/10.1111/j.1741-3729.2002.00130.x

Wegscheider, S. (1981). *Another chance: Hope and health for the alcoholic family*. Science and Behavior Books.

INDEX

Note: **Bold** page numbers refer to tables and *Italic* page numbers refer to figures.